Nutrition Science: Health and Disease

Nutrition Science: Health and Disease

Editor: Gracelyn Pine

STATES
ACADEMIC PRESS
www.statesacademicpress.com

States Academic Press,
109 South 5th Street,
Brooklyn, NY 11249, USA

Visit us on the World Wide Web at:
www.statesacademicpress.com

ISBN: 978-1-63989-389-8 (Hardback)

Cataloging-in-Publication Data

Nutrition science : health and disease / edited by Gracelyn Pine.
p. cm.
Includes bibliographical references and index.
ISBN 978-1-63989-389-8
1. Nutrition. 2. Health. 3. Diseases. 4. Diet in disease.
5. Nutritionally induced diseases. I. Pine, Gracelyn.

TX353 .N88 2022
641.3--dc23

Table of Contents

Preface

Nutrition science is the science that studies the biological process of nutrition. It tries to understand nutrients and other substances in food, and their role in the maintenance, growth, reproduction, health and disease of an organism. Nutrition science focuses on dietary concerns and health issues surrounding food, eating and medicine. It also includes studies on molecular interactions, metabolic and signaling pathways, physiology, pathology, and toxicology. Studies related to the behavioral and social factors associated with food choices also fall under nutrition science. It is a multidisciplinary field rooted in chemistry, biology and the social sciences. The many areas of specialization within this field are food and wellness, community nutrition, exercise science, and nutrition education. The book studies, analyses and upholds the pillars of nutrition science and its utmost significance in modern times. It covers in detail some existent theories and innovative concepts revolving around this field. This book on nutrition science is a collective contribution of a renowned group of international experts.

This book is the end result of constructive efforts and intensive research done by experts in this field. The aim of this book is to enlighten the readers with recent information in this area of research. The information provided in this profound book would serve as a valuable reference to students and researchers in this field.

At the end, I would like to thank all the authors for devoting their precious time and providing their valuable contribution to this book. I would also like to express my gratitude to my fellow colleagues who encouraged me throughout the process.

Editor

1

Antidiabetic Potential of Plants Used in Bulgarian Folk Medicine and Traditional Diet

Milka Nashar, Yoana D. Kiselova-Kaneva and Diana G. Ivanova

Abstract

The idea of this chapter is that currently available antidiabetic drugs specifically target several points of the T2D pathophysiology but they do not cover all aspects of the disease. In addition, many adverse effects of synthetic antidiabetic agents have been reported. The suggested manuscript is an overview of the available scientific literature focused on antiobesity and antidiabetic potential of selected 42 medicinal and edible plants of the Bulgarian flora. Most of the reports reveal the effect of extracts or their active components on specific biochemical mechanisms. Mechanistic data about hypoglycemic and hypolipidemic action are presented for some of the plants. An essential part of this review is dedicated to the target mechanisms behind the effects of the selected plant species. The authors hope that this review will serve as a starting point for future investigations with a contribution to the prevention and therapy of diabetes.

Keywords: medicinal plants, diabetes, folk medicine, traditional diet

Introduction

Diabetes is an endocrine disease related to impaired glucose metabolism due to either impaired insulin secretion or decreased sensitivity to its function, classified, respectively, as type 1 diabetes (T1D) and type 2 diabetes (T2D). Over time, chronic hyperglycemia can cause secondary micro- and macrovascular complications affecting the functions of the eyes, kidneys, peripheral nerves, and arteries. According to recent alarming data, the number of adults living with diabetes has almost quadrupled since 1980 to 2014. This dramatic rise is largely due to the number of T2D sufferers [1].

Although some of the characteristics of the modern lifestyle (obesity, stress, low physical activity) are considered to be risk factors with regard to the occurrence of diabetes, it should be noted that cases of the disease are described in written sources dating back to 3500 years [2–4]. Also, records exist from ancient Egypt, India, and Persia, indicating a long history of medicinal use of plants for treatment of conditions associated with diabetes [5]. Historical and archeological sources indicate that Thracians, the most ancient tribes on the territory of Bulgaria, were familiar with the healing power of the plants [6]. Over the years, empirical data about healing properties of plants used in Bulgarian folk medicine and traditional nutrition have been collected in several reference books [7–10]. Although plants have been used to treat diabetes for centuries, the number of species with completely clarified antidiabetic mechanisms of action is still limited.

Table 1. *References in support of potentially antidiabetic properties of 42 selected plants.*

No.	Plant	Common name	Used parts	References
1	*Achillea millefolium* L. (Asteraceae)	White yarrow	Aerial parts	[13–20]
2	*Agrimonia eupatoria* L. (Rosaceae)	Agrimony	Aerial parts	[21–31]
3	*Alchemilla vulgaris* L. (Rosaceae)	Lady's Mantle	Stalk	[21, 32, 33]
4	*Arctium lappa* L. (Asteraceae)	Burdock	Root	[21, 34–36]
5	*Arctostaphylos uva-ursi* L. (Ericaceae)	Bearberry	Leaves	[37, 38]
6	*Asparagus officinalis* L. (Liliaceae)	Sparrow grass	Stalk	[39–41]
7	*Berberis vulgaris* L. (Berberidaceae)	Barberry	Fruits	[42–44]
8	*Betula* sp. (Betulaceae)	Birch	Leaves	[45, 46]
9	*Cichorium intybus* L. (Asteraceae)	Blue daisy, blue dandelion	Stalk, root	[13, 14, 21, 47]
10	*Cotinus coggygria* Scop. (Anacardiaceae)	Smoke tree, sumach	Leaves	[25, 48]
11	*Cydonia vulgaris* Pers. (Rosaceae)	Quince	Leaves	[49–51]
12	*Foeniculum vulgare* Mill. (Apiaceae)	Dill	Fruits	[52–54]
13	*Fragaria vesca complex* (Rosaceae)	Wild strawberry	Leaves	[33, 55, 56]
14	*Galega officinalis* L. (Fabaceae)	Goat's rue	Stalk	[21, 57–59]
15	*Hypericum perforatum* L. (Hypericaceae)	St. John's wort	Stalk	[25, 60, 61]
16	*Juglans regia* L. (Juglandaceae)	Walnut	Leaves	[62–69]
17	*Juniperus communis* L. (Cupressaceae)	Juniper	Fruits	[13, 14, 21, 31]
18	*Lavandula angustifolia* Mill. (Liliaceae)	Lavender	Flower	[21, 25, 70, 71]
19	*Melissa officinalis* L. (Liliaceae)	Melissa, lemon balm	Stalk	[25, 58, 71, 72]
20	*Mentha piperita* L. (Liliaceae)	Mint	Leaves	[33, 71]
21	*Morus nigra* L. (Moraceae)	Mulberry	Leaves, fruits, root bark, heartwood	[13, 14], 76–82

23	*Ononis spinosa* L. (Lamiaceae)	Spiny restharrow	Root	[62]
24	*Origanum vulgare* L. (Liliaceae)	Marjoram	Stalk	[25, 83–85]
25	*Pelargonium sp.* (Geraniaceae)	Pelargonium	Leaves	[86, 87]
26	*Phaseolus vulgaris* L. (Fabaceae)	Bean	Pods	[13, 14, 21, 88–91]
27	*Plantago major* L. (Plantaginaceae)	Broadleaf plantain	Leaves	[62]
28	*Polygonum aviculare* L. (Polygonaceae)	Prostrate knotweed, birdweed, pigweed	Stalk	[26]
29	*Rheum officinale* Baill. (Polygonaceae)	Rhubarb	Root	[92, 93]
30	*Rosa canina* L. (Rosaceae)	Rose hip	Fruits	[55, 94–96]
31	*Rosa damascena auct.* non-Mill. (Rosaceae)	Oil rose	Flower	[97–98]
32	*Rubus sp.* diversae	Blackberry	Leaves	[21, 25, 100, 101]
33	*Salvia officinalis* L. (Liliaceae)	Garden sage	Leaves	[19, 47, 102–106]
34	*Sambucus ebulus* L. (Caprifoliaceae)	Dwarf elderberry	Fruits	[33, 107–110]
35	*Sambucus nigra* L. (Caprifoliaceae)	European black elderberry	Flower	[34, 111–113]
36	*Taraxacum officinale* Wigg. (Asteraceae)	Dandelion	Root stalk	[19, 21, 34, 81, 114]
37	*Thymus* sp. diversae (Liliaceae)	Thyme	Stalk	[19, 77]
38	*Tilia platyphyllos* Scop. (Tiliaceae)	Lime tree	Flower	[37, 115]
39	*Urtica dioica* L. (Urticaceae)	Nettle	Stalk	[34, 67, 116–120]
40	*Vaccinium myrtillus* L. (Ericaceae)	Blueberry	Leaves and fruits	[13, 14, 21, 81]
41	*Veronica officinalis* L. (Scrophulariaceae)	Veronica, speedwell, Paul's betony	Stalk	[121, 122]
42	*Zea mays* L. (Poaceae)	Corn	Silk	[21, 123]

Currently available antidiabetic drugs could specifically target several points of the T2D pathophysiology, but they do not cover all aspects of the disease [11, 12]. In addition, many adverse effects of synthetic antidiabetic agents have been reported [11].

Therefore, it is not surprising that in recent years, the scientific interest is focused on identifying naturally derived compounds and preparations with hope to address more aspects of the disease without undesirable side effects.

This chapter is an overview of the available scientific literature focused on antiobesity and antidiabetic potential of selected 42 medicinal and edible plants of the Bulgarian flora. Most of the reports reveal the effect of extracts or their active components on specific biochemical mechanisms. Mechanistic data for hypoglycemic and hypolipidemic action are presented for some of the plants (references summarized in **Table 1**). An essential part of this review is dedicated to the target mechanisms behind the effects of the selected plant species.

Without claiming exhaustiveness, the authors hope that this review will serve as a starting point for future investigations with a contribution to the prevention and therapy of diabetes.

Effects of plants and plant-derived compounds on glucose homeostasis

Inhibition of digestive enzymes and glucose absorption in the intestine

Carbohydrates are an essential part of the human diet and are the main energy source of the body. Starch, sucrose, lactose, and glycogen are the main utilizable carbohydrates in human diet. After the action of salivary and pancreatic α-amylase, the digestion products of starch and glycogen along with disaccharides are further digested in the small intestine epithelium, where the membrane-bound enzyme α-glucosidase, as well as various disaccharidases (saccharase, maltase, lactase), catalyze the release of glucose, fructose, and galactose. Monosaccharides are absorbed through the walls of the small intestine and reach the liver by the portal vein.

Inhibition of digestive enzymes is one possible approach to control early-stage hyperglycemia. Inhibition of α-amylase and α-glucosidase can significantly delay the increase in glucose concentration in the postprandial phase [124–127].

For a significant part of the plants presented in **Table 1**, data on the inhibitory effect of their extracts or active components on digestive enzymes in different experimental approaches were reported (**Table 2**). In vitro studies have found that aqueous extracts of basil and walnut leaves exert an inhibitory effect on α-amylase and α-glucosidase as well as on some disaccharidases without affecting insulin secretion and glucose transport proteins [63, 79]. Both studies suggest that polyphenols play a major role in the observed effects, as an extremely rich content of these active compounds in the two extracts is found. Another study [128] demonstrated a strong inhibitory activity of walnuts on the activity of α-amylase and disaccharidases.

Except aqueous extract of thyme, the extracted essential oil of the plant also exhibits an inhibitory effect on the amylase and glucosidase; Paddy et al. [19] and Pongpiriyadacha et al. [46] found that birch extract significantly reduced blood glucose levels after oral administration of sucrose to rats, a result demonstrating the inhibitory action of the extract on α-glucosidase. The same extract in an in vitro study had a concentration-dependent inhibitory effect on α-glucosidase, saccharase, and maltase.

Effects on glucose homeostasis in the liver

The liver has an essential role in maintenance of glucose homeostasis by controlling the utilization of excess glucose after meal for glycogen synthesis or secretion of free glucose into the circulation through glycogenolysis and gluconeogenesis (GNG) in fasting periods. Insulin and glucagon have a major regulatory role in the activity of these processes. In the periods when the nutrients do not enter the body, all the glucose coming into the circulation is delivered by the liver [129]. Upon food intake, increased glucose levels stimulate secretion of insulin, which has an inhibitory effect on hepatic mechanisms delivering free glucose.

In diabetic patients, this regulation is impaired, and even an increased activity of the key enzymes of gluconeogenesis and glycogenolysis is detected [130, 131].

Galega officinalis has been used from ancient times to alleviate polyuria in diabetic patients. Its active ingredients guanidine and gelagine have been shown to inhibit the enzyme fructose-1,6-bisphosphatase and glucose-6-phosphatase (**Table 2**).

Fructose-1,6-bisphosphatase is a rate-limiting enzyme in GNG, and its activity has been reported to be pathologically elevated in experimental models of insulin resistance (IR) and obesity [132]. Therefore, inhibition of the enzyme could be a promising target to overcome the chronic hyperglycemia and to maintain normoglycemic status during fasting periods. The search for new GNG inhibitors of natural origin may be of great importance in the control of diabetes, especially for patients intolerant to synthetic therapeutics [11].

Glucose-6-phosphatase is a key enzyme in GNG and glycogenolysis, catalyzing the last step—release of free glucose from the liver.

Several plants from our list are described to exert their hypoglycemic action by inhibiting enzymes from GNG (**Table 2**). According to folk medicine, *Melissa* sp. has pronounced spasmolytic and antibacterial action and a slight anxiolytic effect [7]. Scientific data from recent years reveal the antidiabetic potential of the plant ([72]. It was demonstrated that chronic administration of neral and geranial essential oils to db/ db mice had significant hypoglycemic effect, due to their stimulatory and, respectively, inhibitory effects on the gene expression of glucokinase and glucose-6-phosphatase.

Table 2. *Mechanisms of action of selected plants in respect of their antidiabetic potential; ↑-activation, ↓-inhibition.*

Metabolic pathway/ mechanism	Effects on molecular targets	Plant No.	Type of studies
Carbohydrate digestion and absorption	↓ α-amylase	1, 3, 6, 8, 22, 26, 30, 31, 33, 36, 37, 39	Spectrophotometrical assessment of enzyme inhibition; STZ-induced diabetes; kinetics of enzyme inhibition
	↓ α-glucosidase	1, 6, 8, 22, 26, 30, 31, 33, 36, 37	Spectrophotometrical assessment of enzyme inhibition; glucose oxidase-based method

	↓ Disaccharidases	16, 22	Intestinal sucrase and maltase in rats with alloxan-induced diabetes
	↓ Glucose absorption	1, 17, 33, 36, 37	Intestinal cell cultures; diabetic rodents
GNG	PEPCK	16, 19, 21	Gene expression in hepatocytes of diabetic rodents
	Fructose-1,6-bisphosphatase	14	Experimental and clinical studies with metformin
	Glucose-6 phosphatase	14, 19	Gene expression in hepatocytes of diabetic rodents; experimental and clinical studies with metformin
Glycogen synthesis	Glucokinase	16, 19	Gene expression in hepatocytes of diabetic rodents
	Glycogen synthase	2, 6, 35	STZ-induced diabetes in rats; mice muscle cell cultures
Polyol pathway	Aldose reductase	5, 24, 42	Diabetic rodents; in vitro enzyme activity in rats lences
Glucose uptake in IDTs	GLUT-4 translocation	1, 16, 18, 19, 20,, 26, 33, 36, 37, 41	Glucose uptake in C2C12 myotubes; gene expression in 3T3-L1 cell culture
Insulin secretion	SUR1 and Ca^{2+} channels	1, 2, 4, 6, 9, 16, 28	$[Ca^{2+}]$ and [insulin] in pancreatic beta cells
Lipid metabolism	↓ TAG	1, 2, 13, 16, 26, 30, 34	Rats with alloxan- or STZ-induced diabetes; human intervention studies 3T3-L1 cell cultures
	↓ VLDL	1	Rats with alloxan- or STZ-induced diabetes
	↓ HMG-CoA reductase	4, 9, 20, 22, 31, 39	Macrophage and 3T3-L1 cell cultures
	↓ Total cholesterol	1, 2, 16, 33, 34	Rats with alloxan- or STZ-induced diabetes; human intervention studies
	↓ LDL	1, 2, 34	Rats with alloxan- or STZ-induced diabetes; human intervention studies
	↑ HDL	16, 34, 36	Rats with alloxan- or STZ-induced diabetes; human intervention studies; cholesterol fed rabbits
	↑ HDL/LDL ratio	2, 34	Human intervention studies

*Plant numbers are in the order as they are listed in **Table 1**.*

The enzyme glucokinase, also called the "glucose sensor," has a key role in the pancreas and liver to maintain glucose homeostasis. Due to the fact that the enzyme has a high Km value for glucose, its role is to provide an excess of glucose (by phosphorylation to glucose-6-phosphate) to activate insulin secretion and glycogen synthesis. The search for active compounds that can stimulate the enzyme is a relatively new concept in the pharmacological approaches to diabetes treatment [11], and probably the role of medicinal plants as sources of such activators is yet to be explored.

The key enzyme for glycogen synthesis is glycogen synthase. *Agrimonia eupatoria* L., *Asparagus officinalis* L., and *Sambucus nigra* L. have shown a stimulating effect on the enzyme activity, but the mechanisms behind this effect remain unclear. Treatment with agrimony and sparrow grass extracts has resulted in increased amount of glycogen in the muscles and liver of rats with streptozotocininduced diabetes [23, 39]. Elderberry aqueous extract applied to isolated mouse muscle cells stimulated both glucose transport and oxidation as well as glycogen synthesis [111]. Similarly, in cells and animal studies, it was found that preparations and active compounds from *Morus* sp. have inhibitory effects on gene expression of all regulatory GNG enzymes, including phosphoenolpyruvate carboxykinase (PEPCK) [133, 134].

Inhibition of polyol pathway of glucose metabolism

The most serious problems resulting from diabetes mellitus are the complications due to increased blood glucose levels. The body has several options to metabolize the excess glucose. Among them, the polyol pathway is of utmost importance for the development of diabetic complications. Catalyzed by the aldose reductase enzyme, glucose is converted to sorbitol, an osmotically active metabolite which accumulates and damages the cells [135]. It has been shown that inhibition of aldose reductase is preventive against the development of micro- and macrovascular diabetic complications [136, 137].

For three of the selected medicinal plants, data exist about their inhibitory effect on aldose reductase (**Table 2**). Treatment of diabetic mice with ursolic acid isolated from the bearberry resulted in a reduction in fructose and sorbitol levels in the kidneys [38]. Active components of oregano (caffeic and rosmarinic acid) and of maize hair (hirsutrin) have proven in their in vitro inhibitory action on aldose reductase activity in rat lenses [83, 123]. Research on potential enzyme inhibitors has so far not led to the development of therapeutics of general usage [138]. Although scarce, data on such activity of medicinal plants is promising in future quests for such a therapeutic approach.

Effects of glucose transport in insulin-dependent tissues

Insulin modulates several metabolic pathways by activating the phosphatidylinositol-3-kinase (PI3K) cascade, including intracellular translocation of the GLUT-4 transport protein for glucose in skeletal and adipose tissues. In diabetes, the transfer of GLUT-4 towards plasma membrane cannot be accomplished. The hypoglycemic properties of some medicinal plants are due to the ability of their active components to promote the translocation of GLUT-4 to the plasma membrane, resulting in a decrease in blood glucose concentration [20, 90, 106, 139].

Hypoglycemic potential based on this mechanism has been reported primarily for essential oils of lavender, lemon balm, and mint [71, 72]. Luteolin, the flavan derived from *Veronica officinalis*, was shown to activate both the expression and translocation of the glucose transport protein [140].

Hypoglycemic activity of plants: putative mechanisms

Much of the data with regards to the antidiabetic activity of the plants were obtained using models of pharmacologically induced diabetes in experimental animals. The most commonly used diabetes-inducing agents are streptozotocin (STZ) and alloxan [141]. Both compounds have destructive effects on pancreatic β cells by different mechanisms. STZ enters the β cells through the transport protein GLUT-2 and damages DNA, resulting in overexpression of DNA repair systems and thus leading to depletion of cell stores of ATP and oxidized nicotinamide dinucleotide (NAD+) [142, 143]; alloxan, transported by GLUT-2, depletes the thiol groups in the cells, establishing a permanent redox cycle with the dialuric acid (its reduced form). This process leads to the accumulation of ROS and hence to the destruction of β cells, which in general have very limited store of endogenous antioxidants [144].

The models of in vivo induced diabetes are informative in terms of the hypo- glycemic and insulin-like effects of plant extracts. For example, such was the effect of the aqueous oregano extract applied over a period of several weeks to rats with STZ-induced diabetes. In this study, the established potential of the extract to lower blood sugar and glycated hemoglobin was comparable to that of the antidiabetic drug glibenclamide [84]. In another similar in vivo study, the plant extract exhibited an insulin-like effect normalizing blood glucose levels without affecting plasma basal insulin levels [145]. Similar data was also obtained about black mulberry leaf extract [74]. However, in addition to the hypoglycemic effect, an increase in the insulin levels was reported, which may be attributed to the protective and possibly stimulatory action of the plant on β cells' function. Data on the antidiabetic properties of *Phaseolus vulgaris* exist in folk medicine of different ethnic groups [146]. At present, many scientific studies confirm the hypoglycemic and hypolipidemic potential of the plant (predominantly of the pod extract), both in experimentally induced diabetes and in human intervention studies [147–149]. *Vaccinium myrtillus* fruits had beneficial effect on obese subjects in a 6-week intervention study as measured by improved insulin sensitivity, inflammatory biomarker levels, and lipid profile [150]. *Zea mays* hair extracts, as recommended by folk medicine as an antidiabetic remedy, was shown to reduce blood sugar and glycated hemoglobin levels, to stimulate β cells' function and increase serum insulin levels in an experimental model of diabetes [151, 152]. Hypoglycemic and insulin-like effects have also been reported for *Taraxacum officinale* roots, for fruits and flowers of *Sambucus nigra*, stalks of *Alchemilla vulgaris* and *Achillea millefolium*, roots from *Arctium lappa* and *Urtica dioica*, *Cydonia vulgaris* leaves, and other plants presented in **Table 1**.

Effects of plants on insulin secretion

There are two mechanisms by which medicinal plants or their active components possibly stimulate insulin secretion [153]:

- Plant active compounds bind to sulfonylurea binding site 1 (SUR1) of K^+-ATP channels resulting in channel closure and membrane depolarization.
- Direct activation of Ca^{2+} channels.

Sulfonylurea derivatives, such as glibenclamide, are applied for treatment of T2D to stimulate translocation of insulin-containing secretory granules to plasma membrane and exocytosis of insulin in the extracellular matrix [11]. Medicinal plants with an effect on insulin secretion are presented in **Table 2**.

It should be noted that according to most of the studies, the stimulatory activity of medicinal plants on insulin secretion is attributed to their antioxidative potential and ability to prevent SZT- and alloxan-induced beta cell injury in experimental models of diabetes.

Plants that affect lipid metabolism

Defined as abnormal accumulation of adipose tissue, obesity is a major health problem worldwide [154]. As a condition that accompanies obesity, dyslipidemia is believed to be a basic factor for the development of obesity-related diseases such as T2D, cardiovascular diseases (CVD), and atherosclerosis [155]. Dyslipidemia is characterized by increased triacylglycerol (TAG) and total cholesterol levels and unfavorable changes in HDL-/LDL-cholesterol ratio [156, 157].

Many plants that are considered to have antidiabetic potential have beneficial effects on the lipid profile in addition to their hypoglycemic activities [158, 159]. These properties are attributed to their naturally occurring secondary metabolites, such as bioflavonoides. Anthocyanin extracts and anthocyanin-rich diet can improve the parameters of lipid profile and therefore are considered to have anti-obesity and anti-atherogenic effects in humans and in rodents [160–164].

Sambucus ebulus (dwarf elderberry) is a plant widely used in Bulgarian folk medicine in various pathological conditions. Its fruits are rich in anthocyanins. Studies report that anthocyanin extracts can reduce body mass and adipose tissue volume in rats fed with high-fat and high-fructose diet [160, 165–167]. There are reports describing the also hypoglycemic activity of the *S. ebulus* fruits in rats on high-fat and high-fructose diet [168, 169].

A 30-day human intervention study with *S. ebulus* fruit tea decreased significantly TAG, total cholesterol, and LDL-cholesterol levels. Slight increase of HDL and significant increase in HDL/LDL ratio were found ([110].

Low HDL levels are recognized as an independent risk factor for the development of cardiovascular diseases [170]. Inhibition of cholesteryl ester transfer protein (CETP) is a probable cause for the increased HDL-cholesterol levels, and LDL- cholesterol levels decrease upon anthocyanin treatment [171]. Anthocyanins can decrease quantity and the activity of CETP in plasma of dyslipidemic patients [161].

The scientific data cited above are in support to the folk medicine reports about the healing properties of *S. ebulus* fruit preparations.

Likewise, lipid profile improving properties have been reported for *Agrimonia eupatoria* (agrimony). Its effect on lipid profile was estimated in our study in a model of metabolic disturbances in rats on high-fructose diet. Intake of 40% aqueous-ethanol extract prevented fat accumulation in the liver and adipose tissue and normalized levels of serum lipids [167].

In addition, we performed a human intervention study with 30-day agrimony tea consumption. As a result, increased levels of HDL cholesterol were established, and LDL-cholesterol levels remained unchanged at the same time [29]. These results reveal good potential of agrimony to improve lipid profile, which is important in prophylaxis of CVD and diabetes.

It can be assumed that polyphenols play a role in the mechanisms by which the plant manifests its effects. It is known that diet rich in polyphenols may improve lipid profile in individuals with normal or compromised health status [172, 173]. Polyphenol preparations and polyphenol-rich extracts have also the potential to improve lipid profile [174–177]. As it was already mentioned, *S. ebulus* fruits are a rich source of polyphenols and especially of anthocyanins [33, 108]. Also, it was found that the aqueous and aqueous alcoholic extracts of agrimony have a high polyphenol content [25, 178], although their exact polyphenol composition has not yet been identified. Polyphenols have limited bioavailability; however, many of the products of their intestinal metabolism overcome the intestinal barrier and reach the tissues where they exert their biological effects [179].

Some of the selected plants (**Table 1**) can exert their effects by inhibiting the activity of the rate-limiting enzyme in cholesterol synthesis—HMG-CoA reductase [99]. Cholesterol is the most abundant sterol in the human body and is essential for the normal functioning of the cells. Cholesterol homeostasis is of great importance for the health status. Apart from being a risk factor for atherosclerosis, increased plasma cholesterol levels are often an accompanying parameter of the metabolic disturbances, such as diabetes. Despite being applied for decades, HMG-CoA reductase inhibitors have adverse and unwanted effects, such as myopathy, liver insufficiency, etc. [99].

Even more, in a case of strictly controlled LDL-cholesterol levels by statins, not always TAG and HDL-cholesterol levels are sensitive to the therapy, and there is still a chance that CVD risk would remain high [180]. Interventions with *S. ebulus* and *A. eupatoria* tea resulted in significantly increased HDL/LDL ratio; beneficial effects of these plants on plasma TAG and total cholesterol levels were established, so it is likely that the plants improve all parameters of the lipid profile. This makes them promising sources of active compounds with a potential to prevent and supplement the therapy of T2D and CVD.

In addition to the above, scientific data about the beneficial effects of rosehip, strawberries, and raspberries on lipid metabolism and inflammation exist (**Table 1**). These plants are rich in the glycoside flavonoid tiliroside, which was shown to inhibit postprandial inflammation, to play a role in the prevention of obesity, hyperinsulinemia, and hyperlipidemia. Its action is associated with elevated levels of adiponectin and also facilitated fatty acids oxidation in the liver and skeletal muscles [181]. Strawberry anthocyanin pelargonidin sulfate and pelargonidin-3-O-glycoside reduced postprandial inflammation and increased insulin sensitivity in overweight individuals [56]. Polyphenols extracted from strawberry decreased postprandial LDL oxidation and enhanced lipid metabolism in a high-fat intervention with overweight individuals with hyperlipidemia [182]. Six of the plants listed in **Table 1** (*Arctium lappa, Cichorium intybus, Mentha piperita, Ocimum basilicum, Rosa damascena, Urtica dioica*) had also inhibitory effect of HMG-CoA reductase. Among them, the extract of *R. damascena* was found to be the most potent one [99].

The discovery of new effective and safe in long-term application therapeutics is essential for the control and prevention of obesity-related diseases. In this respect, the potential of medicinal and edible plants is still to be explored.

Conclusions

The summarized scientific data give a concept about the mechanisms behind the healing effects of plants traditionally used in Bulgarian folk medicine and traditional diet. The selected plants and their active compounds could exert their hypoglycemic and antiobese effects by affecting simultaneously several molecular markers in various processes from carbohydrate and lipid metabolism. Moreover, along with their insulin-like properties, many of the plants can stimulate the insulin secretion. This makes them invaluable in prevention and therapy of socially significant diseases such as diabetes and cardiovascular diseases. Despite the capacity of biotechnology methods to develop new therapeutics, it may be worth to turn a look at the natural resources which potential is still unrevealed.

Author details

Milka Nashar*, Yoana D. Kiselova-Kaneva and Diana G. Ivanova Medical University of Varna, Varna, Bulgaria

*Address all correspondence to: nacharbg@yahoo.com

References

[1] WHO Report. Definition and diagnosis of diabetes mellitus and intermediate hyperglycemia. 2006. ISBN: 9241594934

[2] Ahmed AM. History of diabetes mellitus. Saudi Medical Journal. 2002;**23**:373-378

[3] Eknoyan G, Nagy J. A history of diabetes mellitus or how a disease of the kidneys evolved into a kidney disease. Advances in Chronic Kidney Disease. 2005;**12**:223-229

[4] Lasker SP, McLachlan CS, Wang L, Ali SMK, Jelinek HF. Discovery, treatment and management of diabetes. Journal of Diabetology. 2010;**1**:1

[5] Eddouks M, Zeggwagh NA. Hypoglycemic Plants: Folklore to modern evidence review. In: Eddouks M, Chattopadhyay D, editors. Phytotherapy in the management of diabetes and hypertension. Bentham Science Publishers, Sharjah, U.A.E.; 2012:164-192. ISBN: 978-1-60805-567-8

[6] Teodorov E. Ancient-Thracian Heritage in Bulgarian Folklore. Academic Publishing House of Bulgarian Academy of Sciences "Professor Marin Drinov", Sofia, Bulgaria; 1999. ISBN: 9544304983

[7] Dimkov P. Bulgarian Folk Medicine. Vol. 1. Sofia, Bulgaria; BASPRESS: Publishing House of Bulgarian Academy of Sciences; 1977

[8] Dimkov P. Bulgarian Folk Medicine. Vol. 2. BASPRESS: Publishing House of Bulgarian Academy of Sciences, Sofia, Bulgaria; 1978

[9] Dimkov P. Bulgarian Folk Medicine. Vol. 3. BASPRESS: Publishing House of Bulgarian Academy of Sciences, Sofia, Bulgaria; 1979

[10] Nedelcheva A. Medicinal plants from an old Bulgarian medical book. Journal of Medicinal Plants Research. 2012;**6**(12):2324-2339

[11] Verspohl EJ. Novel pharmacological approaches to the treatment of type 2 diabetes. Pharmacological Reviews. 2012;**64**:188-237

[12] Tahrani A. Novel therapies in type 2 diabetes: Insulin resistance. Practical Diabetes. 2017;**34**(5):161-166

[13] Petlevski R, Hadzija M, Slijepcevic M, Juretic D. Effect of 'antidiabetis' herbal preparation on serum glucose and fructosamine in NOD mice. Journal of Ethnopharmacology. 2001;**75**(2-3):181-184

[14] Petlevski R, Hadžija M, Slijepčević M, Juretić D, Petrik J. Glutathione S-transferases and malondialdehyde in the liver of NOD mice on short-term treatment with plant mixture extract P-9801091. Phytotherapy Research. 2003;**17**(4):311-314

[15] Yazdanparast R, Ardestani A, Jamshidi S. Experimental diabetes treated with *Achillea santolina*: Effect on pancreatic oxidative parameters. Journal of Ethnopharmacology. 2007;**112**(1):13-18

[16] Saeidnia S, Gohari AR, Mokhber- Dezfuli N, Kiuchi F. A review on phytochemistry and medicinal properties of the genus *Achillea*. Daru. 2011;**19**(3):173-186

[17] Mustafa KG, Ganai BA, Akbar S, Dar MY, Masood A. β-Cell protective efficacy, hypoglycemic and hypolipidemic effects of extracts of *Achillea millifolium* in diabetic rats. Chinese Journal of Natural Medicines. 2012;**10**(3):0185-0189

[18] Zolghadri Y, Fazeli M, Kooshki M, Shomali T, Karimaghayee N, Dehghani M. *Achillea millefolium* L. hydro-alcoholic extract protects pancreatic cells by down regulating IL- 1β and iNOS gene expression in diabetic rats. International Journal of Molecular and Cellular Medicine. 2014;**3**(4):255-262

[19] Paddy V, van Tonder JJ, Steenkamp V. In vitro antidiabetic activity of a polyherbal tea and its individual ingredients. British Journal of Pharmaceutical Research. 2015;**6**(6):389-401

[20] Chávez-Silva F, Cerón-Romeroa L, Arias-Durána L, Navarrete-Vázqueza G,Almanza-Pérezb J, Román-Ramosb R, et al. Antidiabetic effect of *Achillea millefollium* through multitarget interactions: α-glucosidases inhibition, insulin sensitization and insulin secretagogue activities. Journal of Ethnopharmacology. 2018;**212**:1-7

[21] Bailey CJ, Day C. Traditional plant medicines as treatments for diabetes. Diabetes Care. 1989;**12**(8):553-564

[22] Kubinova R, Jankovska D, Bauerova V. Antioxidant and alpha- glucosidase inhibition activities and polyphenol content of five species of *Agrimonia* genus. Acta Fytotechnica et Zootechnica. 2012;**2**:38-41

[23] Gray AM, Flatt PR. Actions of the traditional anti-diabetic plant, *Agrimony eupatoria* (agrimony): Effects on hyperglycaemia, cellular glucose metabolism and insulin secretion. The British Journal of Nutrition. 1998;**80**(1):109-114

[24] Al-Snafi AE. The pharmacological and therapeutic importance of *Agrimonia eupatoria*—A review. Asian Journal of Pharmacy and Technology. 2015;**5**(2):112-117

[25] Ivanova D, Gerova D, Chervenkov T, Yankova T. Polyphenols and antioxidant capacity of Bulgarian medicinal plants. Journal of Ethnopharmacology. 2005;**96**:45-150

[26] Bnouham M, Abderrahim Z, Mekhfi H, Tahri A, Legssyer A. Medicinal plants with potential antidiabetic activity—A review of ten years of herbal medicine research (1990-2000). International Journal of Diabetes and Metabolism. 2006;**14**:1-25

[27] Ivanova D, Tasinov O, Vankova D, Kiselova-Kaneva Y. Antioxidative potential of *Agrimonia eupatoria* L. Science and Technology. 2011;**1**(1):20-24

[28] Patel DK, Prasad SK, Kumar R, Hemalatha S. An overview on antidiabetic medicinal plants having insulin mimetic property. Asian Pacific Journal of Tropical Biomedicine. 2012;**2**(4):320-330

[29] Ivanova D, Vankova D, Nashar M. *Agrimonia eupatoria* tea consumption in relation to markers of inflammation, oxidative status and lipid metabolism in healthy subjects. Archives of Physiology and Biochemistry. 2013;**119**(1):32-37

[30] Kuczmannová A, Balažová A, Racanská E, Kameníková M, Fialová S, Majerník J, et al. *Agrimonia eupatoria* L. and *Cynara cardunculus* L. water infusions: Comparison of anti-diabetic activities. Molecules. 2016;**21**:564

[31] Alam F, Shafique Z, Amjad ST, Asad A. Enzymes inhibitors from natural sources with antidiabetic activity: A review: New targets for antidiabetic treatment. Phytotherapy Research. 2019;**33**(1):41-54

[32] Neagua E, Pauna G, Albua C, Radu GL. Assessment of acetylcholinesterase and tyrosinase inhibitory and antioxidant activity of *Alchemilla vulgaris* and *Filipendula ulmaria* extracts. Journal of the Taiwan Institute of Chemical Engineers. 2015;**52**:1-6

[33] Kiselova Y, Ivanova D, Chervenkov T, Gerova D, Galunska B, Yankova T. Correlation between the in vitro antioxidant activity and polyphenol content of aqueous extracts from Bulgarian herbs. Phytotherapy Research. 2006;**20**:961-965

[34] Swanston-Flatt SK, Day C, Flatt PR, Gould BJ, Bailey CJ. Glycaemic effects of traditional European plant treatments for diabetes. Studies in normal and streptozotocin diabetic mice. Diabetes Research. 1989;**10**(2):69-73

[35] Chan YS, Cheng LN, Wu JH, Chan E, Kwan YW, Lee SM, et al. A review of the pharmacological effects of Arctium lappa (burdock). Inflammopharmacology. 2011;**19**(5):245-254

[36] Xu Z, Wang X, Zhou M, Ma L, Deng Y, Zhang H, et al. The antidiabetic activity of total lignan from Fructus Arctii against alloxan-induced diabetes in mice and rats. Phytotherapy Research. 2008;**22**(1):97-101

[37] Slanc P, Doljak B, Kreft S, Lunder M, Janes D, Strukelj B. Screening of selected food and medicinal plant extracts for pancreatic lipase inhibition. Phytotherapy Research. 2009;**23**(6):874-877

[38] Wang P, Mariman E, Renes J, Keijer J. The secretory function of adipocytes in the physiology of white adipose tissue. Journal of Cellular Physiology. 2008;**216**:3-13

[39] Zhao J, Zhang W, Zhu X, Zhao D, Wang K, Wang R, et al. The aqueous extract of *Asparagus officinalis* L. by-product exerts hypoglycaemic activity in streptozotocin-induced diabetic rats. Journal of the Science of Food and Agriculture. 2011;**91**(11):2095-2099

[40] Hafizur RM, Kabir N, Chishti S. *Asparagus officinalis* extract controls blood glucose by improving insulin secretion and β-cell function in streptozotocin-induced type 2 diabetic rats. The British Journal of Nutrition. 2012;**108**(9):1586-1595

[41] Zhang W, Wu W, Wang Q , Chen Y, Yue G. The juice of asparagus by-product exerts hypoglycemic activity in streptozotocin-induced diabetic rats. Journal of Food Biochemistry. 2014;**38**(5):509-517

[42] Meliani N, Amine Dib ME, Allali H, Tabti B. Hypoglycaemic effect of *Berberis vulgaris* L. in normal and streptozotocin-induced diabetic rats. Asian Pacific Journal of Tropical Biomedicine. 2011;**1**(6):468-471

[43] Hajzadeh MAR, Rajaei Z, Shafiee S, Alavinejhad A, Samarghandian S, Ahmadi M. Effect of barberry fruit (*Berberis vulgaris*) on serum glucose and lipids in streptozotocin-diabetic rats. Pharmacology Online. 2011;**1**:809-817

[44] Arumugama G, Manjulab P, Paari N. A review: Anti diabetic medicinal plants used for diabetes mellitus. Journal of Acute Disease. 2013;**2**(3):196-200

[45] Ahmad R, Srivastava SP, Maurya R, Rajendran SM, Arya KR, Srivastava AK. Mild antihyperglycaemic activity in *Eclipta alba, Berberis aristata, Betula utilis, Cedrus deodara, Myristica fragrans and Terminalia chebula*. Indian Journal of Science and Technology. 2008;**1**(5):1-6. DOI: 10.17485/ijst/2008/v1i5/29348

[46] Pongpiriyadacha Y, Nuansrithong P, Chantip D. Antidiabetic activity of the methanolic extract from *Betula alnoides* Buch-Ham. ex G. Don. Journal of Applied Sciences Research. 2013;**9**(12):6185-6188

[47] Abd El-Ghany MA, Nagib RM, Mamdouh SM. Anti-diabetic effect of some herbs and fruit against streptozotocin induced diabetic rats. Global Veterinaria. 2014;**12**(4):541-549

[48] Savikin K, Zdunic G, Jankovic T, Stanojkovic T, Juranic Z, Menkovic N. In vitro cytotoxic and antioxidative activity of *Cornus mas* and *Cotinus coggygria*. Natural Product Research. 2009;**23**(18):1731-1739

[49] Aslan M, Orhan N, Orhan DD, Ergun F. Hypoglycemic activity and antioxidant potential of some medicinal plants traditionally used in Turkey for diabetes. Journal of Ethnopharmacology. 2010;**128**(2):384-389

[50] Khoubnasabjafari M, Jouyban A. A review of phytochemistry and bioactivity of quince (*Cydonia oblonga* Mill.). Journal of Medicinal Plant Research: Planta Medica. 2011;**5**(16):3577-3594

[51] Sajid SM, Zubair M, Waqas M, Nawaz M, Ahmad Z. A review on quince (*Cydonia oblonga*): A useful medicinal plant. Global Veterinaria. 2015;**14**(4):517-524

[52] Abou El-Soud N, El-Laithy N, El-Saeed G, Wahby KM, Morsy F, Shaffie N. Antidiabetic activities of *Foeniculum vulgare* Mill. essential oil in streptozotocin-induced diabetic rats. Macedonian Journal of Medical Sciences. 2011;**4**(2):139-146

[53] Rathera MA, Dara BA, Sofia SN, Bhata BA, Qurishi MA. Foeniculum vulgare: A comprehensive review of its traditional use, phytochemistry, pharmacology, and safety. Arabian Journal of Chemistry. 2016;**9**:S1574-S1583

[54] Hilmi Y, Abushama MF, Abdalgadir H, Khalid A, Khalid H. A study of antioxidant activity, enzymatic inhibition and in vitro toxicity of selected traditional sudanese plants with anti-diabetic potential. BMC Complementary and Alternative Medicine. 2014;**14**:149

[55] Marles RJ, Farnsworth NR. Antidiabetic plants and their active constituents. Phytomedicine. 1995;**2**(2):137-189. DOI: 10.1016/ S0944-7113(11)80059-0

[56] Edirisinghe I, Banaszewski K, Cappozzo J, Sandhya K, Ellis CL, Tadapaneni R, et al. Strawberry anthocyanin and its association with postprandial inflammation and insulin. The British Journal of Nutrition. 2011;**106**(6):913-922. DOI: 10.1017/ S0007114511001176

[57] Lemus I, García R, Delvillar E, Knop G. Hypoglycaemic activity of four plants used in Chilean popular medicine. Phytotherapy Research. 1999;**13**(2):91-94

[58] Andrade-Cetto A. Effects of medicinal plant extracts on gluconeogenesis. Botanics: Targets and Therapy. 2012;**2**:1-6

[59] Hunter RW, Hughey CC, Lantier L, Sundelin EI, Peggie M, Zeqiraj E, et al. Metformin reduces liver glucose production by inhibition of fructose- 1-6-bisphosphatase. Nature Medicine. 2018;**24**:1395-1406

[60] Husain GM, Chatterjee SS, Singh PN, Kumar V. Hypolipidemic and antiobesity-like activity of standardised extract of *Hypericum perforatum* L. in rats. ISRN Pharmacology. 2011;**2011**:505247. 7 p. DOI: 10.5402/2011/505247

[61] Tian J, Tao R, Zhang X, Liu Q, He Y, Su Y, et al. Effect of *Hypericum perforatum* L. extract on insulin resistance and lipid metabolic disorder in high-fat-diet induced obese mice. Phytotherapy Research. 2015;**29**(1):86-92

[62] Çoban T, Çitoglu GS, Sever B, Iscan M. Antioxidant activities of plants used in traditional medicine in Turkey. Pharmaceutical Biology. 2003;**41**(8):608-613

[63] Teimori M, Montasser Kouhsari MS, Ghafarzadegan R, Hajiaghaee R. Study of hypoglycemic effect of *Juglans regia* leaves and its mechanism. Journal of Medicinal Plants. 2010;**9**(Suppl 6):57-65

[64] Taha NA, Alwadaan MA. Utility and importance of walnut, *Juglans regia* Linn: A review. African Journal of Microbiology Research. 2011;**5**(32):5796-5805

[65] Hosseini S, Huseini HF, Larijani B, Mohammad K, Najmizadeh A, Nourijelyani K, et al. The hypoglycemic effect of *Juglans regia* leaves aqueous extract in diabetic patients: A first human trial. Daru. 2014;**22**(1):19

[66] Pitschmann A, Zehl M, Atanasov AG, Dirsch VM, Heiss E, Glasl S. Walnut leaf extract inhibits PTP1B and enhances glucose-uptake in vitro. Journal of Ethnopharmacology. 2014;**152**(3):599-602

[67] Rahimzadeh M, Jahanshahi S, Moein S, Moein MR. Evaluation of alpha-amylase inhibition by *Urtica dioica* and *Juglans regia* extracts. Iranian Journal of Basic Medical Sciences. 2014;**17**(6):465-469

[68] Khoramdelazad H, Pourrashidi A, Hasanshahi G, Vazirinejad R, Hajizadeh M, Mirzaei M, et al. Effect of the Iranian walnut (*Juglans regia*) leaves extract on gene expression of gluconeogenic and glycogenolytic enzymes in stz-induced diabetic rats. International Journal of Current Research in Biosciences and Plant Biology. 2015;**2**(5):47-55

[69] Panth N, Paudel KR, Karki R. Phytochemical profile and biological activity of *Juglans regia*. Journal of Integrative Medicine. 2016;**14**(5):359-373

[70] Issa A, Mohammad M, Hudaib M, Tawah K, Abu Rjai T, Oran S, et al. A potential role of *Lavandula angustifolia* in the management of diabetic dyslipidemia. Journal of Medicinal Plant Research: Planta Medica. 2011;**5**(16):3876-3882

[71] Yen HF, Hsieh CT, Hsieh TJ, Chang FR, Wang CK. In vitro anti-diabetic effect and chemical component analysis of 29 essential oils products. Journal of Food and Drug Analysis. 2015;**23**:124-129

[72] Chung MJ, Cho SY, Bhuiyan MJH, Kim KH, Lee SJ. Anti-diabetic effects of lemon balm (*Melissa officinalis*) essential oil on glucose- and lipid- regulating enzymes in type 2 diabetic mice. British Journal of Nutrition. 2010;**104**:180-188

[73] Volpatoa GT, Calderona IMP, Sinzatoa S, Camposa KE, Rudgea MVC, Damascenoa DC. Effect of *Morus nigra* aqueous extract treatment on the maternal–Fetal outcome, oxidative stress status and lipid profile of streptozotocin-induced diabetic rats. Journal of Ethnopharmacology. 2011;**138**:691-696

[74] Abd El-Mawla AMA, Mohamed KM, Mostafa AM. Induction of biologically active flavonoids in cell cultures of *Morus nigra* and testing their hypoglycemic efficacy. Scientia Pharmaceutica. 2011;**79**:951-961

[75] Pasheva M, Nashar M, Tasinov O, Ivanova D. Effects of mulberry heartwood extract on genes related to lipid metabolism. Scripta Scientifica Pharmaceutica. 2015;**2**(1):34-39

[76] Agrawal P, Rai V, Singh RB. Randomized placebo-controlled, single blind trial of holy basil leaves in patients with noninsulin-dependent diabetes mellitus. International Journal of Clinical Pharmacology and Therapeutics. 1996;**34**(9):406-409

[77] Lee SJ, Umano K, Shibamoto T, Lee KG. Identification of volatile components in basil (*Ocimum basilicum* L.) and thyme leaves (*Thymus vulgaris* L.) and their antioxidant properties. Food Chemistry. 2005;**91**:131-137

[78] Zeggwagh NA, Sulpice T, Eddouks M. Anti-hyperglycaemic and hypolipidemic effects of *Ocimum basilicum* aqueous extract in diabetic rats. American Journal of Pharmacology and Toxicology. 2007;**2**(3):123-129

[79] El-Beshbishy H, Bahashwan S. Hypoglycemic effect of basil (*Ocimum basilicum*) aqueous extract is mediated through inhibition of α-glucosidase and α-amylase activities: An in vitro study. Toxicology and Industrial Health. 2012;**28**(1):42-50

[80] Ugwu MN, Umar IA, Utu-Baku AB, Dasofunjo K, Ukpanukpong RU, Yakubu OE, et al. Antioxidant status and organ function in streptozotocin-induced diabetic rats treated with aqueous, methanolic and petroleum ether extracts of *Ocimum basilicum* leaf. Journal of Applied Pharmaceutical Science. 2013;**3** (4 Suppl 1):S75-S79

[81] Rouhi-Boroujeni H, Rouhi- Boroujeni H, Heidarian E, Mohammadizadeh F, Rafician-Kopaei A. Herbs with anti-lipid effects and their interactions with statins as a chemical anti- hyperlipidemia group drugs: A systematic review. ARYA Atherosclerosis. 2015;**11**(4):244-251

[82] Choudhury H, Pandey M, Hua CK, Mun CS, Jing JK, Kong L, et al. An update on natural compounds in the remedy of diabetes mellitus: A systematic review. Journal of Traditional and Complementary Medicine. 2018;**8**(3):361-376

[83] Veeresham C, Rao AR, Asres K. Aldose reductase inhibitors of plant origin. Phytotherapy Research. 2013;**28**:317-333. DOI: 10.1002/ptr.5000

[84] Mohamed NA, Nassier OA. The antihyperglycaemic effect of the aqueous extract of *Origanium vulgare* leaves in streptozotocin-induced diabetic rats. Jordan Journal of Biological Sciences. 2013;**6**(1):31-38

[85] Vujicic M, Nikolic I, Kontogianni VG, Saksida T, Charisiadis P, Orescanin- Dusic Z, et al. Methanolic extract of *Origanum vulgare* ameliorates type 1 diabetes through antioxidant, anti- inflammatory and anti-apoptotic activity. The British Journal of Nutrition. 2015;**113**(5):770-782

[86] Boukhris M, Bouaziz M, Feki I, Jemai H, El Feki A, Sayadi S. Hypoglycemic and antioxidant effects of leaf essential oil of *Pelargonium graveolens* L. in alloxan induced diabetic rats. Lipids in Health and Disease. 2012;**11**:81

[87] Saraswathi J, Venkatesh K, Baburao N, Hilal MH, Rani AR. Phytopharmacological importance of *Pelargonium* species. Journal of Medicinal Plants Research. 2011;**5**(13):2587-2598

[88] Tormo MA, Gil-Exojo I, Romero de Tejada A, Campillo JE. Hypoglycaemic and anorexigenic activities of an alpha- amylase inhibitor from white kidney beans (*Phaseolus vulgaris*) in Wistar rats. The British Journal of Nutrition. 2004;**92**(5):785-790

[89] Carai MAM, Fantini N, Loi B, Colombo G, Riva A, Morazzoni P. Potential efficacy of preparations derived from Phaseolus vulgaris in the control of appetite, energy intake, and carbohydrate metabolism. Diabetes, Metabolic Syndrome and Obesity. 2009;**2**:145-153

[90] Fatima A, Agrawal P, Singh PP. Herbal option for diabetes: An overview. Asian Pacific Journal of Tropical Disease. 2012;**2**:S536-S544

[91] Etxeberria U, de la Garza AL, Campión J, Martínez JA, Milagro FI. Antidiabetic effects of natural plant extracts via inhibition of carbohydrate hydrolysis enzymes with emphasis on pancreatic alpha amylase. Expert Opinion on Therapeutic Targets. 2012;**16**(3):269-297

[92] Kemper KJ. Rhubarb root (Rheum officinale or *R. palmatum*). The Center for Holistic Pediatric Education and Research. Longwood Herbal Task Force. Available from: http://www.mcp.edu/ herbal/default.htm

[93] Gao Q , Qin WS, Jia ZH, Zheng JM, Zeng CH, Li LS, et al. Rhein improves renal lesion and ameliorates dyslipidemia in db/db mice with diabetic nephropathy. Planta Medica. 2010;**76**(1):27-33

[94] Cosima C, Roufogalis BD, Müller- Ladner U, Chrubasik S. A systematic review on the *Rosa canina* effect and efficacy profiles. Phytotherapy Research. 2008;**22**:725-733

[95] Orhan N, Aslan M, Hosbas S, Deliorman OD. Antidiabetic effect and antioxidant potential of *Rosa canina* fruits. Pharmacognosy Magazine. 2009;**5**:309-315

[96] Asghari B, Salehi P, Farimani MM, Ebrahimi SN. α-Glucosidase inhibitors from fruits of *Rosa canina* L. Rec. Journal of Natural Products. 2015;**9**:3276-3283

[97] Boskabady MH, Shafei MN, Saberi Z, Amini S. Pharmacological effects of *Rosa damascene*. Iranian Journal of Basic Medical Sciences. 2011;**14**(4):295-307

[98] Gholamhoseinian A, Fallah H, Sharifi far F. Inhibitory effect of methanol extract of *Rosa damascena* Mill. flowers on alpha-glucosidase activity and postprandial hyperglycemia in normal and diabetic rats. Phytomedicine. 2009;**16**(10):935-941

[99] Gholamhoseinian A, Shahouzehi B, Sharifi-Far F. Inhibitory activity of some plant methanol extracts on 3-hydroxy- 3-methylglutaryl coenzyme a reductase. International Journal of Pharmacology. 2010;**6**(5):705-711

[100] Bispo K, Piovezan M, García-Seco D, Amusquivar E, Dudzik D, Ramos- Solano B, et al. Blackberry (*Rubus* sp. var. Loch Ness) extract reduces obesity induced by a cafeteria diet and affects the lipophilic metabolomic profile in rats. Journal of Food and Nutritional Disorders. 2014;**3**:4

[101] Zia-Ul-Haq M, Riaz M, De Feo V, Jaafar HZE, Moga M. *Rubus fruticosus* L.: Constituents, biological activities and health related uses. Molecules. 2014;**19**:10998-11029

[102] Eidi M, Eidi A, Zamanizadeh H. Effect of *Salvia officinalis* L. leaves on serum glucose and insulin in healthy and streptozotocin-induced diabetic rats. Journal of Ethnopharmacology. 2005;**100**(3):310-313

[103] Lima CF, Andrade PB, Seabra RM, Fernandes-Ferreira M, Pereira-Wilson C. The drinking of a *Salvia officinalis* infusion improves liver antioxidant status in mice and rats. Journal of Ethnopharmacology. 2005;**97**:383-389

[104] Alarcon-Aguilar FJ, Roman-Ramos R, Flores-Saenz JL, Aguirre-Garcia F. Investigation on the hypoglycaemic effects of extracts of four Mexican medicinal plants in normal and alloxan- diabetic mice. Phytotherapy Research. 2002;**16**:383-386

[105] Lima CF, Azevedo MF, Araujo R, Fernandes-Ferreira M, Pereira-Wilson C. Metformin-like effect of *Salvia officinalis* (common sage): Is it useful in diabetes prevention? The British Journal of Nutrition. 2006;**96**:326-333

[106] Moradabadi L, Montasser Kouhsari S, Fehresti Sani M. Hypoglycemic effects of three medicinal plants in experimental diabetes: Inhibition of rat intestinal α-glucosidase and enhanced pancreatic insulin and cardiac glut-4 mRNAs expression. Iranian Journal of Pharmaceutical Research. 2013;**12**(3):387-397

[107] Shokrzadeh M, Saravi S. The chemistry, pharmacology and clinical properties of *Sambucus ebulus*: A review. Journal of Medicinal Plant Research: Planta Medica. 2010;**4**(2):095-103

[108] Tasinov O, Kiselova–Kaneva Y, Ivanova D. Antioxidant activity, total polyphenol content and anthocyanins content of *Sambucus ebulus* L. aqueous and aqueous—Ethanolic extracts depend on the type and concentration of extragent. Science & Technologies. 2012;**2**(1):37-41

[109] Tasinov O, Kiselova-Kaneva Y, Ivanova D. *Sambucus ebulus* L. fruit aqueous infusion modulates GCL and GPx4 gene expression. Bulgarian Journal of Agricultural Science. 2013;**19**(Supplement 2):143-146

[110] Tasinov O. Investigation of antioxidant, antiobesity and antidiabetic action of Sambucus ebulus fruit extracts in vitro and in vivo [thesis]. 2015

[111] Gray AM, Abdel-Wahab YH, Flatt PR. The traditional plant treatment, *Sambucus nigra* (elder), exhibits insulin- like and insulin-releasing actions in vitro. The Journal of Nutrition. 2000;**130**(1):15-20

[112] Ciocoiu M, Miron A, Mares L, Tutunaru D, Pohaci C, Groza M, et al. The effects of Sambucus nigra polyphenols on oxidative stress and metabolic disorders in experimental diabetes mellitus. Journal of Physiology and Biochemistry. 2009;**65**(3):297-304

[113] Badescu L, Badulescu O, Badescu M, Ciocoiu M. Mechanism by *Sambucus nigra* extract improves bone mineral density in experimental diabetes. Evidence-based Complementary and Alternative Medicine. 2012;**2012**:848269

[114] Yarnell E, Abascal K. Dandelion (*Taraxacum officinale* and *T. mongolicum*). Journal of Integrative Medicine. 2009;**8**(2):35-38

[115] European Medicines Agency of EU. Committee on Herbal Medicinal Products. Assessment report on Tilia cordata Mill., Tilia platyphyllos Scop., Tilia x vulgaris Heyne or their mixtures, flos. 2012. Document 337067/2011, Available from: www.ema.europa.eu

[116] Das M, Sarma BP, Rokeya B, Parial R, Nahar N, Mosihuzzaman M. Antihyperglycemic and antihyperlipidemic activity of *Urtica dioica* on type 2 diabetic model rats. Journal of Diabetology. 2011;**2**:2

[117] Mobaseri M, Aliasgarzadeh A, Bahrami A, Zargami N, Tabrizi A. Efficacy of the total extract of *Urtica dioica* on the glucose utilization by the human muscle cells. Journal of Clinical and Diagnostic Research. 2012;**6**:437-440

[118] Ahangarpour A, Mohammadian M, Dianat M. Antidiabetic effect of hydroalcholic *Urtica dioica* leaf extract in male rats with fructose-induced insulin resistance. Iranian Journal of Medical Sciences. 2012;**37**(3):181-186

[119] Qujeq D, Tatar M, Feizi F, Parsian H, Faraji AS, Halalkhor S. Effect of *Urtica dioica* leaf alcoholic and aqueous extracts on the number and the diameter of the islets in diabetic rats. International Journal of Molecular and Cellular Medicine. 2013;**2**(1):21-26

[120] Kianbakht S, Khalighi-Sigaroodi F, Dabaghian FH. Improved glycemic control in patients with advanced type 2 diabetes mellitus taking *Urtica dioica* leaf extract: A randomized double-blind placebo-controlled clinical trial. Clinical Laboratory. 2013;**59**(9-10):1071-1076

[121] Gründemann C, Garcia- Käufer M, Sauer B, Stangenberg E, Könczöl M, Merfort I, et al. Traditionally used *Veronica officinalis* inhibits proinflammatory mediators via the NF-κB signalling pathway in a human lung cell line. Journal of Ethnopharmacology. 2013;**145**(1):118-126

[122] Crişan G, Tămaş M, Miclăuş V, Krausz T, Sandor V. A comparative study of some Veronica species. Revista Medico-Chirurgicală a Societăţii de Medici şi Naturalişti din Iaşi. 2007;**111**(1):280-284

[123] Kim TH, Kim JK, Kang YH, Lee JY, Kang IJ, Lim SS. Aldose reductase inhibitory activity of compounds from *Zea mays* L. BioMed Research International. 2013;**2013**:727143. 8 pages. DOI: 10.1155/2013/727143

[124] Layer P, Zinsmeister AR, DiMagno EP. Effects of decreasing intraluminal amylase activity on starch digestion and postprandial gastrointestinal function in humans. Gastroenterology. 1986;**91**(1):41-48

[125] Bischoff H. Pharmacology of alpha-glucosidase inhibition. European Journal of Clinical Investigation. 1994;**24**(Suppl 3):3-10

[126] Park MH, Ju JW, Park MJ, Han JS. Daidzein inhibits carbohydrate digestive enzymes in vitro and alleviates postprandial hyperglycemia in diabetic mice. European Journal of Pharmacology. 2013;**712**(1-3):48-52

[127] Hamden K, Mnafgui K, Amri Z, Aloulou A, Elfeki A. Inhibition of key digestive enzymes related to diabetes and hyperlipidemia and protection of liver-kidney functions by trigonelline in diabetic rats. Scientia Pharmaceutica. 2013;**81**(1):233-246

[128] Fukuda T, Ito H, Yoshida T. Effect of the walnut polyphenol fraction on oxidative stress in type 2 diabetes mice. BioFactors. 2004;**2**:251-253

[129] Tan B, Ong K. Influence of dietary polyphenols on carbohydrate metabolism. In: Watson RR, Preedy VR, Zibadi S, editors. Polyphenols in Human Health and Disease. Vol. 2, Academic Press Elsevier Inc, London, UK; 2014. pp. 95-111. ISBN: 978-1239-8471-2

[130] Firth RG, Bell PM, Marsh HM, Hansen I, Rizza RA. Postprandial hyperglycemia in patients with non-insulin-dependent diabetes mellitus. Role of hepatic and extrahepatic tissues. The Journal of Clinical Investigation. 1986;**77**(5):1525-1532

[131] Guyton A, Hall J. Textbook of Medical Physiology. 11th ed. Philadelphia: Elsevier; 2006. pp. 836-839

[132] Visinoni S, Fam BC, Blair A, Rantzau C, Lamont BJ, Bouwman R, et al. Increased glucose production in mice overexpressing human fructose-1,6-bisphosphatase in the liver. American Journal of Physiology. Endocrinology and Metabolism. 2008;**295**:E1132-E1141

[133] Tiana S, Tanga M, Zhao B. Current anti-diabetes mechanisms and clinical trials using *Morus alba* L. Journal of Traditional Chinese Medical Sciences. 2016;**3**(1):3-8

[134] Rodrigues EL, Marcelino G, Silva GT, Figueiredo PS, Garcez WS, Corsino J, et al. Nutraceutical and medicinal potential of the *Morus* species in *Metabolic dysfunctions*. International Journal of Molecular Sciences. 2019;**20**(2):301

[135] Dvornik E, Simard-Duquesne N, Krami M, Sestanj K, Gabbay KH, Kinoshita JH, et al. Polyol accumulation in galactosemic and diabetic rats: Control by an aldose reductase inhibitor. Science. 1973;**182**:1146-1148

[136] Suzen S, Buyukbingol E. Recent studies of aldose reductase enzyme inhibition for diabetic complications. Current Medicinal Chemistry. 2003;**10**:1329-1352

[137] Vikramadithyan RK, Hu Y, Noh HL, Liang CP, Hallam K, Tall AR, et al. Human aldose reductase expression accelerates diabetic atherosclerosis in transgenic mice. The Journal of Clinical Investigation. 2005;**115**:2434-2443

[138] Forbes JM, Cooper ME. Mechanisms of diabetic complications. Physiological Reviews. 2013;**93**:137-188

[139] Ebrahimi E, Shirali S, Afrisham R. Effect and mechanism of herbal ingredients in improving diabetes mellitus complications. Jundishapur Journal of Natural Pharmaceutical Products. 2017;**12**(1):e31657

[140] Ong KW, Hsu A, Song L, Huang D, Tan BK. Polyphenols rich *Verinoca amygdalina* shows anti-diabetic effects in streptozotocin-induced diabetic rats. Journal of Ethnopharmacology. 2011;**133**(2):598-607

[141] Fröde TS, Medeiros YS. Animal models to test drugs with potential antidiabetic activity. Journal of Ethnopharmacology. 2008;**115**(2):173-183

[142] Mythili MD, Vyas R, Akila G, Gunasekaran S. Effect of streptozotocin on the ultrastructure of rat pancreatic islets. Microscopy Research and Technique. 2004;**63**(5):274-281

[143] Eleazu CO, Eleazu KC, Chukwuma S, Essien UN. Review of the mechanism of cell death resulting from streptozotocin challenge in experimental animals, its practical use and potential risk to humans. Journal of Diabetes and Metabolic Disorders. 2013;**12**:60

[144] Szudelski T. The mechanism of alloxan and streptozotocin action in cells of the rat pancreas. Physiology Research. 2001;**50**:536-546

[145] Lemhadri A, Zeggwagh NA, Maghrani M, Jouad H, Eddouks M. Anti-hyperglycaemic activity of the aqueous extract of *Origanum vulgare* growing wild in Tafilalet region. Journal of Ethnopharmacology. 2004;**92**(2-3):251-256

[146] Helmstädter A. Beans and diabetes: *Phaseolus vulgaris* preparations as antihyperglycemic agents. Journal of Medicinal Food. 2010;**13**(2):251-254. DOI: 10.1089/jmf.2009.0002

[147] Venkateswaran S, Pari L. Antioxidant effect of *Phaseolus vulgaris* in streptozotocin-induced diabetic rats. Asia Pacific Journal of Clinical Nutrition. 2002;**11**(3):206-209

[148] Pari L, Venkateswaran S. Effect of an aqueous extract of *Phaseolus vulgaris* on the properties of tail tendon collagen of rats with streptozotocin-induced diabetes. Brazilian Journal of Medical and Biological Research. 2003;**36**:861-870

[149] Celleno L, Tolaini MV, D'Amore A, Perricone NV, Preuss HG. A dietary supplement containing standardized *Phaseolus vulgaris* extract influences body composition of overweight men and women. International Journal of Medical Sciences. 2007;**4**(1):45-52

[150] Stull AJ, Cash KC, Johnson WD, Champagne CM, Cefalu WT. Bioactives in blueberries improve insulin sensitivity in obese, insulin-resistant men and women. The Journal of Nutrition. 2010;**140**(10):1764-1768

[151] Guo J, Liu T, Tan L, Liu Y. The effect of corn silk on glycemic metabolism. Nutrition and Metabolism. 2009;**6**:47

[152] Zhao W, Yina Y, Yua Z, Liub J, Chenc F. Comparison of anti-diabetic effects of polysaccharides from corn silk on normal and hyperglycemia rats. International Journal of Biological Macromolecules. 2012;**50**(4):1133-1137

[153] Prabhakar PK, Doble M. Mechanism of action of natural products used in the treatment of diabetes mellitus. Chinese Journal of Integrative Medicine. 2011;**17**(8):563-574

[154] WHO Technical Report Series 894. Obesity: Preventing and Managing The Global Epidemic. Geneva: WHO; 2004. Available from: https://www.who. int/nutrition/publications/obesity/ WHO_TRS_894/en/

[155] Klop B, Elte JWF, Cabezas MC. Dyslipidemia in obesity: Mechanisms and potential targets. Nutrients. 2013;**5**(4):1218-1240

[156] Peterson AL, McBride PE. A review of guidelines for dyslipidemia in children and adolescents. Wisconsin Medical Society. 2012;**111**(6):274-281

[157] Miller M. Dyslipidemia and cardiovascular risk: The importance of early prevention. QJM: An International Journal of Medicine. 2009;**102**(9): 657-667. DOI: 10.1093/qjmed/hcp065

[158] Mopuri R, Islam MS. Medicinal plants and phytochemicals with anti-obesogenic potentials: A review. Biomedicine & Pharmacotherapy. 2017;**89**:1442-1452

[159] de Freitas Junior LM, de Almeida EB Jr. Medicinal plants for the treatment of obesity: Ethnopharmacological approach and chemical and biological studies. American Journal of Translational Research. 2017;**9**(5):2050-2064

[160] Titta L, Trinei M, Stendardo M, Berniakovich I, Petroni K, Tonelli C, et al. Blood orange juice inhibits fat accumulation in mice. International Journal of Obesity. 2010;**34**(3):578-588

[161] Qin Y, Xia M, Ma J, Hao Y, Liu J, Mou H, et al. Anthocyanin supplementation improves serum LDL- and HDL- cholesterol concentrations associated with the inhibition of cholesteryl ester transfer protein in dyslipidemic subjects. The American Journal of Clinical Nutrition. 2009;**90**(3):485-492. DOI: 10.3945/ajcn.2009.27814

[162] Basuny AMM, Arafat SM, El-Marzooq MA. Antioxidant and antihyperlipidemic activities of anthocyanins from eggplant peels. Journal of Pharma Research & Reviews. 2012;**2**(3):50-57

[163] Hansen AS, Marckmann P, Dragsted LO, Finné Nielsen IL, Nielsen SE, Grønbaek M. Effect of red wine and red grape extract on blood lipids, haemostatic factors, and other risk factors for cardiovascular disease. European Journal of Clinical Nutrition. 2005;**59**(3):449-455

[164] Broncel M, Kozirog M, Duchnowicz P, Koter-Michalak M, Sikora J, Chojnowska-Jezierska J. Aronia melanocarpa extract reduces blood pressure, serum endothelin, lipid, and oxidative stress marker levels in patients with metabolic syndrome. Medical Science Monitor. 2010;**16**(1):CR28-CR34

[165] Tsuda T, Horio F, Uchida K, Aoki H, Osawa T. Dietary cyanidin 3-O-beta-D-glucoside-rich purple corn color prevents obesity and ameliorates hyperglycemia in mice. The Journal of Nutrition. 2003;**133**(7):2125-2130

[166] Kwon SH, Ahn IS, Kim SO, Kong CS, Chung HY, Do MS, et al. Anti- obesity and hypolipidemic effects of black soybean anthocyanins. Journal of Medicinal Food. 2007;**10**(3):552-556

[167] Bratoeva K, Bekyarova G, Kiselova Y, Ivanova D. Effect of Bulgarian herb extracts of polyphenols on metabolic disorders—Induced by high-fructose diet. Trakia Journal of Sciences. 2010;**8**(2):56-60

[168] Grace MH, Ribnicky DM, Kuhn P, Poulev A, Logendra S, Yousef GG, et al. Hypoglycemic activity of a novel anthocyanin-rich formulation from lowbush blueberry, *Vaccinium angustifolium* aiton. Phytomedicine. 2009;**16**(5):406-415

[169] Takikawa M, Inoue S, Horio F, Tsuda T. Dietary anthocyanin-rich bilberry extract ameliorates hyperglycemia and insulin sensitivity via activation of AMP-activated protein kinase in diabetic mice. The Journal of Nutrition. 2010;**140**(3):527-533

[170] Watson RT, Kanzaki M, Pessin JE. Regulated membrane trafficking of the insulin-responsive glucose transporter 4 in adipocytes. Endocrine Reviews. 2004;**25**(2):177-204

[171] Inazu A, Brown ML, Hesler CB, Agellon LB, Koizumi J, Takata K, et al. Increased high-density lipoprotein levels caused by a common cholesteryl- ester transfer protein gene mutation. The New England Journal of Medicine. 1990;**323**(18):1234-1238

[172] Baba S, Osakabe N, Kato Y, Natsume M, Yasuda A, Kido T, et al. Continuous intake of polyphenolic compounds containing cocoa powder reduces LDL oxidative susceptibility and has beneficial effects on plasma HDL-cholesterol concentrations in humans. The American Journal of Clinical Nutrition. 2007;**85**(3):709-717

[173] Marnewick JL, Rautenbach F, Venter I, Neethling H, Blackhurst DM, Wolmarans P, et al. Effects of rooibos (*Aspalathus linearis*) on oxidative stress and biochemical parameters in adults at risk for cardiovascular disease. Journal of Ethnopharmacology. 2011;**133**(1):46- 52. DOI: 10.1016/j.jep.2010.08.061

[174] Yugarani T, Tan BK, Das NP. The effects of tannic acid on serum and liver lipids of RAIF and RICO rats fed on high fat diet. Comparative Biochemistry and Physiology. Comparative Physiology. 1993;**104**(2):339-343

[175] Al-Assafa S, Phillips GO, Williams PA. Studies on acacia exudate gums. Part I: The molecular weight of *Acacia senegal* gum exudate. Food Hydrocolloids. 2005;**19**(4):647-660

[176] Bornhoeft J, Castaneda D, Nemoseck T, Wang P, Henning SM, Hong MY. The protective effects of green tea polyphenols: Lipid profile, inflammation, and antioxidant capacity in rats fed an atherogenic diet and dextran sodium sulfate. Journal of Medicinal Food. 2012;**15**(8):726-732. DOI: 10.1089/jmf.2011.0258

[177] Basu A, Fu DX, Wilkinson M, Simmons B, Wu M, Betts NM, et al. Strawberries decrease atherosclerotic markers in subjects with metabolic syndrome. Nutrition Research 2010;**30**(7):462-469

[178] Kiselova-Kaneva Y. Total antioxidant capacity and polyphenol content correlation in aqueous-alcoholic plant extracts used in phytotherapy. Scripta Scientifica Medica. 2004;**3**:11-13

[179] Pandey KB, Rizvi SI. Plant polyphenols as dietary antioxidants in human health and disease. Oxidative Medicine and Cellular Longevity. 2009;**2**(5):270-278

[180] Freitas WM, Quaglia LA, Santos SN, de Paula RC, Santos RD, Blaha M, et al. Low HDL cholesterol but not high LDL cholesterol is independently associated with subclinical coronary atherosclerosis in healthy octogenarians. Aging Clinical and Experimental Research. 2015;**27**(1):61-67. DOI: 10.1007/s40520-014-0249-4

[181] Goto T, Teraminami A, Lee JY, Ohyama K, Funakoshi K, Kim YI, et al. Tiliroside, a glycosidic flavonoid, ameliorates obesity-induced metabolic disorders via activation of adiponectin signaling followed by enhancement of fatty acid oxidation in liver and skeletal muscle in obese-diabetic mice. The Journal of Nutritional Biochemistry. 2012;**23**(7):768e776

[182] Burton-Freeman B, Linares A, Hyson D, Kappagoda T. Strawberry modulates LDL oxidation and postprandial lipemia in response to high-fat meal in overweight hyperlipidemic men and women. Journal of the American College of Nutrition. 2010;**29**(1):46-54

2

Undernutrition Risk Assessment in Elderly People: Available Tools in Clinical Practice

Isabel Sospedra, Aurora Norte, José Miguel Martínez-Sanz, Enrique de Gomar, José Antonio Hurtado Sánchez and María José Cabañero-Martínez

Abstract

Undernutrition is a public health problem all over the world. More than 30 million people are currently affected by undernutrition in Europe, mainly hospitalized or elderly people. Undernutrition has several medical consequences and in the elderly can be associated with adverse clinical symptoms, contributing to frailty, morbidity, hospitalization, and mortality. These medical situations highlight the importance of an early detection and diagnosis, the objective being to prevent or treat undernutrition. This is why the implementation of a complete nutritional assessment in clinical practice is important. Nutritional screenings are essential tools to identify patients that will likely benefit from nutrition therapy. There are currently several screening methods to identify nutritional risk or malnutrition. However, the lack of a standard has aroused controversy about the best tool to use. Our objective is to describe the screening tools available for the elderly.

Keywords: elderly, undernutrition, malnutrition assessment, malnutrition biomarkers

Introduction

Scientific evidence suggests that nutritional status has a great impact on the health and functional status of older people. In addition, during the aging process there are a series of changes that can have a negative impact on nutritional status. These biological, physiological, social, and psychological changes, together with a higher prevalence of morbidities, further increase the susceptibility of the elderly to malnourishment [1]. The etiology of malnutrition is multifactorial in the elderly. The literature indicates that the elderly are at risk of nutritional deficiencies due to changes in body composition, the digestive system, and the regulation of fluids and electrolytes, sensory alterations, increased likelihood of chronic diseases, poly medication, and hospitalization. But also, social changes—such as retirement, less family responsibility, loneliness, widowhood, or lower purchasing power—increase the risk of inadequate nutrition. Although certain autonomy is maintained, the functional capacity is modified, which makes the daily tasks of life—such as shopping, preparing food, or moving from one place to another—difficult. In addition, the coexistence of physical and mental illnesses may increase or decrease nutritional requirements or may limit the individual's ability to obtain adequate nutrition, thereby increasing the risk of malnutrition [2, 3]. This is why the evaluation of the nutritional risk in this type of population is of the utmost importance.

Nutritional parameters related to undernutrition

The assessment of the nutritional status is the step previous to dietary- nutritional treatment [4]. It is a global evaluation that includes the nutritional status of the individual as well as the severity of the underlying disease, due to the relationship between them. It establishes a methodology to obtain information about the current and past situation of the elderly person in relation to their diet, body composition, and functional and health status [5, 6]. In addition, it will help in the detection of nutritional risk or malnutrition. Two steps can be established in this assessment process: a first step of screening the nutritional risk or malnutrition, and a second step of complete nutritional assessment to identify the causes and consequences of malnutrition. The second step would be carried out when a nutritional risk or malnutrition has been detected [4, 5, 7].

As there is no single marker or nutritional tool that is useful for all types of individuals or physiological or pathological situations and is easily reproducible, predictable, and reliable, correct nutritional assessment involves the use of different nutritional parameters in order to perform an evaluation of the nutritional status that is as complete as possible, according to the subject with which we are dealing; in this case, the geriatric population. In addition, the social and cultural aspects of the patient must also be taken into account, because these data provide information on their resources and ability to prepare food, as well as sociocultural, religious, or personal nutritional habits that may affect the intake and nutritional status. Among the different factors or parameters related to malnutrition that can be assessed in the elderly, we find health status, social and clinical conditions, anthropometry, dietary habits and dietary intake, lifestyle, blood biochemistry, etc. [5, 6]. These factors or parameters and their relationship with malnutrition are described below.

General health status self-assessment

Perceived health status is one of the most consolidated indicators and is easy to enquire about in health surveys. It is a feasible tool and has been studied in recent years because it is useful as a global indicator of the level of population health. Some of the factors that lead to a poor self-perception of the state of health in the elderly are age, female sex, comorbidity, not receiving treatments, and little accessibility to other health services [8].

Social condition

Many aspects of the individual's life are covered here. Some of the causes that can lead to an inadequate consumption of food and, therefore, to malnutrition, are isolation, the loss of loved ones in charge of organizing meals, difficulties in buying or cooking, poor pensions, or changes in feeding when moving to a geriatric residence. It is important to know where the individual lives and with whom, the main career's situation, characteristics of the home, the level of income, their leisure activities, etc. [9].

Clinical condition

This is data from the clinical evaluation performed by a medical professional. It will be necessary to know if the individual suffers or has suffered from any disease, as well as the drugs he or she has taken or is taking for said disease(s). Regarding the intake of drugs, it is important to gather information about the dosage and interactions between food and drugs [5].

Anthropometry

Anthropometric measurements provide information about the morphological dimensions of individuals. It is a non-invasive, low cost, and portable method, when compared to techniques requiring more complex devices. The anthropometric parameters include weight, height, skin folds, diameters, lengths, and girth. Some of these have been related to malnutrition: specifically, weight loss in a short period of time (1–6 months) with respect to usual weight, low percentile of the triceps skin fold, and decrease in body mass index (BMI) [6, 9].

Dietary intake and eating attitudes

Food intake is a process that varies according to the day of the week, month, or season of the year. Other factors that influence food intake are food preferences and aversions, the person preparing the meals, feeling full (before and during meals), and the ease or difficulty of food intake and/or food preparation, among others. Information concerning these factors is relevant to evaluate food intake [6]. To determine the intake of food and liquids, methods that give similar results if they are repeated in the same situation are required; that is, instruments that offer better reproducibility or precision (agreement of results when the same dietary evaluation method is administered more than once, and on different occasions, to the same individual or group). Currently, there are prospective or retrospective methods, such as the dietary diary, 24-hour recall, and food consumption frequency questionnaire (CFCA), among others. The use of two or more methods can give a better and more accurate estimate of the habitual diet of the individual who has been interviewed, since the disadvantages of one method are offset by the advantages of the other. In addition, it is necessary to use a food composition database to obtain information on energy and nutritional intake (macro and micronutrients), thereby allowing comparison with the recommendations for the intake of energy, carbohydrates, proteins, lipids, and micronutrients [5, 6, 10].

Blood biochemistry

Some of the blood biochemical parameters are biomarkers related to nutritional status. In spite of the fact that most nutritional risk screenings aimed at the elderly population do not contemplate biochemical parameters, they are included in the screening of hospitalized patients. Decreases in the values of some of these biochemical parameters (albumin, lymphocytes, cholesterol, etc.) are important in the detection and assessment of protein malnutrition [6, 9–11]. These parameters are described below:

- Albumin: this protein is easily determined due to its long half-life (20 days), but has limitations as a nutritional marker. Changes in blood volume, different pathological situations, or any degree of aggression can produce a decrease in its plasma values, although its decrease is related to an increase in the occurrence of complications and mortality [6, 10].

- Prealbumin: this is a protein with a half-life of 2 days that decreases in some situations of malnutrition, infection, or liver failure and increases upon renal failure. It should be interpreted with caution if used as a nutritional marker; despite this, it is considered a good indicator for assessing acute nutritional changes [9].
- Protein binding retinol: this is a protein with a half-life of 10 hours, whose levels increase with vitamin A intake or renal failure, and are decreased by liver disease, infection, or severe stress. Due to its sensitivity to stress and renal function, it is considered of little clinical use [9].
- Lymphocytes: these are related to immunity and nutritional status. Total lymphocytes are related to protein depletion and loss of immune defenses as a result of malnutrition [10, 11].
- Total cholesterol: in malnourished patients with renal and kidney failure and malabsorption syndrome, low cholesterol levels are associated with an increase in mortality. A decrease in their values to below 150 mg/dl is related to malnutrition [10, 11].

Nutritional screening tools available for elderly people

A wide range of nutritional screening tools have been developed. The screening tools used most commonly, have been developed in several countries specifically for elderly people, are Australian Nutrition Screening Initiative (ANSI) [12], Ayrshire Nutrition Screening Tool (ANST) [13], Canadian Nutrition Screening Tool (CNST) [14], Chinese Nutrition Screen (CNS) [15], Council of Nutrition Appetite Questionnaire (CNAQ) [16], Simplified Nutritional Appetite Questionnaire (SNAQ) [16], Short Nutritional Assessment Questionnaire (SNAQ) [17], Short Nutritional Assessment Questionnaire for the Residential Care (SNAQ RC) [18], Malaysian Tool (MT) [19], Malnutrition Risk Screening Tool-Hospital (MRSTH) [20], Mini Nutritional Assessment (MNA) [21], Mini Nutritional Assessment Short Form (MNA-SF) [22], Minimal Eating Observation and Nutrition Form Version II (MEONF-II) [23], Nursing Nutrition Screening Assessment (NNSA) [24], Nursing Nutritional Assessment (NNA) [25], Nutrition Screening Initiative (NSI "DETERMINE") [26], Nutritional Form for the Elderly (NUFFE) [27], Nutritional Risk Assessment Tool (NRAT) [28], Seniors in the Community Version I (SCREEN I) [29], Seniors in the Community Version II (SCREEN II) [30], South African Screening Tool (SAST) [31], The Burton Score (TBS) [32] and Geriatric Nutrition Risk Index (GNRI-NRI) [33] (**Table 1**). All of them contain several domains, and the parameters included most frequently are those concerning anthropometry, dietary intake, and clinical condition. Among the anthropometric parameters, the most used value is weight change, being the only anthropometric item reported in some of the protocols. Dietary intake comprises information about the quantity and the quality of the food consumed by the patient and, in particular, regarding their appetite and frequency of meals. Some of the instruments also include an item about fluid intake, which is an important aspect to be considered in elderly people. Aspects related to diseases and functional status are the items included most frequently in the clinical condition domain.

Concerning the clinical setting used to develop and/or validate the instrument, the three main contexts found are community, hospital, and long-term care facilities (including nursing homes and residential facilities). Among these settings, the self-administration form is used only in the community or in long-term care facilities. However, in hospitals the administration form used most frequently is filled in by qualified health personnel. The number of items comprising the presented tools ranges from 2 (CNST) to 18 (MNA). Taking into account that the respondents are elderly people, the interviews performed by health professionals seem to be the best option, as well as tools with a low number of items, to minimize the burden of the interviewee.

Table 1. *Anthropometric parameters related to malnutrition.*

Parameter	Definition	Range	Equation
% Habitual weight loss	Weight variation with respect to the usual weight	Mild: 85–95% Moderate: 75–84% Severe: <75%	% Habitual weight loss = (actual weight (kg)/habitual weight (kg)) × 100
Body mass index (BMI)	Relationship between weight and height	Mild: 17–18.4 kg/m^2 Moderate: 16–16.9 kg/m^2 Severe: <16 kg/m^2	BMI = weight (kg)/height (m^2)
Triceps skinfold	Vertical skinfold in the middle back of the arm	Mild: percentile 10–15 Moderate: percentile 5–10 Severe: percentile <5	Review percentiles of the population of origin

In order to have the appropriate arguments for using one or other of the screening methods, the main psychometric parameters that should be considered are the sensitivity and specificity of the test. Among the selected tools the sensitivities ranged from 0.32 for the ANSI [34] to 99% for the MNA [22] and the specificities of the tools ranged from 0.38% for the SCREEN I [29] to 0.96% for the MRSTH [20]. Only for five of these instruments Receiver Operating Characteristic (ROC) curves, as a combined measure of sensitivity and specificity, has been informed [16, 17, 22, 29, 30]. The tool which has shown the best values for both, sensitivity and specificity is MNA and its short form (MNA-SF) and, consequently are the nutritional screening tests most commonly used (**Table 2**).

Characteristics of nutritional screening: advantages and limitations

All the screening tools described here were designed specifically for elderly people; however, there is a set of screenings developed for other populations, mainly adults, which could be used also for aged people. This supposes an advantage if different populations need to be compared. Nevertheless, these instruments could lose content validity in comparison with specific aged-population tools. Among the different forms of data collection, face to face interview has been demonstrated to be the most suitable form for this age group. A low number of items are also recommended in order to reduce the burden of the respondent [35]. The domains included in each tool can influence the validity of the evaluations.

The use of parameters that examine aspects related to the patient's perception could be less appropriate for elderly patients. The frequent sensorial and cognitive problems of these patients make the collection of accurate data more difficult [36].

Table 2. *Summary of nutritional screening tools.*

Nutrition screening tool	Parameters	Specific	No. of items	Setting	Administration	Nutritional score
ANSI [12]	Anthropometry	Weight change	12	Community	Self-administered Administered by family members or caregivers	Range: 0–29 0–3: good 4–5 moderate nutritional risk 6 or more: high nutritional risk
	Social condition	Loneliness Food access				
	Clinical condition	Functional status Disease Oral problems Drugs				
	Dietary intake	Frequency of meals and food intake Fluid intake				
	Life style	Alcohol intake				
ANST [13]	Anthropometry	Weight change	6	Hospital	Nursing staff	Range: 0–18 6 or less: moderate risk 7 or more: high risk
	Clinical condition	Disease				
	Dietary intake	Frequency of meals Fluid intake Appetite				
CNST [14]	Anthropometry	Weight change	2	Hospital	Dietitians	Range: 0–2 0–1: no risk 2: nutrition risk
	Dietary intake	Food frequency intake				

Nutrition screening tool	Parameters	Specific	No. of items	Setting	Administration	Nutritional score
CNS [15]	Anthropometry	Weight change	16	Hospital Long-term care facilities	Professional not indicated	Range: 0–32 ≤16: malnourished 17–19: risk >19: normal
	Social condition	Loneliness				
	Clinical condition	Functional status Disease Drugs Skin status				
	Dietary intake	Appetite Food intake Frequency of meals Fluid intake				
	Emotional status	Happiness				
	Self-assessment	Health status				
CNAQ [16]	Dietary intake	Frequency of meals Appetite	8	Long-term care facilities Community	Self-administered	Range: 8–40 ≤28: significant risk of at least 5% weight loss within 6 months
	Emotional status	Sadness				
	Eating attitudes	Food tastes Feel full, hungry or nauseated				
SNAQ [16]	Dietary intake	Frequency of meals Appetite	4	Long-term care facilities Community	Self-administered	Range: 4–20 ≤14: significant risk of at least 5% weight loss within 6 months
	Eating attitudes	Food tastes Feeling of fullness				
SNAQ [17]	Anthropometry	Weight change	3	Hospital	Nursing staff Dietitians	Range: 0–5 ≥2: moderate malnourishment ≥3: severe malnourishment
	Dietary intake	Appetite Supplemental drinks or tube feeding				

Nutrition screening tool	Parameters	Specific	No. of items	Setting	Administration	Nutritional score
SNAQRC [18]	Anthropometry	Weight change BMI	3 + 1 (BMI)	Long-term care facilities	Self-administered Administered by family members or care workers Trained care works for anthropometric measures	Traffic light system Red score: high risk of undernourishment Orange score: moderate risk of undernourishment Green score: no risk
	Clinical condition	Functional status				
	Dietary intake	Appetite				
MT [19]	Anthropometry	Weight change	11	Rural community	Interviewer (professional not indicated)	Two sections: A (range: 0–7): undernutrition: ≥4 high risk of undernutrition B (range: 0–5): dietary inadequacy: ≥2 high risk of consuming an inadequate diet
	Social condition	Food access				
	Clinical condition	Functional status Disease Oral problems				
	Dietary intake	Frequency of meals and food intake Appetite				
	Life style	Smoking				
MRSTH [20]	Anthropometry	Weight change Arm circumference Calf circumference	5	Hospital	Health care professionals	Range: 0–8 ≥5: high risk of malnutrition
	Social condition	Food access				
	Clinical condition	Functional status				

Nutrition screening tool	Parameters	Specific	No. of items	Setting	Administration	Nutritional score
MNA [21]	Anthropometry	Weight change BMI Arm circumference Calf circumference	18	Long-term care facilities Community Hospital	Health care professionals	Range: 0–30 ≥24: well nourished 17–23: at risk of malnutrition <17: malnourished
	Clinical condition	Functional status Disease				
	Dietary intake	Frequency of meals and food intake Fluid intake Appetite				
	Self-assessment	Nutritional problems Health status				
MNA-SF [22]	Anthropometry	Weight change BMI	6	Long-term care facilities Community Hospital	Health care professionals	Range: 0–14 ≥12: normal-no need for further assessment ≤11: possible malnutrition-continue assessment
	Clinical condition	Functional status Disease				
	Dietary intake	Appetite				
MEONF-II [23]	Anthropometry	Weight change BMI (or calf circumference)	6	Hospital	Nursing staff	Range: 0–8 0–2: low risk of undernutrition 3–4: moderate risk of undernutrition ≥5: high risk of undernutrition
	Clinical condition	Functional status Oral problems Clinical signs				
	Dietary intake	Appetite				
NNSA [24]	Anthropometry	Weight change	5	Hospital	Nursing staff Dietitians	Range: 0–100 <65: high risk 65–79: moderate risk 80–100: minimal risk
	Clinical condition	Functional status Disease				
	Dietary intake	Frequency of meals and food intake				

Nutrition screening tool	Parameters	Specific	No. of items	Setting	Administration	Nutritional score
NNA [25]	Anthropometry	Weight change	9	Hospital	Nursing staff Dietitians	Range: 9–36 <18: low risk 19–27: moderate risk 28–36: high risk
	Clinical condition	Functional status Disease				
	Dietary intake	Appetite Frequency of meals				
NSI "DETERMINE" [26]	Anthropometry	Weight change	10	Community	Self-administered Administered by family members or caregivers	Range: 0–21 0–2: good 3–5: moderate nutritional risk 6 or more: high nutritional risk
	Social condition	Loneliness Food access				
	Clinical condition	Functional status Disease Oral problems Drugs				
	Dietary intake	Frequency of meals and food intake				
	Life style	Alcohol intake				
NUFFE [27]	Anthropometry	Weight change	15	Long-term care facilities	Nursing staff	Range: 0–30 Norwegian version cut-offs: <6: low risk 6–10: medium risk ≥11: high risk
	Social condition	Loneliness Food access				
	Clinical condition	Functional status Disease Oral problems Drugs				
	Dietary intake	Frequency of meals and food intake Appetite Dietary intake changes Portion size				
	Self-assessment	Health status				

Nutrition screening tool	Parameters	Specific	No. of items	Setting	Administration	Nutritional score
NRAT [28]	Anthropometry	Weight change	9	Community	Nursing staff Dietitians	Range: 0–26 0–6: little or no risk 7–16: probable risk ≥17: malnourished
	Clinical condition	Functional status Oral problems				
	Dietary intake	Frequency of meals Appetite				
	Eating attitudes	Feeling of fullness				
	Self-assessment	Health status Thinness				
SCREEN I [29]	Anthropometry	Weight change	15	Community	Self-administered Interviewer (professional not indicated)	Not specified
	Social condition	Food access Loneliness				
	Clinical condition	Functional status Oral problems				
	Dietary intake	Frequency of meals and food intake Fluid intake Appetite Supplemental drinks Dietary intake changes				
SCREEN II [30]	Anthropometry	Weight change	17	Community	Self-administered Dietitians	Range: 0–64 Cut-offs not specified
	Social condition	Food access Loneliness				
	Clinical condition	Functional status Oral problems				
	Dietary intake	Frequency of meals and food intake Fluid intake Appetite Supplemental drinks Dietary intake changes Quality of meals				

Nutrition screening tool	Parameters	Specific	No. of items	Setting	Administration	Nutritional score
SAST [31]	Anthropometry	Arm circumference	10	Community Long-term care facilities	Trained fieldworkers	Range: 0–23 **Men** <9.5: malnourished 9.5–14.5: risk of malnutrition >14.5: well nourished **Women** <9.5: malnourished 9.5–16: risk of malnutrition >16: well nourished
	Social condition	Functional status				
	Clinical condition	Disease				
	Dietary intake	Frequency of meals and food intake				
	Self-assessment	Health status				
TBS [32]	Anthropometry	Weight change BMI	7	Hospital	Nursing staff Dietitians	Range: 6–28 0–5: well nourished 6–10: moderately nourished 11–15: poorly nourished ≥16: very poorly nourished
	Social condition	Age Sex				
	Clinical condition	Functional status Symptoms Skin risk areas				
	Dietary intake	Appetite				
GNRI-NRI [33]	Anthropometry	Knee height Usual weight	No items	Hospital	Professional not indicated	Grades of nutrition-related risk: <82: major risk 82 to <92: moderate risk 92 to ≤98: low risk >98: no risk
	Social condition	Age				
	Biochemistry	Albumin				

The inclusion of objective parameters, such as anthropometric measurements or clinical data, helps to avoid this disadvantage. However, the collection of such data, especially for parameters derived from biochemical analyses, involves a high cost and cannot be achieved in all settings.

The absence of a Gold Standard criterion to validate this kind of instrument supposes a disadvantage. This is a reason for the ongoing development of new, appropriate parameters. Although most of these tools are widely used, none of them has been compared to standard criteria used to evaluate nutritional status.

Conclusions

There is no single nutritional marker that can predict or diagnose malnutrition; rather, the state of health, social and clinical conditions, anthropometry, eating habits, and blood chemistry of the elderly person under consideration—in relation to their specific situation (health, illness, hospitalization, or institutionalization)— must be taken into account. Therefore, the tools described here that include various dimensions are currently the most recommended.

Author details

Isabel Sospedra, Aurora Norte, José Miguel Martínez-Sanz*, Enrique de Gomar, José Antonio Hurtado Sánchez and María José Cabañero-Martínez

Nursing Department, Faculty of Health Sciences, University of Alicante, Alicante, Spain

*Address all correspondence to: josemiguel.ms@ua.es

References

[1] Ahmed T, Haboubi N. Assessment and management of nutrition in older people and its importance to health. Clinical Interventions in Aging. 2010;**5**:207-216

[2] Brownie S. Why are elderly individuals at risk of nutritional deficiency? International Journal of Nursing Practice. 2006;**12**(2):110-118

[3] Rathnayake KM, Wimalathunga M, Weech M, Jackson KG, Lovegrove JA. High prevalence of undernutrition and low dietary diversity in institutionalised elderly living in Sri Lanka. Public Health Nutrition. 2015;**18**(15):2874-2880

[4] García de Lorenzo A, Álvarez Hernández J, Planas M, Burgos R, Araujo K. Consenso multidisciplinar sobre el abordaje de la desnutrición hospitalaria en España. Nutrición Hospitalaria. 2011;**26**(4):701-710

[5] Mahan LK, Escott-Stump S, Raymond JL. Krause Dietoterapia. España: Elsevier; 2012. 1263 p

[6] Salas-Salvadó J. Nutrición y dietética clínica. España: Elsevier; 2008. 702 p

[7] Álvarez J, Río JD, Planas M, García Peris P, García de Lorenzo A, Calvo V, et al. Documento SENPE-SEDOM sobre la codificación de la desnutrición hospitalaria. Nutrición Hospitalaria. 2008;**23**(6):536-540

[8] Vergara DMC, Arango DC. Percepción del estado de salud y factores asociados en adultos mayores. Revista de Salud Pública. 2015;**17**(2):171-183

[9] Gómez Candela C, Reuss Fernández JM. Manual de recomendaciones nutricionales en pacientes geriátricos. Editores Médicos; 2004. 364 p

[10] Ravasco P, Anderson H, Mardones F. Métodos de valoración del estado nutricional. Nutrición Hospitalaria. 2010;**25**:57-66

[11] Ignacio de Ulíbarri J, González- Madroño A, de Villar N, González P, González B, Mancha A, et al. CONUT: Una herramienta para controlar el estado nutritivo. Primera validación en una población hospitalaria. Nutrición Hospitalaria. 2005;**20**(1):38-45

[12] Lipski PS. Australian nutrition screening initiative. Australasian Journal on Ageing. 1996;**15**(1):14-17

[13] Mackintosh MA, Hankey CR. Reliability of a nutrition screening tool for use in elderly day hospitals. Journal of Human Nutrition and Dietetics. 2001;**14**(2):129-136

[14] Laporte M, Keller HH, Payette H, Allard JP, Duerksen DR, Bernier P, et al. Validity and reliability of the new Canadian Nutrition Screening Tool in the "real-world" hospital setting. European Journal of Clinical Nutrition. 2015;**69**(5):558-564

[15] Woo J, Chumlea WC, Sun SS, Kwok T, Lui HH, Hui E, et al. Development of the Chinese nutrition screen (CNS) for use in institutional settings. The Journal of Nutrition, Health & Aging. 2005;**9**(4):203-210

[16] Wilson M-MG, Thomas DR, Rubenstein LZ, Chibnall JT, Anderson S, Baxi A, et al. Appetite assessment: Simple appetite questionnaire predicts weight loss in community-dwelling adults and nursing home residents. The American Journal of Clinical Nutrition. 2005;**82**(5):1074-1081

[17] Kruizenga HM, Seidell JC, de Vet HCW, Wierdsma NJ, van Bokhorst-de Van der Schueren MAE. Development and validation of a hospital screening tool for malnutrition: The short nutritional assessment questionnaire (SNAQ). Clinical Nutrition (Edinburgh, Scotland). 2005;**24**(1):75-82

[18] Kruizenga HM, de Vet HCW, Van Marissing CME, Stassen EEPM, Strijk JE, van Bokhorst-de Van der Schueren MAE, et al. The SNAQ(RC), an easy traffic light system as a first step in the recognition of undernutrition in residential care. The Journal of Nutrition, Health & Aging. 2010;**14**(2):83-89

[19] Shahar S, Dixon RA, Earland J. Development of a screening tool for detecting undernutrition and dietary inadequacy among rural elderly in Malaysia: Simple indices to identify individuals at high risk. International Journal of Food Sciences and Nutrition. 1999;**50**(6):435-444

[20] Sakinah H, Suzana S, Noor Aini MY, Philip Poi JH, Shahrul Bahyah K. Development of a local malnutrition risk screening tool-hospital (MRST-H) for hospitalised elderly patients. Malaysian Journal of Nutrition. 2012;**18**(2):137-147

[21] Guigoz Y, Vellas B, Garry PJ. Assessing the nutritional status of the elderly: The mini nutritional assessment as part of the geriatric evaluation. Nutrition Reviews. 1996;**54**(1 Pt 2): S59-S65

[22] Rubenstein LZ, Harker JO, Salvà A, Guigoz Y, Vellas B. Screening for undernutrition in geriatric practice: Developing the short-form mini- nutritional assessment (MNA-SF). The Journals of Gerontology. Series A, Biological Sciences and Medical Sciences. 2001;**56**(6):M366-M372

[23] Westergren A, Norberg E, Vallén C, Hagell P. Cut-off scores for the minimal eating observation and nutrition form— Version II (MEONF-II) among hospital inpatients. Food & Nutrition Research. 2011;**55**:7289

[24] Pattison R, Corr J, Ogilvie M, Farquhar D, Sutherland D, Davidson HIM, et al. Reliability of a qualitative screening tool versus physical measurements in identifying undernutrition in an elderly population. Journal of Human Nutrition and Dietetics. 1999;**12**(2):133-140

[25] McCall R, Cotton E. The validation of a nursing nutritional assessment tool for use on acute elderly wards. Journal of Human Nutrition and Dietetics. 2001;**14**(2):137-148

[26] Posner BM, Jette AM, Smith KW, Miller DR. Nutrition and health risks in the elderly: The nutrition screening initiative. American Journal of Public Health. 1993;**83**(7):972-978

[27] Söderhamn U, Söderhamn O. Developing and testing the nutritional form for the elderly. International Journal of Nursing Practice. 2001;**7**(5):336-341

[28] Ward C, Little B, Perkins C, et al. Development of a screening tool for assessing risk of undernutrition in patients in the community. Journal of Human Nutrition and Dietetics. 1998;**11**(4):323-330

[29] Keller HH. The SCREEN I (seniors in the community: Risk evaluation for eating and nutrition) index adequately represents nutritional risk. Journal of Clinical Epidemiology. 2006;**59**(8):836-841

[30] Keller HH, Goy R, Kane S-L. Validity and reliability of SCREEN II (seniors in the community: Risk evaluation for eating and nutrition, Version II). European Journal of Clinical Nutrition. 2005;**59**(10):1149-1157

[31] Charlton KE, Kolbe-Alexander TL, Nel JH. Development of a novel nutrition screening tool for use in elderly South Africans. Public Health Nutrition. 2005;**8**(5):468-479

[32] Russell L, Taylor J, Brewitt J, Ireland M, Reynolds T. Development and validation of the Burton score: A tool for nutritional assessment. Journal of Tissue Viability. 1998;**8**(4):16-22

[33] Bouillanne O, Morineau G, Dupont C, Coulombel I, Vincent J-P, Nicolis I, et al. Geriatric nutritional risk index: A new index for evaluating at-risk elderly medical patients. The American Journal of Clinical Nutrition. 2005;**82**(4):777-783

[34] Patterson AJ, Young AF, Powers JR, Brown WJ, Byles JE. Relationships between nutrition screening checklists and the health and well-being of older Australian women. Public Health Nutrition. 2002;**5**(1):65-71

[35] Isaksson U, Santamäki-Fischer R, Nygren B, Lundman B, Åström S. Supporting the very old when completing a questionnaire: Risking bias or gaining valid results? Research on Aging. 2007;**29**(6):576-589

[36] Walters SJ, Munro JF, Brazier JE. Using the SF-36 with older adults: A cross-sectional community- based survey. Age and Ageing. 2001;**30**(4):337-343

3

General Nutritional Problems in the Different Countries of the Four Continents - Our Challenges Now and Forthcoming Time

Gyula Mózsik and Mária Figler

Introduction

The right for nutrition is a major principle in the Universal Declaration of Human Rights announced in 1948 [1]. *The Declaration of Social Progress and Development* of 1969 specified the major aim as "the elimination of hunger and malnutrition and the guarantee of the right to proper nutrition" [2]. The Universal Declaration of Human Rights accepted in 1974 makes it clear that "Everyone has the right to get rid of starvation and malnutrition in order to use and preserve their physical and mental capacities" [3]. The Declaration of 1992 also recognized "access to safe food suitable for nutrition" as a universal right.

Every day globally about 40,000 people die from malnutrition and the diseases associated with it, which are also responsible for the death of 5 million children according to FAO, the Food and Agricultural Organization of the United Nations report of 2004.

From time to time, efforts are made by the developed world to eliminate the extreme poverty prevailing in the developing countries. Radical changes, however, can only be achieved by effective measures at the local level.

Up until the nineteenth century, famines most commonly originated from the natural disasters. At present, in most of the cases, they are caused by people; suffice with Ethiopia, Cambodia, the former Yugoslavia, Rwanda, or Haiti. In the era when we are capable of handling famine, a lot more than ever before, such situations prove to be a big shame of mankind.

Undernutrition and malnutrition

Malnutrition (undernutrition) is a pathological condition where energy deficiency or lack of energy or absolute or relative lack of at least one nutrient is present [4]. More than one of the factors playing a part in the development of malnutrition may be present in hospitalized individuals or in those living in social institutions offering prolonged stay. Starvation in the child's organism may range from occasional or rare mild undernutrition through severe deficiency in growth to life hazard.

Starvation (inanition) is the condition where the bodyweight decreases due to the lack or low level of food intake, the body grows thinner and weaker, and the metabolism of essential nutrients shows a value lesser than normal.

"Quantitative" starvation means that the individual for some reason consumes too little food. Insufficient energy uptake leads to weight loss even in the short run. The regenerating mechanisms of the organism are capable of preventing only the effect of moderate undernutrition, while weight loss also leads to reduced spontaneous and voluntary activity.

"Qualitative" starvation is less conspicuous, while its importance is high, since in this case, the intake of vitally important nutrients (such as vitamins and minerals) is insufficient, especially in childhood and babyhood.

Specialists most commonly encounter protein and energy deficiency resulting in protein-energy malnutrition. In this case, the fatty tissue disappears, the organism can resist infections to a lesser extent, and chronic diarrhea may also occur. If the energy balance in the organism is upset for a long time (i.e., the daily energy uptake is less than the energy use), emaciation may develop. If the body weight is 15–20% less than the optimal and the amount of fatty tissue reserve also gets reduced or disappears, cachexia can be established, while in cases when the organism uses up the muscle proteins in addition to fat reserves, marasmus is diagnosed.

Obesity

It seems the most cruel and absurd thing that the world struggling with famines needs to fight obesity at the same time. In history, this is the first time when there are more obese people than those suffering from undernutrition. In the United States alone, every year, more than 300,000 people die due to obesity, while 100 billion dollars are spent on the treatment of the disease and the related consequences. Overweight and obesity are two endemics that are not restricted to the population of rich countries. There are more than 300 million obese people in the world, of them 115 million live in the developing countries [5].

According to the World Health Organization, it is among the top 10 most severe diseases. Plenty of people suffer from its complications and even more from the esthetic and social consequences. The incidence of cancer increases with the pathological obesity of the population, while both obesity and individual types of tumors are preventable. The simplest recipe of slimming diets: eat less and move more. If we consume just 500 kcal less daily, it results in 0.5 kg weight loss, which is 2 kg in the month. Body weight reducing therapies are built on four pillars: slimming diet, exercise, behavior change, and medication. A long-lasting effect can be achieved by the combined application of these four possibilities [6].

The effects of overweight and obesity are well documented. Obesity studies typically reveal association with cardiovascular diseases, cerebrovascular diseases diabetes, gall stones, goiter, and a number of cancers (e.g., breast, colon, ovary, and prostate cancer) endocrine disturbances, renal disturbances, liver damages, pulmonary disturbances, and joint diseases.

Health industry

The composition, quality, and quantity of the food consumed and the frequency of food intake have crucial effect on our general feeling, well-being, and diseases. A healthy adult consumes half a ton of food per annum. Nowadays, information on the role of nutritional factors in developing diseases gains more and more importance. The explanation is simple: there is a whole industry that focuses on health preservation, optimal body weight, and well-being. The products promoting healthy way of living need to be advertised, whereas the value of programs arousing public interest is unfortunately determined by the number of viewers of such programs and the chances for placing commercials in them, rather than their usefulness for the society.

In the civilized world, preferences are to be given to foods which, in addition to their nutritional value, have obvious biological usefulness; therefore, beside the level of microelements vitamin, fiber and flavonoid content of foods to be consumed should be taken into account. The quality of foods also counts, so the qualitative approach should gain priority over the quantity-centered nutrition; mass media plays an important part.

For national economies, the treatment of obesity-related conditions is a great challenge which takes up an increasing part of health care expenditure. Obese people suffer three to four times more often and intensely from depression and anxiety than their fellow citizens with optimal body weight.

Since both obesity and the development of some malignant tumors are preventable, the greatest issue and challenge for health care providers is the number of pathologically obese European citizens. Besides public health specialists parents and those in charge of children's education also share this responsibility. We, Hungarians, would not die 10 years earlier than our European fellow humans if we valued health, cared for ourselves and others, and increased our knowledge on health preservation [7].

Ethical issues

Safe food supply does not sheerly mean that we have a sufficient amount of food at our disposal but the diversity of this food at reasonable price is also important. Families need income covering the cost of sufficient and diverse food for each family member.

Apart from that it is also important for individuals to have access to relevant information about the nutrients and food. It is a fact that the amount of corn grown all over the world could provide 3000 kcal of energy for each man, woman, and child, whereas the optimal value is 2300 kcal per person. Food production exceeds the growth of population by 16%.

The real problem is caused by distribution. For many people, appropriate food is unaffordable -this is how starvation becomes a global problem. Since it is widely known that the amount of foodstuff is sufficient, increasing the production provides no solution for the problem. In spite of the fact that climate factors and various natural disasters have a huge influence on the agricultural production, there are economic, social, cultural, and political issues behind starvation and malnutrition. Intensive cultures are accused with damaging the environment and endangering natural resources,—water and soil—with fertilization and inconsiderate use of chemicals. The intensification of agricultural cultivation of the land maybe defined as the increase in the proportion of industrial products as compared to the cultivated agricultural area. By now, agricultural technology has become independent of the land, its own natural basis. By destroying the environment, we will not have the chance for producing appropriate and sufficient foodstuff.

Globally every day 40,000 people die from undernutrition and the related diseases. Every fourth child in the Earth suffers from undernutrition and annually 11 million infants below 1 year of age die from undernutrition, 2 billion people suffer from chronic undernutrition [8], while the amount of foodstuff produced could profoundly satisfy all people's needs.

"If the order of values gets disturbed and good is mixed with bad, then individuals and groups take sheerly their own interests and not those of others into account. Safe food supply of the world is endangered by the greediness of the rich and the spread of inappropriate methods of production—the excessive increase of the productivity of soils and the use of excessive amounts of pesticides" [3]. This is what we need to change until it is not too late.

Our challenges now and forthcoming time

Besides these aforementioned facts, the nutritional problems from the viewpoint of science need to cover other "real scientific problems" namely characteristics of the different foods and food preparations: toxicological approach, clinical nutrition behaviors (chemical constituents, their stabilities utilization, physical-chemical properties, food preparation forms, etc.).

Sorry to say, the toxicological problems of the different food or food components are not sufficiently studied in over the world.

In our previous studies, we deeply analyzed the capsaicin problems and were very surprised that no human clinical toxicological examination was found independently in the literature during the human population of the last 7000–9000 years [9–11] by the international authorities asked different toxicological data and by the measurements given internationally accredited institutes. We received these data from the different authorities, and Hungarian authorities gave permission to carry out observations with capsaicin for 1 month period (Phase I). However, we would like to use capsaicin for human therapy we need to give farther toxicological data (two species of animals—rats and Beagle dogs for 6 months, and thereafter in human beings).

From this book, the changes of different physical-chemical properties of the food produced by different preparation are absolutely absent; meanwhile, these data are important in the utilization of different foods or food preparations.

For the objective analysis of the foods, we need to use objective methods as we did during drug therapy [11].

In case of drug preparation, we need to give the international authorities so-called Drug Master File (DMF). In case of capsaicin, the DMF has to be present in the following details: (1) specification of the capsicum species, (2) climatic regulations in places of capsicum cultivation, (3) chemical treatments of capsicum plants during their cultivation, (4) detailed treatment of capsicum plants (their collection, drying, extraction storages, etc.), (5) analytical results supporting the chemical composition of the plant origin of capsaicinoids extract, (6) chemical stability of natural capsaicin (capsaicinoids), (7) analytical results showing the possible contamination of natural compounds with organic phosphates, pesticides, fusarium, and aflatoxins, and (8) international certification (including the Food and Drug Administration, FDA) on the capsaicin (capsaicinoids) content of the natural preparation. Aforementioned data need to be given by internationally accredited laboratories. These data are collected in the DMF.

Sorry to say, similar qualification systems do not exist in case of foods regardless of using much higher portions in the everyday life (Food Master File, FMF). These are in under discussion by the international organizations.

The qualification of the foods would be necessary to be done firstly in human beings, of course, with respect to the actual physiological (pathophysiological) parameters of the human organs [12].

Our challenges now and in the forthcoming decades are the solutions of these aforementioned problems. Our biggest challenge is that although the number of human population increases exponentially, increase of food supply does not happen exponentially.

Our Take Home Message is

"TO BE OR NOT TO BE"

(William Shakespeare, 1564–1616)

Acknowledgements

The editors thank the excellent cooperation of the contributors during the book edition.

Author details

Gyula Mózsik[1]* and Mária Figler[2]

1 First Department of Medicine, University of Pécs, Hungary

2 Second Department of Medicine, The Institute of Dietitian and Nutritional Science, University of Pécs, Hungary

*Address all correspondence to: gyula.mozsik@gmail.com

References

[1] UN. The Universal Declaration of Human Rights. 10th December 1948. 217 A (III) 25. 1.

[2] UN. Declaration on Social Progress and Development. General Assembly resolution. 2542 (XXIV) of 11 December 1969. Part II, 10b

[3] Cor Unum Papal Council Starvation in the world. Challenge for all of us: Solidarity Development (Éhezés a világban. Kihívás mindannyiunk számára: a szolidáris fejlődés) URL: https://katolikus.hu/ kereses/%C3%A9hez%C3%A9s%20 a%20vil%C3%A1gban (22 July, 2008)

[4] Varga P. Theory and Practice of Clinical Nutrition (A klinikai táplálás elmélete és gyakorlata). Budapest: Melania; 1998

[5] Brown P. Culture and the evolution of obesity. Human Nature. 1991;**2**:31-57

[6] Ádány R, editor. Health condition of Hungarian Population in the millennium (A magyar lakosság egészségi állapota az ezredfordulón). Budapest: Medicina; 2003

[7] Kopp M, Csoboth C. Self- harming behaviours among Hungarian population (Önkárosító magatartásformák a magyar népesség körében.). Hungarian Oncology. 2001;**45**(2):139-141

[8] WHO. Nutrition for health and development: A Global Agenda for Combating Malnutrition. 2002

[9] Mózsik Gy, Dömötör A, Past T, Vas V, Perjési P, Kuzma M, et al. Capsaicinoids: From the plant cultivation to the production of the human medical drug. Akadémiai Kiadó, Budapest, 2009 (ISBN 978 963 05 8694 8)

[10] Gy M, OME A-S, Takeuchi K, editors. Capsaicin-Sensitive Neural Afferentation and the Gastrointestinal Tract: From Bench to Bedside. Rijeka: InTech Open Science/Open minds; 2014. DOI: 10.5772/57289. (ISBN 978-953-51-1631-8)

[11] Gy M, editor. Introductory chapter: the general problems of human clinical nutritional and pharmacological observation of capsaicin in human beings and patients. In: Capsaicin and its Human Therapeutic Development. London: InTech Open; 2018. pp. 3-9. DOI: 10.5772/intechopen.73124 (Print ISBN 978-1-78923-520-3; Online ISBN 978-1-78923-521-0)

[12] Mózsik G, Figler M. Metabolic Ward in Human Clinical Nutrition and Dietetics. Kerala: Research Signpost; 2005. ISBN 81-308-0035-7

4

Food Additives in Food Products: A Case Study

Aleksandra Badora, Karolina Bawolska, Jolanta Kozłowska-Strawska and Jolanta Domańska

Abstract

Socioeconomic progress, diseases, and the constantly changing pace of life and lifestyles of consumers worldwide require food to be improved and tailored to meet the needs of purchasers. The produced food is functional, convenient, and enriched. This is achieved, i.e. with food additives. Nowadays, food additives are very widespread in the human diet, but not all of them are synthetic and invasive on human health. All food additives, and their application and dosage, are subject to strict regulations. The purpose of this work was to investigate which food additives are the most common in our everyday diet and how they affect our health.

Keywords: food additives, preservatives, sweeteners, colours

Introduction

The history of food additives goes back to ancient times. As great civilisations developed, populations grew and so did the demand for food. In ancient Egypt, where the climate was not conducive to food storage, especially due to the heat, people started looking for ways to extend the usability life of products. Common practices included the addition of salt, drying in the sun, curing/corning, meat and fish smoking, pickling, and burning sulphur during vegetable preservation. The earliest preservatives included sulphur dioxide (E220), acetic acid (E260), and sodium nitrite (E250), while turmeric (E100) and carmine (E120) were among the first colours. Food preservation was also of immense importance during numer- ous armed conflicts. Both during the Napoleonic wars in Europe and during the American Civil War, seafarers and soldiers needed food. Limited access to fresh food at the front motivated the armed forces to transport their food with them. This is when cans were introduced for food preservation purposes. In the subsequent centuries, ammonium bicarbonate (E503ii), also known as salt of hartshorn, used as a rising agent for baked goods, and sodium hydroxide solution (E524), used in the production of salty sticks, rose to prominence [1, 2].

The nineteenth century saw considerable advancements in the fields of chemistry, biology, and medicine. A name that needs to be mentioned here is Louis Pasteur, a French scientist, who studied microbiology, among other things. He was the first to prove that microorganisms were responsible for food spoilage. At the same time, new chemical compounds were discovered that were able to inhibit the growth of microbes. Some substances, such as picric acid, hydrofluoric acid, and their salts, often had disastrous consequences when added to food. Insufficient knowledge of toxicology resulted in consumer poisonings and even deaths [1, 3]. At that time, food preservation was the number one priority, which was achieved, for instance, by using salicylic acid, formic acid (E236), benzoic acid (E210), boric acid (E284), propionic acid (E280), sorbic acid (E200) and its potassium salt (E202), and esters of p-hydroxybenzoic acid. Later, food concerns also focused on improving the organoleptic properties of their products and started to enhance food with colours, flavours, and sweeteners, without first researching their effects on human health. For example, such practices involved the use of synthetic colours used in fabric dyeing. This desire to make money on beautiful-looking products led to adulterating food with copper and iron salts, which have a negative impact on the human body. It was as late as in 1907 that the United States studied 90 of the synthetic colours used at that time for food dyeing and found only 7 to be acceptable for further use. Detailed studies and strict regulations on the use of food additives were created almost a century later [1, 4].

Globally, food safety is ensured by the World Health Organization (WHO) and the Food and Agriculture Organization (FAO). In 1962, these organisa tions established a special agenda—the Codex Alimentarius Commission. The Commission has prepared and updated the Codex Alimentarius, which is not a legal Act per se, but provides a reference for standards on raw materials and food products, acceptable contamination levels, hygienic processing, research methods, and food additives for almost all countries worldwide [5]. In the European Union, the body responsible for improving human health protection and food safety risk mitigation, as well as for taking care of purchaser interests, is the European Food Safety Authority (EFSA). It is a scientific agency established in 2002 pursuant to the Regulation of the European Parliament and of the Council of 28 January 2002. European legislation is based on the Codex Alimentarius but conducts its own complementary research. Therefore, the list of food additives permitted by the European Union is different from the American one [5].

The primary legal Act governing food in Poland is the Food and Nutrition Safety Act of 25 August 2006 (as amended). It specifies the requirements applicable to food and nutrition, concerning product labelling, hygienic conditions throughout the production process, and product replacement rules, as well as requirements concerning the use of food additives. The key document that pertains specifically to food additives is the Regulation of the European Parliament and of the Council of 16 December 2008 on food additives. The EU-approved list of food additives is presented in the Commission Regulation (EU) of 11 November 2011 [4, 5].

A **food additive** (additional substance) is any substance that is not a food in itself or an ingredient in food, but when added to a product for processing purposes, it becomes part of the food [5]. The following are not considered to be food additives: ingredients in food or chemicals to be used in other products, i.e. in particular sweeteners, such as monosaccharides, disaccharides, and oligosaccharides; substances with flavouring, dyeing, and sapid properties (such as dried fruit); glazing and coating substances, which are not intended to be consumed; and chewing gum bases, dextrin, modified starch, ammonium chloride, edible gelatine, milk protein and gluten, blood plasma, casein, and inulin. The law forbids the use of food additives in unprocessed food, honey, non-emulsified oils and fats of an animal or vegetable origin, butter, milk, fermented milk products (unflavoured, with living bacteria cultures), natural mineral and spring water, unflavoured leaf tea, coffee, sugar, dry pasta, and unflavoured buttermilk [5]. Any marketed additive must comply with the requirements of the European Food Safety Authority, i.e. it has to be technologically justified. It must not put consumers' life or health at risk; its use should not mislead the purchaser; its acceptable daily intake (ADI), or *quantum satis*, the smallest amount which is needed to achieve a specific processing objective for the substance, must be calculable; and, last but not least, such an additive must not adulterate the product it is to be added to. Producers are also required to include information on any food additives on product labelling [6, 7].

EU legislation has approved approximately 330 food additives for use. The primary objectives behind the use of additives are to extend the shelf life and freshness of products, prevent product quality impairment, make the product more attractive to customers, achieve the desired texture, ensure specific product functionality, facilitate production processes, reduce production costs, and enrich the nutritional value of products. In order to harmonise, effectively identify any additives, and ensure smooth exchange of goods, each food additive has its own, standardised, code. This code is consistent with the International Numbering System (INS) and comprises the letter "E" and three or four digits. There are several food additive classifications. One is based on the regulation and differentiates between colours (approx. 40), sweeteners (approx. 16), and other additives (approx. 277) [8, 9].

Additional substances can also be categorised on the basis of code numbers:

1. Colours—E100–E199
2. Preservatives and acidity regulators—E200–E299
3. Antioxidants and synergists—E300–E399
4. Stabilising, thickening, emulsifying, coating, and bulking substances—E400–E499
5. Other substances—E500 and above

Food additives can also be divided into four major groups, based on their processing purpose. These are substances that prevent food spoilage, those which improve sensory features, firming additives and excipients. The most numerous group among additives that slow down food spoilage are **preservatives**. These are either natural or synthetic chemical compounds added to food to restrict as much as possible the biological processes that take place in the product, e.g. the development of microflora and pathogenic microbes, and the effects of enzymes that affect food freshness and quality. In food products, preservatives change the permeability of cytoplasmic membranes or cell walls, damage the genetic system, and deactivate some enzymes. Food is preserved using antiseptics or antibiotics. The former

are synthetically produced simple compounds that often have natural correlates, and they make up no more than 0.2% of the product. Antibiotics, or substances produced by microorganisms, are used in very small, yet effective, doses. The effectiveness of preservatives depends primarily on their effect on a specific type of microorganism, which is why it is vital to select the appropriate preservative based on the microbes found in the product (bacteria, mould, or yeast). Other factors that determine the effectiveness of preservatives include the pH value (a low pH is desirable), temperature, the addition of other substances, and the chemical composition of the product. Preservatives constitute an alternative to physical and biological product freshness stabilisation methods, such as drying, pickling, sterilising, freezing, cooling, and thickening. Consumer objections concerning the widespread use of chemical preservatives and their effects on human health have motivated producers to develop new food preservation procedures. These include radiation, packaging, and storing products in a modified atmosphere, using aseptic technology. Products that are most commonly preserved include ready-made dishes and sauces, meat and fish products, fizzy drinks, and ready-made deserts [9, 10].

Other substances used as preservatives are **acids** and **acidity regulators**. These substances lower the pH level and slow down the growth of enzymes, which hampers the development of microbes. They are used mainly in the production of marinades. For a specific acid or acidity regulator to fulfil its role as a preservative, it needs to be added in highly concentrated form, but acetic acid, for instance, can irritate mucous membranes when its concentration exceeds 3%. Acids and acidity regulators are also used to enhance flavour (usually in fruit or vegetable products, or beverages, to bring out their sour taste) or to facilitate gelatinisation and frothing during food processing [11, 12].

Not only microorganisms but also oxygen is responsible for food spoilage. Products such as oils, fats, and dry goods (flour, semolina) oxidise when they come into contact with atmospheric oxygen. Fat oxidisation (rancidification) occurs in oils, lard, flour, and milk powder. The browning of fruit, vegetables, and meat, on the other hand, is the result of non-fat substance oxidisation. These oxidisation processes can be slowed down or eliminated completely using **antioxidants**. There are natural and synthetic antioxidants and synergists. Synthetic antioxidants are primarily esters (BHA, BHT, propyl gallate). These are used to stabilise fats used to fry, e.g. crisps and chips. The most common natural antioxidants are tocopherols, i.e. vitamin E. Other antioxidants include phenolic compounds, such as flavonoids and phenolic acids. Synthetic antioxidants are more potent and resistant to processing. Synergists are substances that support and extend the functioning of antioxidants. They can form complexes with heavy metal ions, which retard the oxidisation process. The most frequently used synergists are EDTA, citric acid, and ascorbic acid. Antioxidants do not pose a risk to human health. In fact, they can be beneficial. Antioxidants prevent unfavourable interactions between free radicals and tissue and slow down ageing processes and the development of some diseases [12, 13].

In order to extend the freshness of consumer goods, products are also packaged in a modified atmosphere. As part of this process, the oxygen content inside the packaging is reduced and replaced with other **gases**, such as nitrogen, argon, helium, and hydrogen. Furthermore, products in the form of aerosol sprays, such as whipped cream, have nitrous oxide, butane, or propane added to them. All these gases are also food additives with their own E codes [5, 11].

The organoleptic properties of consumer goods are very important to consumers. Visual appeal is considered to be as important as taste or smell. This is where **food colours** come into play.

These are used to add colour to transparent products (e.g. some beverages), intensify or bring out product colour (beverages, sweets), preserve or reproduce colours that have faded as a result of processing, ensure that all product batches have a specific colour, and provide the products that are diluted after purchase with strong colour. In order to add colour to a product, manufacturers use natural, nature-identical, synthetic, and inorganic colours. Natural colours are produced from edible plant parts (fruits, flowers, roots, leaves) and from animal raw materials, such as blood, chitinous exoskeletons of insects, and muscle tissue. New technologies have also made it possible to obtain colours from algae, fungi, and mould. Natural colouring substances include carotenoids that provide a spectrum of yellow and orange colours (carrot, citrus fruit skin), flavonoids that give products blue and navy-blue colours (grapes, currants, chokeberry, elder), betalains that give products a red colour (beetroot, capsicum), and chlorophyll that lends green colours (salad, parsley), as well as riboflavin (vitamin B_2), curcumin, and caramel. Natural colours are desirable for consumers, as they do not show any negative effects on health. However, a significant drawback to using natural colours is that they are very sensitive to environmental factors, such as pH, ambient temperature, oxygen content, or sun exposure, which is why they are not durable when it comes to processing and storage. Moreover, the cost of obtaining such colouring substances is rather high. The list of additives contains 17 natural colours, and their market share in 2012 was approx. 31% and was subject to an upward trend [6, 8].

Synthetic food colours are very competitive compared to natural ones. They offer a wide spectrum of colours, including those that are not available in nature, provide strong colouring, and are resistant to environmental factors, so they do not fade during processing. Furthermore, they are not expensive to produce, which contributes to low end-product prices. Synthetic colours can be divided into organic and inorganic, with organic constituting the considerable majority in terms of food colouring. In the past, chemical colours were made of coal, while now crude oil is used for this purpose. EU law approves 15 synthetic colours, including the so-called Southampton colours. A study conducted in 2007 in the United Kingdom (in Southampton, hence the name) showed the particularly negative effects of six colours on children's health [10]. Specifically, tartrazine (E102), quinoline yellow (E104), sunset yellow (E110), azorubine (E122), cochineal red (E124), and Allura red AC (E129) were found to cause hyperactivity. As a result, since 2010, manufacturers which add at least one of their products have been required to provide label information about their negative effects on concentration and brain functioning in children. Acceptable daily doses of these colours have also been reassessed and updated. Moreover, research conducted on lab animals has shown that the long-term use of synthetic colours, and especially the three that account for 90% of the use of all synthetic colours (Allura red, tartrazine, and sunset yellow), can cause cancer, allergies, and chromosome mutations. Products that are most often synthetically coloured include candy, wine gums, readymade desserts, and refreshing beverages [8, 10].

During consumption, one can experience product taste, smell, and consistency. These three sensations are referred to as palatability and are caused by **flavours.** Taste is experienced by taste buds located in the tongue. Adult individuals have approximately 10,000 such receptors. There are four primary tastes, namely, salty, sweet, bitter, and sour. There is also an additional type, referred to as *umami*, which is Japanese for "savoury, meaty". This taste experience is provided by monosodium glutamate. Smell is experienced through volatile compounds that go directly through the nasal or oral cavity and throat to smell receptors. Taste and smell provide a ready source of information on whether the product is fresh, whether it has specific characteristics, and whether it has been adulterated. Flavours are mixtures of many compounds, in which the specific characteristic smell is produced by a single compound or several indispensable compounds. These are added to enhance the taste or smell of the product or to give something the flavour or aroma that has been lost during product processing [6, 7, 11]. There are natural, nature-identical, and synthetic flavours. Natural flavours are obtained from parts of fruits and vegetables, spices, and their flavouring compounds, such as lactones (found in fruits and nuts), terpenes (in essential oils, found in almost every plant), and carbonyl compounds (fermented dairy products). Nature-identical flavours are compounds originally found in a given raw material that can be recreated in the lab. Synthetic flavours are compounds that have been chemically created and produced and do not have their equivalent in nature. Similarly to natural colours, natural flavours are easily degraded during processing, and their extraction is costly, which is why the food industry generally uses synthetic substances to provide products with specific taste and odour. Moreover, synthetic compounds are capable of giving products much stronger flavours than natural ones [6–7, 13].

A separate group that enhances the sensory properties of food are **sweeteners**. Formerly, in order to make products sweet, manufacturers used sucrose, commonly known just as sugar, obtained from sugar beet or sugarcane. Now large-scale methods are commonly used, such as chemical production and the extraction of intensively sweetening substances, known as sweeteners, from specific plants. What is characteristic about such substances is that they are much more potent as sweeteners compared to sucrose, and, at the same time, their calorific value is close to zero. Natural sweeteners include glucose-fructose syrup (or syrup based on one of those sugars), thaumatin, neohesperidin DC, stevia, and xylitol. Synthetic sweeteners include acesulfame K, aspartame (and the salts of these two compounds), sucralose, cyclamates, saccharin, and neotame. Sweeteners are used in the production of beverages, juices, dairy products, spirits, sweets, marmalade, and chewing gum [14, 15].

In contrast to sucrose, the majority of synthetic sweeteners do not increase blood sugar level and do not cause tooth decay. These substances are attractive for producers because the cost of their production is low, and even small amounts of such compounds are able to ensure the desired sweetness of the product, so these are economical to use. In addition, most sweetener additives remain functional during processing, although some compounds are not resistant to high temperatures. A study conducted in 2010 on lab animals raises some concerns when it comes to sweetener safety in relation to human health [20]. Its findings showed that regular consumption of sweeteners in large quantities caused obesity and neoplasms in animals. Sweetener additives in consumer goods have been considered safe for humans [10]. Each such additive has a specific ADI value and amount (in milligrammes) that can be added to 1 kg (or 1 dm^3) of product [13–15].

The additives that are vital in terms of processing are **firming additives**. They create or stabilise the desirable product structure and consistency. Firming agents include gelling, thickening, emulsifying, bulking, binding, and rising agents, humectants, and modified starches. The highest status among these substances is enjoyed by hydrocolloids. **Hydrocolloids**, known as gums, are polysaccharides of plant, animal, or microbiological origin. There are natural (guar gum, agar, curdlan), chemically and physically modified (modified starches), and synthetic gums. With their macromolecular structure, they are able to bind water, improve solution viscosity, and create gels and spongiform masses. Hydrocolloids are used as gelling (e.g. in the production of jelly, desserts, pudding, and fruit-flavoured starch jelly), thickening (ready made sauces, vegetable products), water-binding (powdered products to be consumed with water, frozen food), and emulsifying agents (to create oil-in-water-type emulsions). They also act as emulsion stabilisers. Hydrocolloids are considered safe for human health, although some of them can cause allergies. Consumed in large quantities, they can have laxative effects [12].

What is also important in creating product structure are **emulsifiers** and the emulsification method. Emulsifiers are compounds which facilitate emulsification. There are water-in-oil (margarine) and oil-in-water (mayonnaise) type of emulsions. Emulsifiers position themselves at the interface between two different phases to stabilise the emulsion. There are natural emulgents, with lecithin as the most common, and synthetic emulgents (glycerol and its esters) [1]. Product consistency and texture are also adjusted using **modified starches**. Such starches are usually obtained from potatoes or corn (also genetically modified one) with chemically altered composition. Similarly to hydrocolloids, such substances can bind water and produce gels and are also resistant to high temperatures [11, 12]. Modified starches are added to ready-made sauces and dishes (such as frozen pizza), frozen goods, bread, and desserts (also powdered) to thicken and maintain product consistency after thermal processing. In order to enhance starch properties, phosphates are often added during starch modification. The human body needs phosphorus, but its excess can negatively affect the bones, kidneys, and the circulatory system [7, 11, 12].

Nowadays, consumer goods are widely available, and consumers are provided with a broad range of products to choose from. The continuously growing number of world population (approximately 7 billion in 2011) has made supply on the food market exceed demand. This situation is characteristic of countries with a high GDP. Food producers examine consumer behaviour patterns to see what encourages them to make a purchase, and also the purchase itself and its consequences, and then analyse these processes to launch a new product or a substitute for an already existing one. To sum up, the market has provided more food products than consumers are able to purchase, which results in unimaginable food wastage. Each year, approximately 100 million tonnes of food goes to waste in Europe. This quantity does not include agricultural and food waste or fish discards [13].

Materials and methods

The methodology of this study was based on the information contained on the labels. The chemical composition of the investigated food products was presented. Interview with the store's seller concerned the popularity and frequency of sales listed in the product tables. It should be noted that the examined store is representative when it comes to this type of stores in the majority of small towns in southeastern Poland.

This study was based on data on the most frequently chosen consumer goods in a store in a small town in Poland. The town is located in a commune that has 5300 residents. Data were obtained by monitoring the sales over the course of 12 months. These products are presented in **Tables 2–6** and classified into the following categories: (i) meat and fish; (ii) beverages; (iii) condiments; (iv) ready-made sauces, soups, and dishes; and (v) sweets and desserts. The main classification criterion was segregation into primary food groups. The chemical composition of each product, as listed on the packaging, was included in a table and then assessed against the presence of any food additives. Sixteen most common additives were selected in all the investigated products; only chemical compounds that were found in at least four food products were taken into consideration. The most common food additives were highlighted in Holt in the "product composition" column and presented in **Table 1**, together with their E codes. Then, based on the literature, the study described the most common additional substances.

Table 1. *The most common food additives and ingredients.*

Name	Symbol	Number of products
Citric acid	E330	15
Monosodium glutamate	E621	10
Guar gum	E412	8
Sodium nitrite	E250	7
Disodium 5′-ribonucleotides	E635	6
Sodium erythorbate	E316	5
Glucose-fructose syrup	Not considered an additive	5
Soy lecithin	Not considered an additive	5
Maltodextrin	Not considered an additive	5
Triphosphates	E451	4
Xanthan gum	E415	4
Carrageenan	E407	4
Tocopherols	E306	4
Glucose syrup	Not considered an additive	4
Sodium benzoate	E211	4
Ammonia caramel	E150c	4

Results and discussion

Table 1 shows 16 of the most popular substances found in food. The majority of these substances are food additives; four other substances are not considered in the European Union as food additives. The additives that are the most frequently found in the food products examined in this study are citric acid (E330), monosodium glutamate (E621), and guar gum (E412). In Ref. [16] it is reported that the most popular preservatives found in food are the mixture of sodium benzoate and potassium sorbate, or potassium sorbate (E202) and sodium benzoate (E211) used separately, and also ulphur dioxide (E220). Data presented in **Table 1** shows that, compared to citric acid, another preservative, sodium benzoate, is used rarer. No potassium sorbate was found in any of the products examined in this study. In Ref. [13] it can be concluded that the most commonly used preservatives and antioxidants are sorbic acid and its salts (E200-203), benzoic acid and its salts (E210-213), sulfur dioxide (E220), sodium nitrite (E250), lactic acid (E270), citric acid (E330) and tocopherols (E306). The majority of the additives listed in Ref. [13] can be found in **Table 1**.

Table 2 shows 10 meat and fish products and their composition, as specified on the label. Each of the investigated items contained at least 1 of the 16 most common food additives (**Table 1**). As much as 50% of meat and fish products contained four or more of such additives. The highest number of additives (seven) was found in "Z doliny Karol" mortadella. "Masarnia u Józefa" crispy ham and "Lipsko" Śląska sausage contained six different food additives. Seventy percent of the examined products had had sodium nitrite (E250) added. This means that this preservative is frequently added to meat products, as confirmed in Ref. [9]. Other widespread preservatives mentioned in Ref. [9] include lactic acid (E270), sodium benzoate (E211), sorbic acid (E200), and sulphur dioxide (E220). In Ref. [9] it also mentions other additives frequently added to meat and fish products; these include carrageenan, gum arabic, and xanthan gum. In this study, 50% of the examined items contain one or two gums, and carrageenan is present in only three in ten products. A study in Ref. [17] demonstrates that fish products are the second leading food (after edible fats) in terms of preservative content.

Table 3 shows ten non-alcoholic beverages, six of which contain at least one common food additive (**Table 1**). Foreign substances that are most frequently found in this food group are citric acid (E330), sodium benzoate (E211), and glucose- fructose syrup. A study in Refs. [18–19] shows that the most popular sweeteners in non-alcoholic beverages are glucose, fructose, and glucose-fructose syrups. As shown on product label, 100% juice by brands such as "Hortex" and "Tymbark", as well as "Cisowianka" and "Kubuś" mineral waters, is additive free. Pursuant to the Regulation of the European Parliament and of the Council (EC) of 16 December 2008, no food additives may be used in mineral and spring bottled water. The beverage to contain the largest number of additive substances was white orangeade by "Hellena".

Table 4 shows 12 food items, such as ketchup, mustard, herbs and spices, and tomato concentrates, together with their composition. Only four products in this group contain a food additive, of which three are preserved using citric acid (E330). In this group of products, the products to contain the most common additive substances were the ketchup and the Kucharek seasoning by "Prymat". Pursuant to the Regulation of the European Parliament and of the Council (EC) of 16 December 2008, tomato products (such as concentrates) must not contain food colours. They may, however, contain other additives. The ketchup has no colours, but contains other food additives. Studies in Ref. [17] demonstrate that mayonnaises and mustards are the fourth most often preserved product group, with ready-made concentrates ranking seventh. One of the two mustards examined in this paper contained a preservative, and two of the presented tomato concentrates had not had any food additives added to them.

Table 2. *Food additives and ingredients in the studied meat and fish products.*

Product	Ingredients	Product	Ingredients
Szynka krucha (ham) Masarnia u Józefa	Pork ham, salt, pork protein, **carrageenan**, potassium acetate, potassium lactate, smoke flavouring, **monosodium glutamate**, diphosphates, **triphosphates**, flavourings, **sodium erythorbate, tocopherols, sodium nitrite**	Pasztet podlaski (pâté) 155 g Drosed	Water, mechanically separated chicken meat, rapeseed oil, chicken liver and skin, cream of wheat, salt, soy protein, potato starch, dried vegetables, spices, powdered milk, (milk) whey, sugar, **maltodextrin**, plant protein hydrolysate, yeast extract
Kiełbasa śląska (sausage) Lipsko	Pork 60%, pig fat 17%, water, mechanically deboned chicken meat, fibre, pork skin emulsion, potato starch, milk proteins, **triphosphates**, tara gum, **xanthan gum**, sodium erythorbate, aluminium ammonium sulphate, salt, glucose, flavourings, carmine, spice extracts, **maltodextrin, monosodium glutamate**, soy protein, **sodium nitrite**	Łuków przysmak kanapkowy (tinned meat) 300 g	Pork meat 30%, water, beef meat 18%, pig fat, soy protein, salt, beef fat, **triphosphates**, spices, pork gelatine, flavouring, **sodium nitrite**, tinned high-yield luncheon meat
Mortadela doliny (mortadella) Karol	Water, pork 20%, mechanically separated chicken meat 15%, pig fat, pork connective tissue, cream of wheat, acetylated starch, polyphosphates, **triphosphates**, diphosphates, sodium citrate, calcium lactate, sodium lactate, salt, soy protein concentrate, pork protein, wheat fibre, spices (including mustard seeds, corn, and legumes), spice extracts, yeast extract, flavourings, **glucose syrup**, glucose, vinegar, **sodium erythorbate**, ascorbic acid, **guar gum, disodium 5′-ribonucleotides, monosodium glutamate, sodium nitrite**	Agrovit duże porcje konserwa tyrolska (tinned meat) 400 g	Water, mechanically separated chicken meat 23%, pork raw materials 23%, modified (corn) starch, wheat fibre, pea fibre, salt, **carrageenan**, processed Eucheuma seaweed, spices, spice extracts, **monosodium glutamate, sodium erythorbate, sodium nitrite**
Mięso mielone wieprzowe (ground pork) Adrian	Pork meat 65%, pig fat 34%, salt, **xanthan gum, carrageenan**, konjac, starch, **sodium nitrite**	Euro Fish szprot w sosie pomidorowym (sprat in tomato sauce) 170 g	Fish—sprat without heads—tomato sauce, water, tomato concentrate, sugar, rapeseed oil, salt, modified starch, dried onion, **guar gum, xanthan gum**, spice extracts, acetic acid
Parówki (frankfurters) Indykpol	Chicken meat 25.9%, mechanically separated turkey meat 17%, mechanically separated chicken meat 17.3%, water, poultry fat, pork, corn flour, chicken skins, pig fat, pork skins, potato starch, soy protein, salt, spices, spice extracts, flavourings, **monosodium glutamate**, acetylated distarch adipate, **guar gum**, potassium acetate, potassium lactate, diphosphates, ascorbic acid, **sodium erythorbate, sodium nitrite**	Graal Flet z makreli w sosie pomidorowym (mackerel fillet in tomato sauce) 170 g	Mackerel fillets 60%, tomato sauce, water, tomato concentrate, sugar, rapeseed oil, modified starch, spirit vinegar, salt, powdered tomatoes, dried onion, spice extract, spices, **guar gum, xanthan gum**, pepper extract, **maltodextrin**

Table 3. *Food ingredients in the studied non-alcoholic beverages.*

Product	Ingredients	Product	Ingredients
Woda mineralna gazowana (carbonated mineral water) Cisownianka 1.5 L	Natural mineral water, unsaturated with carbon dioxide, moderately mineralised	Woda mineralna niegazowana (non-carbonated mineral water) Kubuś water 0.5 L	Water, cane sugar, apple juice from concentrated apple juice, lemon juice from concentrated lemon juice, flavouring
Sok jabłko (apple juice) 100% 1 L Hortex	100% apple juice from concentrated apple juice	Coca cola 1.5 L	Water, sugar, carbon dioxide, **sulphite ammonia caramel**, phosphoric acid, natural flavourings, including caffeine
Sok multiwitamina (multivitamin juice) 100% 1 L Tymbark	Juices from concentrated apple juice 60% and orange juice 22%, carrot juice from concentrated juice 12%, purées from banana 3%, peach, guava, papaya, juices from concentrated pineapple juice 2%, mango juice 0.5%, passion fruit juice 0.1%, lychee juice 0.05%, cactus fig juice, kiwi fruit juice and lime juice, vitamins A, C, E, B6, and B12, thiamine, riboflavin, niacin, biotin, folic acid, pantothenic acid	Tymbark 2 L jabłko-pomarańcza (apple-orange)	Water, orange juice from concentrated juice 19%, **glucose-fructose syrup**, sugar, peach juice from concentrated juice 1%, lemon concentrate, flavourings, ascorbic acid, carotenes
Volcano 2 L cola	Spring water, carbon dioxide, sulphite ammonia caramel, phosphoric acid, **citric acid**, sodium citrates, flavourings (including caffeine), gum arabic, aspartame, saccharin, **sodium benzoate**, potassium sorbate	Volcano 2 L pomarańcza (orange)	Spring water, carbon dioxide, orange juice 0.3% from concentrated orange juice, **citric acid**, gum arabic, glycerol and plant resin esters, flavouring, cyclamates, saccharin, aspartame, acesulfame K, **sodium benzoate**, potassium sorbate, ascorbic acid, carotenes, beta-apo-8′-carotenal
Hellena 1.25 L oranżada biała (white orangeade)	Sugar, water, **glucose-fructose syrup**, carbon dioxide, **citric acid**, flavouring, **sodium benzoate**	Kubuś marchew, jabłko, pomarańcza, sok (carrot, apple, and orange juice) 330 mL	Purées and juices (59%), water, **glucose-fructose syrup, citric acid**, vitamin C, flavouring

Table 5 shows 12 products categorised into ready-made dishes, soups and sauces, and their chemical composition. Each of these products contains at least one common additive. Citric acid (E330) was added to nearly 67% of the products in this category. Only five in twelve items (including four instant soups and stock cubes) contain the three most popular food additive substances (**Table 1**). A study in Ref. [13] shows that the most common additives in ready-made dishes are citric acid (E330), sunset yellow (E110), guar gum (E412), disodium guanylate (E627), disodium inosinate (E631), and monosodium glutamate (E621).

Table 6 shows 10 food items classified as sweets and desserts. As many as nine products in this group contained at least one of the most common food additives (**Table 1**). Glucose-fructose or glucose syrups were found in six of the examined items. A study in Ref. [19] shows that sweets often include the so-called Southampton colours, such as quinoline yellow and tartrazine. However, the study reports that the amounts of these substances added to sweets are much lower than the maximum values allowed by the applicable law.

Table 4. *Food ingredients in the studied condiments.*

Product	Ingredients	Product	Ingredients
Koncentrat pomidorowy (tomato concentrate) Aro 190 g	30% tomato concentrate	Koncentrat pomidorowy (tomato concentrate) Pudliszki	30% tomato concentrate
Ketchup łagodny (mild ketchup) 470 g	37% tomato concentrate, water, sugar, vinegar, modified starch, salt, **citric acid, sodium benzoate,** thyme, oregano, savoury, sage, coriander, flavouring	Ketchup Pudliszki łgodny (mild ketchup) 480 g	Tomatoes, sugar, vinegar, salt, modified starch, natural flavouring
Musztarda Parczew kremska (Krems mustard) 180 g	Water, mustard seeds, vinegar, sugar, salt, spices	Musztarda Roleski stołowa (table mustard)	Water, mustard seeds, sugar, spirit vinegar, salt, spices, turmeric extract, **citric acid**, natural flavouring
Zioła prowansalskie (Herbes de Provence) Prymat	Basil, marjoram, rosemary, savoury, sage, thyme, oregano, mint	Przyprawa do kurczaka (chicken seasoning) Goleo	Salt, garlic, white mustard seeds, sweet pepper, carrot, coriander, fenugreek, caraway, chilli, turmeric, cinnamon
Przyprawa Tzatziki (tzatziki seasoning) Prymat	Garlic, salt, sugar, onion, **citric acid**, onion extract, dill extract, dill leaves, pepper extract, black pepper	Kucharek Prymat 250 g	Salt, died vegetables, **monosodium glutamate, disodium 5′-ribonucleotides**, sugar, starch, black pepper, riboflavin

Citric acid (E330) is a natural compound found in citrus fruits. It is also the by-product of digestive processes in the human body. However, on the industrial scale, the substance is produced using the *Aspergillus niger* mould. Citric acid isused in food as an acidity regulator, preservative, and flavour enhancer. Outside the food industry, the acid is added to cleaning agents and acts as a decalcifying agent. Citric acid in food is a safe additive and is added to food on the *quantum satis* basis; nevertheless its widespread use constitutes a risk. This substance is found in many food products, such as beverages, juices, lemonades, sweets, ice creams, canned goods, and even bread, so customers consume it in large quantities everyday [20]. When consumed frequently in excess, citric acid can lead to enamel degradation and teeth deterioration. This additive also supports the absorption of heavy metals, which, in turn, might lead to brain impairment. It can also affect the kidneys and liver [13, 15].

Monosodium glutamate (E621) is the most widespread flavour enhancer. It is even considered to be one of the five basic tastes (*umami*). Glutamic acid and its (magnesium, potassium, and calcium) salts lend a meaty flavour to products. The substance was first extracted from algae by a Japanese scientist, but now it is generally produced by biotechnological means using microorganisms that can be genetically modified [6]. Another commonly used flavour enhancer is chemically produced **disodium 5′-ribonucleotides (E635)**. These additives can be found in ready-made dishes, sauces, meat and fish products, instant soups, crisps, and cakes. These flavour enhancers are the not inert in relation to the neurological system [16].

Table 5. *Food ingredients and additives in the studied ready-made dishes, soups, and sauces.*

Product	Ingredients	Product	Ingredients
Rosół drobiowy kucharek (chicken soup) 60 g	Salt, palm fat, partially hydrogenated, starch, **monosodium glutamate, disodium 5′-ribonucleotides**, rapeseed oil, dried vegetables, sugar, flavourings, chicken fat, turmeric, **citric acid**, dried chicken meat	Rosół drobiowy Winiary (chicken soup) 60 g	Salt, **monosodium glutamate, disodium 5′-ribonucleotides**, starch, fully hydrogenated palm fat, flavourings, sugar, chicken fat, spices, dried vegetables, **citric acid**, dried chicken meat
Vifon kurczak Carry (curry chicken)	Noodles (92.1%), wheat flour, plant fat, tapioca, modified starch, acetylated starch, sugar, stabilisers (pentasodium triphosphate, **guar gum**, rising substances: sodium carbonate, potassium carbonate, turmeric), flavouring additives (7.9%) (refined palm oil, salt, sugar), flavour enhancers (**monosodium glutamate**, disodium guanylate, disodium inosinate, dried vegetables (carrot, green onion, coriander), powdered curry (flavour additive content 6%), turmeric, aniseed, clove, coriander seed, cinnamon, pepper, garlic, chilli, lemongrass, flavouring), colour (beta-carotene, antioxidant **tocopherols)**	Amino zupa błyskawiczna gulaszowa (instant goulash soup)	Noodles (85%), wheat flour, palm fat, modified starch, salt, rapeseed oil, **tocopherols**, fatty acid and ascorbic acid esters; flavouring mix: salt, starch, paprika, **monosodium glutamate**, disodium guanylate and disodium inosinate, tomato concentrate, onion, flavourings, palm fat, Cayenne pepper, garlic, caraway, hydrolysed plant protein, dried pork, parsley, **ammonia caramel**
Sos Winiary Italia boloński (Bolognese sauce)	Dried vegetables, modified starch, sugar, salt, spices, flavourings, sunflower oil, **citric acid**, spices, beetroot juice concentrate, olive oil	Sos Winiary pieczeniowy ciemny (dark roasting sauce)	Potato starch, modified starch, salt, dried vegetables, flavourings, sugar, yeast extracts, fully hydrogenated palm fat, palm oil, rice flour, **ammonia caramel**, wheat protein hydrolysate, spices, **citric acid**
Sos Winiary borowikowy (bolete sauce)	Corn starch, wheat flour, powdered cream, palm oil, sunflower oil, **maltodextrin**, dried mushroom, salt, flavourings, lactose, yeast extract, sugar, dried fried onion, dried onion, milk proteins, spices, wheat protein hydrolysate, **ammonia caramel**, bolete extract	Zupa Winiary barszcz biały (white borscht)	Wheat flour, skimmed powdered milk, salt, potato starch, sugar, smoked pig fat, citric acid, dried vegetables, yeast extract, herbs, spices, smoke flavour
Zupa Winiary jak u mamy pieczarkowa (champignon soup)	Corn starch, skimmed powdered milk, wheat flour, powdered cream, dried champignons, yeast extracts, salt, potato starch, dried vegetables, flavourings, sunflower oil, wheat protein hydrolysate, parsley, black pepper, **citric acid**	Łowicz sos boloński (Bolognese sauce) 350 g	Tomatoes, water, vegetables, **glucose-fructose syrup**, apple purée, modified corn starch, salt, sugar, **guar gum**, **citric acid**, rapeseed oil, spices, herbs, flavourings, ground dried parsley, garlic and paprika, leek and carrot extracts
Danie gotowe Flaczki (ready-made tripe) Pamapol	Water, beef rumen 305, wheat flour, carrot, parsley, celeriac, tomato concentrate, onion, salt, pork gelatine, sugar, soy protein hydrolysate, dried vegetables, yeast extract, spices, **disodium 5′-ribonucleotides**, **ammonia caramel**, flavourings, partially hydrogenated palm and rapeseed fats	Pomysł na soczystą karkówkę z ziemniakami (pork shoulder with potatoes seasoning) Winiary	Wheat flour, vegetables, salt, modified starch, yeast extract, herbs, **maltodextrin**, plant oil, spices, flavourings, wheat protein hydrolysate, **citric acid**

This can affect brain cells and lead to headaches, heart palpitations, excessive sweating, listlessness, nausea, and skin lesions. Such anomalies, which could have been caused by the excessive consumption of products rich in glutamates, are referred to as the Chinese restaurant syndrome [20]. Flavour enhancers can also serve a positive function by increasing appetite in the sick or the elderly [20]. Other additional substances commonly found in foodstuffs are polysaccharides:

Table 6. *Food additives and ingredients in the studied sweets.*

Product	Ingredients	Product	Ingredients
Lód Top milker (ice cream) Koral	Skimmed reconstituted milk, sugar, cocoa oil, **glucose syrup**, skimmed powdered milk, mono- and diglycerides of fatty acids, locust bean flour, **guar gum**, powdered cream, natural vanilla, flavourings	Baton 3bit (candy bar)	Sugar, biscuit 14% [wheat flour, sugar, plant fat, powdered whey, **glucose-fructose syrup**, whole powdered milk, salt, rising agents (sodium bicarbonate, ammonium bicarbonate), acidity regulator (**citric acid**), skimmed powdered milk (13. 5% in filling), plant fat, cocoa fat, cocoa paste, powdered whey, plant oil, milk fat, emulsifiers (**soy lecithin**, polyglycerol polyricinoleate), flavourings, salt. Cocoa mass in chocolate—minimum 30%
7 days	Wheat flour, cocoa filling 25% [(sugar, partially hydrogenated plant fats, water, low-fat powdered cocoa 7%, skimmed powdered milk, ethyl alcohol, emulsifier (lactic acid esters of mono- and diglycerides of fatty acids), vanilla flavouring, gelling agent (sodium alginate), preservative (potassium sorbate 0.1%)], margarine [partially hydrogenated plant fats, water, salt, emulsifier (mono- and diglycerides of fatty acids), acidity regulator, flavouring, preservative (potassium sorbate 0.1%)], sugar, stabiliser (mono- and diglycerides of fatty acids), **glucose-fructose syrup**, yeast, skimmed powdered milk, salt, vanilla flavouring, preservative (calcium propionate 0.1%), soy flour, emulsifier (**soy lecithin**)	Lód rożek truskawkowy (ice cream cone) Koral	Skimmed reconstituted milk, cornet 14% [wheat flour, sugar, palm fat, potato starch, emulsifier (**soy lecithin**, wheat fibre, salt), colour (sulphite ammonia caramel], sugar, coconut oil, strawberry sauce 7% [strawberries 42%, sugar, **glucose syrup**, water, thickening agent (hydroxypropyl distarch glycerol), acidity regulator (**citric acid**, flavouring], coating for cornet waterproofing [sugar, coconut and palm fats, reduced-fat powdered cocoa (10–12%), emulsifier (**soy lecithin**)], water, **glucose syrup**, strawberry purée 1%, emulsifier (mono- and diglycerides of fatty acids), stabilisers (**Guar gum**, cellulose gum, **carrageenan**, locust bean flour), acidity regulator (**citric acid**), colours (betanin, annatto, flavourings)
Baton Milky way (candy bar)	Sugar, **glucose syrup**, skimmed powdered milk, cocoa fat, palm fat, cocoa mass, milk fat, lactose, powdered (milk) whey, barley malt extract, salt, emulsifier (**soy lecithin**), powdered egg white, hydrolysed milk protein, natural vanilla extract	Mlekołaki Lubella muszelki (cereal) 250 g	Wholemeal wheat, wheat, and corn flours, sugar, glucose, reduced-fat cocoa, cocoa, barley malt extract, milk chocolate, palm fat, salt, **soy lecithin**, flavourings, vitamin C, niacin, pantothenic acid, vitamin B, riboflavin, thiamine, folic acid, vitamin B12, calcium, iron
Nestlé Corn Flakes 600 g	Corn grits, sugar, salt, glucose, brown sugar, invert sugar syrup, cane sugar molasses, sodium phosphates, niacin, pantothenic acid, riboflavin, vitamin B6, folic acid	Nestlé Frutina 250 g	Wheat flakes (wholemeal wheat, sugar, wheat bran, barley malt extract, invert sugar syrup, salt, cane sugar molasses, **glucose syrup**, sodium phosphates, **tocopherols**), raisins, cut dried apples, sodium metabisulphite, niacin, pantothenic acid, vitamin B6, riboflavin, folic acid, calcium, iron
Lays zielona cebulka (crisps) 150 g	Potatoes, palm oil, sunflower oil, flavouring, powdered onion, powdered milk whey, powdered milk lactose, sugar, powdered milk, **monosodium glutamate**, **disodium 5′-ribonucleotides**, flavourings, powdered milk cheese, **citric acid**, malic acid, annatto, pepper extract, powdered garlic, **maltodextrin**, salt	Star chips paprika (crisps) 170 g	Potatoes, palm fat, flavourings, wheat breadcrumbs, glucose, sugar, **monosodium glutamate**, pepper extract, **citric acid**, salt

Guar gum (E412) and **xanthan gum (E415)**. These are referred to as hydrocolloids, i.e. substances that bind water, are easily soluble in both cold and warm water, and improve mixture viscosity. Guar gum is a polysaccharide obtained from guar, a leguminous plant grown in India and Pakistan [14]. Xanthan gum is a polysaccharide of microbiological origin. On the industrial scale, it is obtained as a result of *Xanthomonas campestris* bacteria fermenting the sugar contained in corn (often genetically modified). Both these additives are approved for use in all food products as thickening, firming, and stabilising agents, on the *quantum satis* basis. Guar gum and xanthan gum can be found mainly in bread, cakes, ready-made sauces and dishes, and powdered food, where they ensure the appropriate consistency.

Moreover, they prevent the crystallisation of water in ice cream and frozen food and the separation of fluids in dairy products and juices. The human body is not capable of digesting, breaking down, or absorbing these gums. These substances swell in the intestines, which can cause flatulence and stomach ache. In addition, guar gum can cause allergies [13–15].

A commonly found preservative is **sodium nitrite (E250)**. It is a salty and white or yellowish crystalline powder, obtained by the chemical processing of nitric acid or some lyes and gases [9]. This additive is generally used in the meat industry to inhibit botulinum toxin and *Staphylococcus aureus* bacteria, slow down fat rancidification, maintain the pink red colour of meat, and provide meat with a specific flavour. It does not, however, prevent the growth of yeast or mould. Sodium nitrite is toxic, oxidising, and dangerous to the environment, so it must not be added to food in its pure form. This additive is used in very small doses (0.5–0.6%) in the form of a mixture with domestic salt [9] in amounts up to 150 mL per L or mg kg^{-1}. When consumed in large quantities, nitrites can cause cyanosis, whose symptoms include blue coloration of the skin, lips, and mucous membranes. During digestion, nitrites are transformed into carcinogenic nitrosamines. Moreover, they are particularly dangerous for children, since they stop erythrocytes from binding oxygen, which can lead to death by suffocation [11].

A common ingredient in food is **maltodextrin**, which in the European Union is not considered as a food additive, but as an ingredient. Therefore, within the community, maltodextrin has no E code, while in Sweden it is considered an additive and identified as E1400 [18]. Maltodextrin is a disaccharide obtained from corn starch, but it is not sweet in taste. Nevertheless, it provides greater sweetness than normal sugar or grape sugar (the glycaemic index of maltodextrin is 120, that of normal sugar is 70, and that of grape sugar is 100). It is used as a thickening agent, stabiliser, bulking agent, and even as a fat substitute in low-calorie products. It is added to products for athletes and children, to instant soups, sweets, and meat products [10]. Maltodextrin does not affect the natural product taste or flavour, while it provides human body with carbohydrates and energy. Due to the fact that glucose particles in maltodextrin are broken down only in the intestines, it can also support metabolism. A negative aspect of its use is tooth decay [10, 18].

What frequently occurs in consumer goods is **glucose-fructose syrup**. Similarly to maltodextrin, it is not considered to be a food additive, but, due to its widespread application, it is important to mention it here. Glucose-fructose syrup, also known as high-fructose corn syrup (HFCS), replaces traditional sugar in many products, such as beverages, sweets, jams, fruit products, and liqueurs, and in the United States and Canada is the dominant sweetener [19]. Sucrose is a disaccharide composed of glucose and fructose, which are joined with alpha-1,4-glycosidic bond, and HFCS contains free fructose and free glucose in specific proportions. The name of this substance depends on the proportion of its ingredients. When the syrup contains more fructose, it is referred to as fructose-glucose syrup [12]. It is obtained mainly from corn starch as a result of acid or enzymatic hydrolysis. Glucose- fructose syrup is much sweeter and cheaper than traditional sugar, it does not crystallise, and it has a liquid form, which makes it functional during processing. Nevertheless, there are some disturbing aspects of using this substance. During the consumption of products with glucose-fructose syrup, the body receives unnatural amounts of fructose, which is broken down in the liver in a manner similar to alcohol. Therefore, its excessive amounts can cause fatty liver and overburden this organ. This has even been named "non-alcoholic fatty liver disease". In addition, heavy consumption of monosaccharides has been found to contribute to obesity, which, in turn, can cause high blood pressure and diabetes. Fructose affects the lipid metabolism and disrupts the perception of hunger and satiety. Labels do not provide the exact HFCS content, but it is estimated that the consumption of a single product with this substance satisfies the acceptable daily monosaccharide intake [5–6, 11, 13].

Another frequently added substance is **sodium erythorbate (E316)**. This synthetic compound is used as an antioxidant and stabiliser in meat and fish products and is useful for ham and sausage pickling [13]. It has similar properties to ascorbic acid, but it is not effective as vitamin C. Sodium erythorbate is considered to be noninvasive in the human body [12–13].

The most widespread natural emulsifier is **soy lecithin**. Etymologically, the word "lecithin" can be traced back to *lekythos*, Greek for egg yolk, but this compound is actually found in any plant or animal cell. Lecithin is produced from eggs, sunflower and rapeseed oils, and soybeans [11–13]. This additive is identified as E322 and is used for the production of mayonnaise, ice creams, margarine, readymade desserts, sauces, and instant soups. Products with added lecithin dissolve in water more easily. EU law does not impose any limits on the use of E322. Only in products for children, lecithin content must not exceed 1 g per L.

Triphosphates (E451), as well as diphosphates and polyphosphates, are used as preservatives, flavour enhancers, stabilisers, and rising and water-binding agents. Triphosphates are produced chemically and have a broad application. They are added to sauces, meats and meat products, desserts, bread, pâtés, fish products, ice creams, and non-alcoholic beverages [21]. The human body needs phosphorus in specific amounts, but the widespread use of phosphoric acids and phosphates in food makes people likely to consume this element in excess. When consumed regularly, increased doses of phosphates can lead to osteoporosis or contribute to kidney dysfunction and affect the circulatory system [13, 21]. A popular hydrocolloid found in food is **carrageenan (E407)**. This substance is extracted from *Eucheuma*, a tribe of red algae. Carrageenan is highly soluble in water and is used as a bulking agent in dietary products, and it is also added to beverages, ice creams, sauces, marmalades, and powdered milk [6, 7]. Carrageenan can be used on the *quantum satis* basis. Usually, it is combined with other hydrocolloids. This additive is not digestible by the human body. There are certain objections concerning the consumption of carrageenan, e.g. it can cause intestinal cancer and stomach ulcers [11–13].

Tocopherols (E306) are commonly known as vitamin E, insoluble in water and soluble in fats. It is used as a preservative, stabiliser, and potent antioxidant in such products as oils, margarines, desserts, meat products, and alcoholic beverages. Tocopherols are produced synthetically or obtained from plant oils, but natural vitamin E is twice as easily absorbed by the human body [21].

Common preservatives include benzoic acid and its salts, of which the most frequently used is **sodium benzoate (E211)**. Negligible amounts of these substances are naturally found in berries, mushrooms, and fermented milk-based drinks. On an industrial scale, it is produced synthetically from toluene obtained from crude oil [3, 12]. What is characteristic of sodium benzoate is that it slows down the growth of mould and yeast, but does not prevent the growth of bacteria, which is why it is often used with other preservatives, such as sulphur dioxide (E220). It is commonly used in products with acidic pH, such as marinades, fruit juices, and products with mayonnaise, such as vegetable salads. Sodium benzoate can cause allergies [6, 13]. Our own study (see "Results and discussion") showed that **ammonia caramel (E150c)** and sulphite ammonia caramel (E150d) are fairly common colours. It adds brown to black colours to products. Under natural conditions, this substance is created when sugar is heated. As a food additive, it is produced chemically using ammonia, as well as phosphates, sulphates, and sulphites (sulphite ammonia caramel is produced) [19]. This substance is approved for use under EU law [5]; however, there are studies that have confirmed that it negatively affects human health. It has been proven that this colour can cause hyperactivity and liver, thyroid, and lung neoplasms and also impair immunity. Ammonia caramel is used to dye non-alcoholic beverages, such as cola and marmalades [10, 11].

The external aspect that is most crucial for buyers when it comes to food selection is its freshness. Buyers assess the best before date against the possibility of consuming the food quickly or storing it for future use. Another determinant is the value of the item. Any consumer will pay attention to the price of the product they buy. Another factor is the product ingredients specified on the packaging. Buyers have been observed to have developed a habit of reading labels before buying anything. Some customers also pay attention to the country of origin or brand [22]. Men and women who are determined to stay fit will also consider nutritional value. The factors that are not considered that are relevant include net product weight, information about any genetically modified raw material content, and notices about any implemented quality management systems. Moreover, consumers are likely to be affected by marketing devices, such as advertisements or special offers, used by producers. A temporary reduction in price, or the opportunity to buy two items for the price of one, encourages customers to make a purchase [3, 4]. What is also vital is whether the food is functional. Many people live at a fast pace, work a lot, or get stuck in traffic jams, and the lack of free time pushes them to buy ready-made dishes to be heated up at home or food that can be prepared in an instant [4, 13, 22].

Nowadays, food additives are very widespread in the everyday human diet, but not all of them are synthetic and invasive to human health. Products which must not contain foreign substances do not contain food additives. The explorations undertaken by this and other studies confirm the widespread use of the investigated additives, except for citric acid, which is less popular an additive than sodium benzoate and potassium sorbate. This study shows that when adopting a healthy lifestyle, consumers can choose from a range of food and pharmaceutical products that either contain a limited amount of unconventional substances or do not contain such substances at all.

Author details

Aleksandra Badora*, Karolina Bawolska, Jolanta Kozłowska-Strawska and Jolanta Domańska

Department of Agricultural and Environmental Chemistry, The University of Life Sciences in Lublin, Lublin, Poland

*Address all correspondence to: aleksandra.badora@up.lublin.pl

References

[1] Toussaint-Samat MA. History of Food. Oxford, United Kingdom: Wiley-Blackwell; 2009. ISBN: 978 1-405-18119-8

[2] Couture L. The history of canned food. Johnson and Wales University School of Arts and Science. Academic Symposium of Underground Scholarship; 2010

[3] Gram L, Ravn L, Rasch M, Bruhn JB, Christensen AB, Givskov M. Food spoilage—Interactions between food spoilage bacteria. International Journal of Food Microbiology. 2002;**78**(1-2): 79-97. PMID: 12222639

[4] Publikacja Komisji Europejskiej. Zrozumieć politykę UE— Bezpieczeństwo Żywności (Understanding EU policy—Food Safety). Urząd Publikacji Unii Europejskiej; 2014 (in Polish)

[5] Rozporządzenie Parlamentu Europejskiego i Rady (WE) z dnia 16 grudnia 2008 r. w sprawie dodatków do żywności [The Regulation of the European Parliament and of the Council (EC) of 16 December 2008 on food additives]. Dz. Urz. L 354 (in Polish)

[6] Sharma S. Food preservatives and their harmful effects. International Journal of Scientific and Research Publications. 2015;**4**(5):1-2. ISSN 2250-3153

[7] Abdulmumeen HA. Food: Its preservatives, additives and applications. International Journal of Chemical and Biochemical Sciences. 2012;**1**:36-45. DOI: 10.13140/2.1.1623.5208

[8] Kobylewski S, Jacobson MF. Food Dyes, A Rainbow of Risks. Washington: Centre for Science in the Public Interest; 2010. Available from: https://cspinet. org/resource/food-dyes-rainbow-risks

[9] Uchman W. Substancje dodatkowe w przetwórstwie mięsa [Additives in Meat Processing]. Poznań: Wydawnictwo Uniwersytetu Przyrodniczego w Poznaniu; 2008 (in Polish)

[10] McCam D, Barrett A, Cooper A, Crumpler D, Dalen L, Grinshaw K, et al. Food additives and hyperactive behavior in 3-years-old and 8/9-years-old children in the community, a randomized, double-blind, placebo-controlled trial. The Lancet. 2007;**370**:1560-1567. DOI: 10.1016/S0140-6736(07)61306-3

[11] Belitz H. Food Chemistry. Berlin: Springer Berlin Heidelbeg; 2009. DOI: 10.1007/978-3-540-69934-7

[12] Wüstenberg T. General overview of food hydrocolloids in cellulose and cellulose derivatives in the food industry. Fundamentals and Applications. 2014;**16**:986-994. DOI: 10.1002/9783527682935.ch01

[13] Report of European Food Safety Authority. Scientific opinion on the safety and efficacy of citric acid when used as a technological additive (acidity regulator). EFSA Journal. 2015;**13**(2):4010. Available from: www. efsa.europa.eu/efsajourna

[14] Tripathy S, Das MK. Guar gum: Present status and applications. Journal of Pharmaceutical and Scientific Innovation. 2013;7(2):24-28. DOI: 10.7897/2277-4572.02447

[15] Sengar GI, Sharma HK. Food caramels: A review. Journal on Food Science and Technology. 2014;**51**(9): 1686-1696. DOI: 10.1007/ s13197-012-0633-z

[16] Husarova V, Ostatnikowa D. Monosodium glutamate toxic effects and their implications for human intake. JMED Research. 2013:**2013**:1-12. DOI: 10.5171/2013.608765

[17] Ratusz K, Maszewska M. Ocena występowania konserwantów w żywności na rynku warszawskim [The Assessment of Preservative Occurrence in Food in Warsaw]. Bromatologia i Chemia Toksykologiczna. 2013;**3**(45):917-922 (in Polish). Available from: https://docplayer.pl/13226410- Ocena-wystepowania-konserwantow-w-zywnosci-na-rynku-warszawskim. html

[18] Chronakis J. On the molecular characteristics, compositional properties and structural—Functional mechanism of maltodextrins. Critical Review in Food Science and Nutrition. 2010;**38**(7):599-637. Available from: http://www.tandfonline.com/page/terms-and-conditions

[19] Jacobson MF. Carcinogenicity and regulation of caramel colorings. International Journal of Occupational and Environmental Health. 2011;**18**(3):254-259. DOI:10.1179/1077352512Z.00000000034

[20] Gahalawat S, Singh M, Farswan A. Chinese restaurant syndrome by MSG: A Myth or Reality. Guru Dron. Journal of Pharmacy Research. 2014;**2**(2):38-41. Available from: http://www.sbspgi.edu.in/downloads/SSR_NAAC.pdf

[21] Zielińska A, Nowak I. Tokoferole i tokotrienole jako witamina E [Tocopherols and tocotrienols as vitamin E]. Chemik. 2014;**7**(68):585-591 (in Polish)

[22] Rudawska E, Perenc J. Tendencje zachowań konsumenckich na regionalnym rynku [Consumer behaviour trends on the regional market]. Szczecin: Wydawnictwo Naukowe Uniwersytetu Szczecińskiego; 2010 (in Polish). ISSN 1640-6818

5

Health Status and Permanent Loss to Follow up of Ellisras Longitudinal Study Subjects: Rural South African Context

Monyeki K. Daniel, Siweya H. James, Kemper C.G. Han and Ramoshaba N. Elfas

Abstract

Noncommunicable diseases (NCDs) are responsible for two out of three deaths worldwide with their profile changing from one country to another. But evidence to sustained these changes are still very limited in rural South African population. The well-characterized Ellisras Longitudinal Study (ELS) provides a unique opportunity of mapping some of these changes in vulnerable adolescent and young adults. The objective is we determined the extent of NCD risk factors derived from anthropometric and blood pressure measurements affected Ellisras Longitudinal Study (ELS) subjects over time for those who died or permanently lost to follow-up. A total of 2238 subjects aged 3–10 years (born between 1994 and 1986) were randomly selected to take part of the Ellisras Longitudinal Study (ELS) in November 1996. The attrition rate of ELS subjects based on death ranges between 0.71 and 3.73% for boys and 0.75 and 4.89% for girls. The prevalence of sever undernutrition ranges from 3.2 to 53%, moderate undernutrition ranges from 9.7 to 28.8%, while mild undernutrition ranges from 17.9 to 59.1% for both males and females. The prevalence of undernutrition was high while hypertension, obesity, and overweight were low in the population. The identification of appropriate NCD indicators for mortality in rural South African population needs more consideration and evaluation.

Keywords: mortality, epidemiology, nutritional status, cause of death, lifestyle

Introduction

Noncommunicable diseases (NCDs) are a group of diseases that share similar risk factors resulting from long exposure to unhealthy diets, smoking, lack of exercise, and possibly stress [1]. Major risk factors are high blood pressure (BP), tobacco addictions, poor lipids profile, and diabetes. These result in high mortality rates due to stroke, heart attacks and nutrition-induced cancers, chronic bronchitis, and many others [1, 2].

NCDs are responsible for two out of three deaths worldwide with their profile changing from one country to the other [3]. Africa is expected to experience the largest increase in NCD-related mortality globally with about 46% of all mortality expected to be attributed to NCDs by 2030 [3, 4]. Exposure to the known risk factors account for about two-thirds of premature NCD deaths with an estimated half of NCD deaths attributed to weak health systems and poverty in sub-Saharan Africa [5]. However, the rising NCD burden will add great pressure to the overstretched health systems and pose a major challenge to the development in Africa given the fragmented literature information and the indigenous knowledge system deep rooted in rural areas of South Africa [6, 7]. While low-cost solutions and high-impact essential NCD interventions delivered through primary healthcare approach have been shown to have impacts on population level, the existing literature shows that the changing profile of NCDs has been inadequate and fragmented [8]. A well-formulated cohort study in Africa could answer major questions relating to the changing magnitude of NCD risk factor profiles in Africa. Furthermore, NCDs are no longer just an issue for older people, there were in fact 16 million deaths from NCDs in people under the age of 17 years in 2005 of which the World Heart Federation has plan to reduce these deaths by 25% in 2025 [9].

Documenting the profiles of NCDs over time will not only assist the policy makers to get to the bottom of the problem but the population will also be aware of their health status as they grow older. The South African National Development Plan vision of reducing NCDs mortality by 28% in 2030 requires a cohort study that focuses on NCDs from younger ages to older ages. The Ellisras Longitudinal Study and the Birth to Twenty Study are among other cohort studies in South Africa which are geared to achieving this goal [10, 11]. The concepts of relying on indigenous knowledge system to combat NCDs among rural South African population will be replaced by well-researched concepts of NCD profiles from young age to adulthood [7].

In South Africa, NCD such as cardiovascular disease (CVD) is the second leading cause of death after HIV accounting for up to 43% of deaths among adults [12]. The Ellisras Longitudinal Study (ELS) from rural areas of Ellisras in South Africa clearly reported that NCD profiles are changing rapidly over time from childhood to young adults.

The attrition rate for the ELS ranges from 2.4 to 70.3% (Table 1) due to migration to urban areas, illness, pregnancy, and death. However, the attrition rate of ELS subjects based on death ranges between 0.71 and 3.73% for boys and 0.75 and 4.89% for girls. Therefore, the aim of the study was to determine the extent of NCD risk factors derived from anthropometric and blood pressure measurements which affected ELS subjects over time who died or permanently lost to follow-up.

Methods

Geographical area

Ellisras is a deep rural area situated within the north-western area of the Limpopo province, South Africa. The population is about 50,000 residing in 42 settlements [13]. These villages are approximately 70 km from the Ellisras town (23°40S 27°44 W), now known as Lephalale, adjacent to Botswana border. The Iscor coal mine, Matimba and Medupi electricity power stations are the major sources of employment for many of the Ellisras residents, whereas the remaining workforce is involved in subsistence farming and cattle rearing, while the minority is in education and civil services [14, 15].

Table 1. *Number and percentages (%) of longitudinal participants and dropouts over the years of measurements.*

Period of measurements	Males		Females		Total	
	N	%	N	%	N	%
November 1996	1201		1054		2255	
May 1997	1106		969		2075	
Dropouts	95	7.9	55	5.2	150	6.7
November 1997	1146		1054		1890	
Dropouts	55	4.5	0	0	55	2.4
May 1998	999		891		1890	
Drop outs	202	16.8	133	12.6	335	14.9
November 1998	1007		894		1901	
Dropouts	194	16.2	130	12.3	324	14.4
May 1999	1033		941		1974	
Dropouts	168	14.0	83	7.9	251	11.1
November 1999	998		920		1918	
Dropouts	217	18.1	117	11.1	334	14.8
May 2000	1006		918		1924	
Dropouts	195	16.2	106	10.1	301	13.3
November 2000	936		877		1813	
Dropouts	265	22.1	147	14.0	412	18.3
May 2001	962		904		1866	
Dropouts	239	19.9	120	11.4	359	15.9
November 2001	914		855		1769	
Dropouts	287	23.9	169	16.0	456	20.2
May 2002	890		823		1713	
Dropouts	311	25.9	201	19.1	512	22.7
May 2003	942		878		1820	
Dropouts	259	21.6	146	13.9	405	18.0
November 2003	911		828		1739	
Dropouts	328	27.3	196	18.6	524	23.2
November 2009	854		800		1654	
Dropouts	347	28.9	224	21.3	571	25.3
November/December 2013	520		541		1061	
Dropouts	681	56.7	483	45.8	1164	51.6
November/December 2015	356		372		728	
Dropouts	845	70.3	652	61.9	1497	66.4

Study design and sampling

This study is part of the ongoing Ellisras Longitudinal Study (ELS), for which the details of the sampling procedure were reported elsewhere [16]. For the purpose of the current study, only the subjects who died were included in the analysis. The cause of death for the majority of the subjects was unknown as it is a family secret given the indigenous knowledge system followed in the Ellisras rural population [6, 7]. A total of 373 boy and 613 girl subjects aged 8–26 years who were permanently lost to follow-up over time (November 1996–December 2015) (see Tables 2 and 3) were included in the analysis.

Anthropometry

All participants underwent a series of anthropometric measurements [weight, height, waist circumference, hip circumference, and skinfold thickness (triceps, subscapular, biceps, and supraspinale)] were taken according to the standard procedures recommended by the International Society of the Advancement of Kinanthropometry (ISAK) from November 1996 to December 2015 [17, 18]. The weight was measured on an electronic scale to the nearest 0.1 kg. Martin anthropometric measurement was used to measure height to the nearest 0.1 cm, and waist circumference measurements were taken to the nearest 0.1 cm, using a soft measuring tape. Skinfold measurements were taken using a slime guide caliber to the nearest 10 mm.

Blood pressure

Using an electronic Micronta monitoring kit, at least three blood pressure (BP) readings of systolic blood pressure (SBP) and diastolic blood pressure (DBP) were taken after the child had been seated for 5 min or longer [19]. The bladder of the device contains an electronic infrasonic transducer that monitors the BP and pulse rate, displaying these concurrently on the screen. This versatile instrument has been designed for research and clinical purposes [19]. In a pilot study, conducted before the survey, a high correlation of 0.93 was found between the readings taken with the automated device and those with a conventional mercury sphygmomanometer. Hypertension, defined as the average of three separate BP readings where the SBP or DBP is ≥95th percentile for age and sex, was determined [20].

Statistical analysis

Descriptive statistics for absolute body size were presented. Body mass index (BMI) was defined as weight (kg)/height x height $(m)^2$. All children (under 18 years) were classified as underweight, normal, overweight, and obese according to Cole et al. [21, 22] cutoff points and the WHO [3] for adults using BMI. Waist-to-height ratio (WHtR) cutoff point of 0.5 was used [23, 24] while cutoff point for the waist circumference [25], waist-to-hip ratio (WHR) was derived from the WHO [3]. Over fatness was defined as the 95% percentile by age and gender for the sum of four skinfolds thickness [26]. The correlation coefficient moment was used to assess the association between NCDs risk factors fat (i.e., sum of four skinfolds, BMI, WC, WHR, WHtR, BP, and pulse rate) at the first measurement and at all repeated measurements by gender. Statistical significance was set at $p < 0.05$. All the statistical analyses were done using the Statistical Package for the Social Sciences (SPSS).

Results

Tables 2 and 3 present the development over time of cardiovascular risk factors derived from anthropometric measurements and blood pressure measurements of Ellisras rural males and

Table 2. *Development over time of absolute body size and blood pressure of Ellisras rural males who dropped out of the study presently due to death aged 7–26 years.*

	November 1996	May 1997	November 1997	May 1998	November 1998	May 1999	November 1999	May 2000	November 2000	May 2001	November 2001	May 2002	May 2003	November 2003	November 2015
N	16	17	42	31	31	33	34	35	28	28	22	23	28	25	8
Age	8.0 (1.29)	8.6 (1.36)	9.2 (1.68)	9.9 (1.59)	10.4 (1.60)	10.6 (1.76)	11.2 (1.74)	11.5 (1.75)	11.8 (1.79)	12.5 (1.73)	13.0 (1.95)	13.5 (1.79)	14.5 (1.76)	14.8 (1.79)	25.9 (2.10)
Ht	125.4 (9.11)	129.6 (8.26)	130.4 (10.48)	132.7 (9.12)	135.0 (8.84)	136.0 (9.61)	138.9 (9.34)	141.9 (10.66)	141.8 (10.14)	145.2 (10.37)	147.1 (10.70)	150.0 (10.79)	153.7 (10.41)	157.8 (10.81)	173.4 (8.54)
Wt	20.5 (3.33)	22.7 (3.51)	23.7 (4.36)	25.8 (4.12)	26.7 (4.52)	27.6 (4.65)	28.4 (5.16)	30.1 (7.18)	30.6 (6.02)	32.4 (8.09)	33.1 (7.01)	35.2 (8.21)	38.0 (9.01)	40.8 (9.75)	71.3 (21.47)
Waist	52.0 (5.43)	54.7 (4.04)	53.4 (4.12)	54.4 (3.96)	55.6 (3.93)	55.9 (4.00)	56.7 (3.35)	57.9 (4.13)	57.5 (4.11)	58.3 (5.27)	58.8 (4.35)	60.1 (5.59)	59.2 (4.39)	60.1 (5.46)	81.5 (21.24)
Hip	56.4 (6.25)	59.2 (5.66)	60.6 (5.22)	61.3 (4.00)	63.4 (4.74)	63.3 (5.19)	64.8 (5.32)	65.4 (6.27)	65.7 (5.95)	66.3 (8.12)	66.2 (5.84)	69.7 (7.69)	69.8 (7.54)	69.6 (7.56)	96.7 (17.11)
BMI	13.1 (1.96)	13.6 (1.63)	13.9 (1.33)	14.6 (1.39)	14.5 (1.27)	14.8 (1.31)	14.6 (1.47)	14.8 (1.92)	15.1 (1.34)	15.1 (2.16)	15.1 (1.60)	15.5 (2.17)	15.8 (2.08)	16.4 (2.27)	24.0 (8.63)
WHtR	0.42 (0.04)	0.42 (0.02)	0.41 (0.03)	0.41 (0.02)	0.41 (0.02)	0.41 (0.02)	0.41 (0.02)	0.41 (0.03)	0.41 (0.02)	0.40 (0.45)	0.40 (0.02)	0.40 (0.03)	0.39 (0.09)	0.38 (0.03)	0.47 (0.13)
WHR	0.92 (0.05)	0.93 (0.08)	0.88 (0.41)	0.90 (0.04)	0.88 (0.05)	0.88 (0.03)	0.88 (0.04)	0.89 (0.05)	0.88 (0.05)	0.89 (0.06)	0.86 (0.05)	0.87 (0.05)	0.85 (0.06)	0.87 (0.05)	0.83 (0.07)
S4sk	19.3 (1.84)	18.9 (2.65)	20.1 (4.35)	21.0 (4.98)	21.7 (3.5)	21.5 (3.18)	19.7 (4.16)	20.6 (4.12)	20.8 (3.32)	24.8 (9.94)	24.2 (10.71)	22.1 (12.75)	22.5 (6.48)	27.6 (12.5)	29.4 (18.72)
SBP (mmHg)	–	–	–	–	–	97.1 (9.26)	99.2 (9.67)	101.9 (12.60)	101.9 (7.97)	93.1 (8.42)	90.9 (8.10)	102.2 (13.0)	105.4 (9.03)	101.6 (12.56)	134.6 (20.88)
DBP (mmHg)	–	–	–	–	–	60.3 (7.51)	61.1 (7.89)	65.60 (9.94)	67.0 (10.12)	62.8 (6.80)	61.0 (7.60)	60.0 (10.27)	67.9 (7.67)	59.9 (9.89)	76.0 (19.6)
Heart rate (beat/min)	–	–	–	–	–	69.9 (12.57)	76.1 (13.60)	80.37 (15.52)	75.61 (11.66)	74.9 (11.2)	74.6 (7.92)	74.0 (10.57)	79.1 (12.95)	75.5 (11.59)	78.8 (18.74)

Ht—height in cm; Wt—weight in kg; BMI—body mass index in kg/m^2; WHtR—waist-to-height ratio; WHR—waist-to-hip ratio; S4sk—sum of four (triceps, subscapular, biceps, and supraspinale) skinfold in mm.

Table 3. *Development over time of absolute body size and blood pressure factors of Ellisras rural females who dropped out of the study presently due to death aged 7–26 years.*

	November 1996	May 1997	November 1997	May 1998	November 1998	May 1999	November 1999	May 2000	November 2000	May 2001	November 2001	May 2002	May 2003	November 2003	November 2015
N	31	28	54	51	51	52	52	47	46	46	47	45	44	45	8
Age	7.6 (1.51)	8.1 (1.53)	8.8 (1.74)	9.3 (1.65)	9.8 (1.65)	10.5 (1.45)	10.9 (1.51)	11.3 (1.54)	11.8 (1.53)	12.3 (1.56)	12.95 (1.43)	13.3 (1.56)	14.20 (1.52)	14.8 (1.54)	26.2 (2.01)
Ht	121.3 (8.40)	123.6 (7.95)	127.6 (10.54)	129.6 (8.62)	132.0 (8.57)	135.9 (8.32)	138.7 (8.82)	142.3 (9.22)	145.2 (8.96)	147.1 (9.46)	150.0 (9.15)	152.6 (8.39)	155.5 (7.94)	158.4 (7.0)	163.0 (8.86)
Wt	19.0 (3.67)	19.8 (2.80)	22.3 (4.69)	23.4 (3.89)	24.7 (4.14)	26.4 (4.25)	27.6 (4.93)	29.6 (5.87)	31.5 (5.83)	33.7 (6.79)	35.7 (7.18)	38.2 (7.62)	40.4 (7.71)	44.1 (7.22)	61.1 (9.25)
Waist	51.0 (4.08)	50.3 (2.74)	51.3 (3.20)	52.3 (3.86)	53.8 (3.56)	55.5 (3.32)	56.0 (3.79)	55.8 (4.57)	56.4 (3.90)	57.8 (4.47)	58.1 (4.09)	60.2 (4.81)	60.1 (5.10)	60.3 (4.90)	79.4 (10.4)
Hip	55.8 (4.59)	58.3 (3.44)	60.4 (5.00)	60.7 (4.04)	63.3 (4.41)	63.1 (8.40)	66.7 (5.20)	68.1 (6.1)	69.5 (6.40)	67.5 (6.22)	71.9 (6.63)	77.0 (8.43)	75.8 (7.73)	77.4 (8.35)	100.4 (6.96)
BMI	12.8 (1.98)	13.0 (1.26)	13.7 (2.09)	13.9 (1.27)	14.1 (1.39)	14.2 (1.38)	14.4 (1.55)	14.5 (1.92)	14.8 (1.56)	15.43 (1.89)	15.75 (2.09)	16.28 (2.29)	16.57 (2.06)	17.53 (2.46)	23.11 (3.75)
WHtR	0.42 (0.04)	0.41 (0.03)	0.40 (0.04)	0.40 (0.03)	0.41 (0.03)	0.41 (0.02)	0.40 (0.02)	0.40 (0.03)	0.4 (0.02)	0.40 (0.04)	0.39 (0.03)	0.39 (0.03)	0.39 (0.03)	0.38 (0.03)	0.49 (0.07)
WHR	0.92 (0.06)	0.86 (0.05)	0.85 (0.05)	0.86 (0.05)	0.85 (0.05)	0.9 (0.43)	0.8 (0.05)	0.8 (0.04)	0.8 (0.04)	0.86 (0.07)	0.81 (0.05)	0.79 (0.58)	0.80 (0.06)	0.78 (0.06)	0.79 (0.06)
S4sk	20.02 (3.16)	19.4 (2.44)	22.1 (5.07)	23.9 (4.88)	24.5 (4.78)	24.1 (4.34)	25.0 (6.40)	26.7 (7.73)	28.5 (7.14)	26.5 (12.23)	27.63 (13.88)	31.92 (8.99)	30.56 (12.90)	34.71 (10.84)	33.8 (10.52)
SBP (mmHg)						99.4 (11.62)	100.4 (10.79)	104.3 (10.67)	103.3 (12.48)	99.1 (7.11)	97.6 (8.63)	104.9 (12.41)	109.5 (9.39)	105.1 (12.3)	106.1 (8.75)
Diastolic BP (mmHg)						61.2 (8.28)	61.9 (9.05)	67.6 (8.74)	67.4 (9.54)	64.8 (6.46)	63.8 (7.10)	61.9 (8.08)	68.7 (6.84)	62.0 (8.05)	70.8 (14.74)
Pulse (beats/min)						79.1 (10.73)	75.3 (13.54)	77.4 (16.00)	82.9 (14.24)	77.8 (11.37)	79.1 (11.16)	84.3 (15.68)	82.8 (12.53)	83.9 (15.52)	92.1 (12.33)

Ht—height in cm; Wt—weight in kg; BMI—body mass index in kg/m^2; WHtR—waist-to-height ratio; WHR—waist-to-hip ratio; S4sk—sum of four (triceps, subscapular, biceps, and supraspinale) skinfold in mm.

females mean aged 7–26 years who died. There was a gradual increase in mean height (125.4 cm SD 9.11), weight (20.5 kg SD 3.33) for males from November 1996 to November 2015 (height = 173.4 cm SD 8.54, weight = 71.3 kg SD 21.47) (Table 2). Females showed a gradual growth increase in mean height (121.3 cm SD 8.40) and mean weight (19.0 kg SD 3.67) from November 1996 to November 2015 (mean height 163.0 = cm SD 8.86) and mean weight 61.1 kg SD 9.25) (Table 3). Similar trend was observed for blood pressure (mean systolic blood pressure = 97.1 mmHg SD 9.26 and mean diastolic blood pressure = 60.3 mmHg SD 7.51) from May 1999 to November 2015 (mean systolic blood pressure = 134.6 SD 20.88 and mean distolic blood pressure = 78.8 mmHg SD 18.74) for males (Table 2). For girls, mean systolic blood pressure (99.4 mmHg SD 11.62) and diastolic blood pressure (61.2 mmHg SD 8.28) increased from November 1996 to November 2015 (mean systolic blood pressure = 106.1 mmHg SD 8.75 and diastolic blood pressure = 70.8 mmHg SD 14.74).

Table 4 shows the development of the prevalence of cardiovascular risk factors of Ellisras rural males and females aged 7–26 who died. The prevalence of sever undernutrition ranges from 3.2 to 53%, moderate undernutrition ranges from 9.7 to 28.8% while mild undernutrition ranges from 17.9 to 59.1% for both males and females. The prevalence of abdominal obesity ranges from 0 to 37.5%, while obesity, overweight, and over fatness was low (ranges from 0 to 12.5%) (Table 4). Table 5 presents moment correlation coefficient for the first measurement and subsequent measurements for the cardiovascular risk factors derived from anthropometric measurements for Ellisras rural males and females over time (November 1996 to November 2015). The correlation coefficient was low and insignificant for males and females for all cardiovascular risk factors over time. The correlation for blood pressure was significant (p ranges from 0.001 to 0.05) for systolic blood pressure (r^2 ranges from 0.42 to 0.95) and diastolic blood pressure (r^2 ranges from 0.28 to 0.77) over time.

Discussions

The current study aimed to determine the extent of NCD risk factors derived from anthropometric and blood pressure measurements which affected ELS subjects over time who died or permanently lost to follow-up. The prevalence of under- nutrition was high while obesity, overweight, abdominal obesity and hypertension was low. However, there was significant positive correlation between systolic and diastolic over time. The data presented the mortality rate owing to NCD in rural communities of Ellisras areas which differs to the urban area counterparts reported by Miranda et al. and Kengne et al. [27, 28]. In Amsterdam, Kemper et al. [29] reported a clear increase in prevalence of obesity from youth to adulthood with a decrease in physical activity. However, undernutrition and low physical activity was high in the Ellisras rural population [30, 31]. This might indicate that undernutrition as an indicator of NCD could be the cause of death or leads to permanent loss of follow-up of the ELS participants.

The burden of NCD in rural South African population is substantial, and patients with this condition make significant demands on the health-care resources. Epide- miological data from South Africa and Tanzania reveal high prevalence of diabetes and hypertension [32, 33]. The burden of NCD is likely to increase in the next coming decade in rural South African population. The projection from Global Burden of Diseases Study suggests that by the year 2020, the proportion of overall burden in Africa due to NCD will increase to 42% among adults aged 15–59 years [34].

Table 4. *Development over time of prevalence cardiovascular risk factors of Ellisras rural males and females who died aged 7–26 years.*

	November 1996	May 1997	November 1997	May 1998	November 1998	May 1999	November 1999	May 2000	November 2000	May 2001	November 2001	May 2002	May 2003	November 2003	November 2015
	% (n)	% (n)	% (n)	% (n)	% (n)	% (n)	% (n)	% (n)	% (n)	% (n)	% (n)	% (n)	% (n)	% (n)	% (n)
Males															
High SBP	–	–	–	–	–	3.0 (1)	2.9 (1)	8.6 (3)	3.6 (1)	–	–	8.7 (2)	–	8.0 (2)	62.5 (5)
High DBP	–	–	–	–	–	–	–	5.7 (2)	7.1 (2)	–	–	4.3 (1)	3.6 (1)	4.0 (1)	25.0 (2)
Hypertension	–	–	–	–	–	–	–	–	–	–	–	–	–	–	25 (2)-
BMI—undernutrition															
BMI—severe	37.5 (6)	17.6 (3)	11.9 (5)	3.2 (1)	3.2 (1)	6.1 (2)	11.8 (4)	5.7 (2)	3.6 (1)	17.9 (5)	9.1 (2)	21.7 (5)	10.7 (3)	20.0 (5)	
BMI—moderate	12.5 (2)	17.6 (3)	28.6 (12)	12.9 (4)	16.1 (5)	21.2 (7)	14.7 (5)	22.9 (8)	17.9 (5)	14.3 (4)	13.6 (3)	8.7 (2)	25.0 (7)	12.0 (3)	
BMI—mild	25.0 (4)	35.3 (6)	31.0 (13)	38.7 (12)	41.9 (13)	24.2 (8)	35.3 (12)	40.0 (14)	39.3 (11)	32.1 (9)	59.1 (13)	34.8 (8)	32.1 (9)	24.0 (6)	
BMI—overweight	–	–	–	3.2 (1)	–	–	–	–	–	–	–	–	–	–	12.5 (1)
BMI—obese	–	–	–	–	–	–	–	–	–	–	–	–	–	–	12.5 (1)
WHtR abdominal	25 (4)	17.6 (3)	9.5 (4)	9.7 (3)	6.5 (2)	6.1 (2)	2.9 (1)	8.6 (3)	3.6 (1)	21.4 (6)	–	8.7 (2)	–	4.0 (1)	25.0 (2)
WHP obese	75.0 (12)	70.6 (12)	38.1 (16)	48.4 (15)	41.9 (13)	30.3 (10)	32.4 (11)	42.9 (15)	32.1 (9)	42.9 (12)	27.3 (6)	30.4 (7)	25.0 (7)	28.0 (7)	12.5 (1)
Over fatness	–	–	7.1 (3)	9.7 (3)	6.5 (2)	9.1 (3)	2.9 (1)	2.9 (1)	3.6 (1)	7.1 (2)	9.1 (2)	8.7 (2)	3.6 (1)	8.0 (2)	12.5 (1)
Females															
High SBP	–	–	–	–	–	5.8 (3)	7.7 (4)	4.3 (2)	6.5 (3)	–	–	4.4 (2)	4.5 (2)	4.4 (2)	–
High DBP	–	–	–	–	–	3.8 (2)	7.7 (4)	8.5 (4)	13.0 (6)	4.3 (2)	2.1 (1)	–	2.3 (1)	–	12.5 (1)
Hypertension	–	–	–	–	–	–	3.8 (2)	–	4.3 (2)	–	–	–	–	–	–

	November 1996	May 1997	November 1997	May 1998	November 1998	May 1999	November 1999	May 2000	November 2000	May 2001	November 2001	May 2002	May 2003	November 2003	November 2015
	% (n)	% (n)	% (n)	% (n)	% (n)	% (n)	% (n)	% (n)	% (n)	% (n)	% (n)	% (n)	% (n)	% (n)	% (n)
BMI—undernutrition															
BMI—severe	48.4 (15)	53.6 (15)	27.8 (15)	21.6 (11)	19.6 (10)	17.3 (9)	17.3 (9)	25.5 (12)	8.7 (4)	6.5 (3)	4.3 (2)	2.2 (1)	4.5 (2)	2.2 (1)	12.5 (1)
BMI—moderate	9.7 (3)	10.7 (3)	14.8 (8)	15.7 (8)	13.7 (7)	28.8 (15)	25.0 (13)	12.8 (6)	21.7 (10)	15.2 (7)	19.1 (9)	13.3 (6)	4.5 (2)	15.6 (7)	–
BMI—mild	19.4 (6)	17.9 (5)	37.0 (20)	39.2 (20)	39.2 (20)	28.8 (15)	32.7 (17)	40.4 (19)	39.1 (18)	37.0 (17)	46.8 (22)	37.8 (17)	47.7 (21)	28.9 (13)	–
BMI—overweight	–	–	–	–	–	–	–	–	–	–	–	–	–	–	25.0 (2)
BMI obese	–	–	1.9 (1)	–	–	–	–	2.1 (1)	–	–	–	–	–	2.2 (1)	–
WHtR abdominal	19.4 (6)	7.1 (2)	7.4 (4)	5.9 (3)	7.8 (4)	5.8 (3)	5.8 (3)	6.4 (3)	2.2 (1)	10.9 (5)	4.3 (2)	4.4 (2)	4.5 (2)	4.4 (2)	37.5 (3)
WHP obese	87.1 (27)	67.9 (19)	64.8 (35)	64.7 (33)	54.9 (28)	73.1 (38)	44.2 (23)	34.0 (16)	32.6 (15)	50.0 (23)	17.0 (8)	11.1 (5)	25.0 (11)	6.7 (3)	12.5 (1)
Overfatness	3.2 (1)	–	3.7 (2)	5.9 (3)	5.9 (3)	–	3.8 (2)	4.3 (2)	4.3 (2)	8.7 (4)	8.5 (4)	6.7 (3)	4.5 (2)	–	12.5 (1)

BMI—body mass index; SBP—systolic blood pressure; DBP—diastolic blood pressure; WHtR—waist-to-height ratio.

Table 5. *Moment correlation coefficient for the first measurement and subsequent measurements for cardiovascular risk factors measured over time among diseases Ellisras Longitudinal Study children.*

	May 1997	November 1997	May 1998	November 1998	May 1999	November 1999	May 2000	November 2000	May 2001	November 2001	May 2002	May 2003	November 2003	November 2015
Waist	0.201	0.316	0.342	0.475	0.613*	0.651*	0.626*	00.775**	−0.031	0.416	0.128	0.542	0.128	−0.180
WHP	−0.103	−0.169	−0.505	0.001	0.085	−0.069	0.185	−0.121	−0.391	−0.195	−0.052	0.291	−0.052	0.877
WHtR	0.118	0.198	0.109	0.313	0.453	0.530	0.599*	0.512	0.176	0.226	0.034	0.315	−0.073	0.676
BMI	0.454	0.411	0.409	0.364	0.271	0.273	0.062	0.194	0.235	0.492	0.521	0.094	0.603	0.785
Sum4sk	−0.076	−0.074	−0.126	−0.289	−0.122	−0.003	−0.349	−0.226	−0.077	−0.139	−0.418	−0.513	−0.417	−0.150
Systolic	–	–	–	–	–	0.21	−0.12	−0.29	−0.00	−0.52	−0.48	0.88	0.45**	−0.30
Diastolic	–	–	–	–	–	−0.22	−0.12	0.37	0.52	0.53	−0.05	0.94	0.05	0.38
Pulse	–	–	–	–	–	0.23	−0.07	0.18	0.26	0.12	−0.19	0.13	−0.19	0.65
Girls														
Waist	−0.071	0.129	−0.228	−0.097	0.131	−0.015	0.280	0.043	−0.188	0.061	−0.136	−0.057	−0.136	0.123
WHR	−0.115	0.088	−0.162	0.030	−0.177	−0.024	0.041	−0.133	−0.181	0.100	−0.191	−0.041	−0.191	−0.468
WHtR	0.373	0.449*	0.142	0.230	0.455*	0.221	0.394*	0.344	0.333	0.210	0.076	0.103	−0.035	0.179
BMI	0.192	0.239	−0.047	0.071	0.021	−0.053	−0.127	−0.010	−0.074	−0.112	−0.112	−0.216	−0.021	0.488
Sum4sk	−0.079	−0.042	−0.030	−0.022	−0.003	−0.129	−0.017	−0.169	−0.182	−0.141	−0.208	−0.202	−00.445*	−00.969**
Systolic	–	–	–	–	–	0.26	−0.10	0.95**	0.14	0.25	00.43**	0.67**	0.42**	0.02
Diastolic	–	–	–	–	–	0.63**	0.28*	0.77**	0.07	0.12	0.012	0.72**	0.08	0.66**
Pulse	–	–	–	–	–	−0.08	0.01	−0.11	−0.12	−0.08	−0.36	−0.20	0.35	0.64**

WHR—waist-to-hip ratio; WHtR—waist-to-height ratio; BMI—body mass index. $^{*}P < 0.05$; $^{**}P < 0.01$

By not taking action on NCDs in sub-Saharan Africa would mean that the development of effective measure for preventing and managing these NCDs will be compromised. Ideal health promotion should reach an individual at school-going age to ensure the adoption of a healthy lifestyle. Community involvement must empower people to promote and adopt a healthy lifestyle throughout their lives and identify and reach appropriate target groups. South Africa's school health curriculum needs to be developed. A health curriculum planning group representing stakeholders of various disciplines, particularly in rural area, needs to revise current curricula to address health promotion issues in all public schools in the rural areas. Education methods used in this curriculum should allow children to make healthy choice while simultaneously increasing their self-esteem. The curriculum should address smoking prevention, abstinence from alcohol usage, establishing healthy eating pattern, and exercise habits that could be sustainable for life time. The community should develop discernment skills to evaluate the impact of the advertising industry on their lives.

Despite the clear pattern of NCD risk that has emerged from the current study, there are some short comings that need to be considered when assessing the overall value of the present data. The small number of subjects could probably provide a biased sample, and these data must be viewed in the light of this situation. The socioeconomic status of the subjects and the cause of death might impact negatively on the major findings of the present study. The early diagnosis and cost-effective management of patients with risk factors and early target organs damage particularly of those with high level of cardiovascular diseases risk is needed [35]. A comprehensive surveillance system should include indicators that monitor both the prevention and health service aspects of the program.

Conclusion

The prevalence of undernutrition was high, while hypertension, obesity, and overweight were low in the population. The blood pressure showed a significant correlation over time, while other NCD risk indicators do not show significant correlation over time. The identification of appropriate NCD indicators for mortality in rural South African population needs more consideration and evaluation. Death information and feasibility and cost of generating such indicators are critical issues as most rural South African population regard the cause of death as a family issue. Death registration information and cost of generating such information are critical issues in moving away from the indigenous knowledge system. More thorough analysis of the variable data will be essential to investigate the quality of the information, and additional information is needed to assess the validity of the indicators.

Author details

Monyeki K. Daniel[1*], Siweya H. James[2], Kemper C.G. Han[3] and Ramoshaba N. Elfas[1]

1 Department of Physiology and Environmental, University of Limpopo, Sovenga, South Africa

2 Faculty of Science and Agriculture, University of Limpopo, Sovenga, South Africa 3 Health and Activity, Amsterdam Public Health Academic Research Institute, Vrije Universiteit, Amsterdam, The Netherlands

*Address all correspondence to: kotsedi.monyeki@ul.ac.za

References

[1] Steyn K. Management of chronic diseases of lifestyle in South African population. Supplement to South African Medical Journal. 1994:49-50

[2] Kemper HCG. Amsterdam Growth and Health Longitudinal Study: A 23 Year Follow Up from Teenager to Adult About Lifestyle and Health. New York: Karger Press; 2004. pp. 1-20

[3] WHO. Non Communicable Diseases Country Profiles. Geneva: World Health Organization; 2014. p. 207

[4] Dalal S, Beunza JJ, Volmink J, Adebamowo C, Bajunirwe F, Njelekela M, et al. Non-communicable diseases in sub-Saharan Africa: What we know now. International Journal of Epidemiology. 2011;40(4):885-901

[5] Nyaaba GN, Stronks K, Aikins AD, Kengne AP, Agyemang C. Tracing Africa's progress towards implementing the non-communicable diseases global action plan 2013–2020: A synthesis of WHO country profile reports. BMC Public Health. 2017;17(1):297

[6] Monyeki KD, Kemper HCG. Longitudinal development and tracking of anthropometric risk indicators for under nutrition of Ellisras rural children in South Africa. In: Muhongo SM, Gudyanga FP, Enow AA, Nyanganyura D, editors. Science, Technology and Innovation for the Socio-Economic Development: Success Stories from Africa. Pretoria: International Council for Science Regional Office for Africa; 2009. pp. 41-56

[7] Monyeki KD, Kemper HCG, Twisk JWR. Trends in obesity and hypertension in South African youth. In: O'Dea JA, Eriksen M, editors. Childhood Prevention—International Research, Controversies and Intervention. Sydney: Oxford University Press; 2010. pp. 152-163

[8] Yeates K, Lohfeld L, Sleeth J, Morales F, Rajkotia Y, Ogedegbe O. A global perspective on cardiovascular disease in vulnerable populations. The Canadian Journal of Cardiology. 2015;31(9): 1081-1093

[9] Yusuf SH, Hawken S, Ounpuu S, Dans T, Avezum A, Lanas F, et al. Effect of potential modifiable risk factors associated with myocardial infarction in 52 countries (the INTERHEART study): A case control study. Lancet. 2005;364: 937-952

[10] Steyn K, de Wet T, Richter L, Cameron N, Levitt NS, Morrell C. Cardiovascular diseases risk factors in 5- year old urban South African children— The birth to ten study. South African Medical Journal. 2000;90:719-726

[11] Monyeki KD, van Lenthe F, Styen NP. Obesity: Does it exist in Ellisras rural community children. International Journal of Epidemiology. 1999;28: 287-292

[12] Biying H, Sernsson P, Sundstrom J, Lind L. Effects of cigarette smoking on cardiovascular-related protein profiles in two community-based cohort studies. Atherosclerosis. 2016;254:52-58

[13] Sidiropoulos E, Jeffery A, Mackay S, Gallocher R, Forgey H, Chips C. South Africa Survey 1995/1996. Johannesburg: South African Institute of Race and Relations; 1996. pp. 234-360

[14] Bradshaw D, Stey K. Poverty and Chronic Disease in South Africa: Technical Report. Cape Town: Medical Research Council; 2001. pp. 38-45

[15] Statistics South Africa. Cause of Death in South Africa 1997–2001: Advance Release of Records of Death, PO309.2.2002. Pretoria, South Africa; 2002

[16] Monyeki KD, Cameron N, Getz B. Growth and nutritional status of rural South African children 3–10 years old: The Ellisras growth study. American Journal of Human Biology. 2000;12(1): 42-49

[17] Norton K, Olds T. Anthropometrica. Sydney: University of New South Wales Press; 1996. pp. 120-267

[18] Tanner JM, Whitehouse RH, Takaishi M. Standards from birth to maturity for height weight, weight velocity: British children, 1965. Archives of Disease in Childhood. 1996;41: 613-635

[19] National High Blood Pressure Education Program Working Group on High Blood Pressure in Children and Adolescents. The fourth report on the diagnosis, evaluation, and treatment of high blood pressure in children and adolescents. Pediatrics. 2004;114: 555-576

[20] National High Blood Pressure Education Program (NHBPEP) Working Group on Hypertension Control in Children and Adolescents. Update on the 1987 task force report on high blood pressure in children and adolescents: A working group report from the National High Blood Pressure Education Program. Pediatrics. 1996;98: 649-658

[21] Cole TJ, Bellizzi MC, Flegal KM, Dietz WH. Establishing a standard definition for child overweight and obesity worldwide: International survey. BMJ. 2000;320:1240-1243

[22] Cole TJ, Flegal KM, Nicholls D, Jackson AA. Body mass index cut offs to define thinness in children and adolescents: International survey. BMJ. 2007;335:194

[23] Ashwell M, Hsieh SD. Six reasons why the waist-to-height ratio is a rapid and effective global indicator for health risks of obesity and how its use could simplify the international public health message on obesity. International Journal of Food Sciences and Nutrition. 2005;56(5):303-307

[24] Ashwell M, Gunn P, Gibson S. Waist-to-height ratio is a better screening tool than waist circumference and BMI for adult cardiometabolic risk factors: Systematic review and meta- analysis. Obesity Reviews. 2012;13: 275-286

[25] Ahmad N, Adam SIM, Nawi AM, Hassan MR, Ghazi HF. Abdominal obesity indicators: Waist circumference or waist-to-hip ratio in Malaysian adults population. International Journal of Preventive Medicine. 2016;7

[26] Twisk JWR, Kemper HCG, van Mechelen W, Post GB, van Lenthe FJ. Body fatness: Longitudinal relationship of body mass index and the sum of skinfolds with other risk factors for coronary heart disease. International Journal of Obesity and Related Metabolic Disorder. 1998;22:915-922

[27] Miranda JJ, Kinra S, Casas JP, Smith GD, Ebrahim S. Non-communicable diseases in low and middle-income countries: Context determinants and health policy. Tropical Medicine & International Health. 2009;13(10): 1225-1234

[28] Kengne AP, Amoah AGB, Mbanya J. Cardiovascular complications of diabetes mellitus in sub-Saharan Africa. Circulation. 2005;112:3592-3601

[29] Kemper HCG, Post GB, Twisk JWR, van Mechelen W. Lifestyle and obesity in adolescent and young adulthood: Results from Amsterdam growth and health longitudinal study. International Journal of Obesity. 1999;22(3):S34-S40

[30] Monyeki KD, Kemper HC. The risk factors for elevated blood pressure and how to address cardiovascular risk factors: A review in paediatric populations. Journal of Human Hypertension. 2008;22:450-459

[31] Matshipi M, Monyeki KD, Kemper H. The relationship between physical activity and plasma glucose level amongst Ellisras rural young adult males and females: Ellisras longitudinal study. International Journal of Environmental Research and Public Health. 2017;14: 198. DOI: 10.3390/ijerph14020198

[32] Unwin N, Setel P, Rashid S, Mugusi F, Mbanya J, Katange H, et al. Non communicable diseases in Sub-Saharan Africa: Where do they feature in the health research agenda? Bulletin of the World Health Organization. 2001;79: 947-953

[33] Sekgala MD, Monyeki KD, Mogale MA, Ramoshaba NE. Performance of blood pressure to height ratio as a screening tool for elevated blood pressure in rural children: Ellisras Longitudinal Study. Journal of Human Hypertension. 2017;31:591

[34] Murray C, Lopez S, editors. The Global Burden of Diseases. Boston, MA: Harvard University Press on behalf of WHO and the World Bank; 1996

[35] Steyn K, Bradshaw D. Non- communicable diseases surveillance in developing countries. Scandinavian Journal of Public Health. 2001;29: 161-165

6

Electrochemical Sensors for Food Safety

Lingwen Zeng, Lei Peng, Dazhi Wu and Baoguo Yang

Abstract

Food safety poses an increasing threat to human health worldwide. The development of analytical methods and techniques to ensure food safety is therefore of great importance. Electrochemical sensors provide unique opportunity to realize sensitive, accurate, rapid, and portable detection for food safety. They have the potential to overcome the restrictions and limitations of traditional methods. In this chapter, we review the progress of electrochemical sensors for the detection of food contaminants including heavy metals, illegal additives, pesticide residues, veterinary drug residues, biological toxins, and foodborne pathogen. Future perspectives and challenges are also discussed.

Keywords: electrochemical sensors, cyclic voltammetry, linear sweep voltammetry, differential pulse voltammetry, square wave voltammetry, food safety, detection

Introduction

Food safety has become a global public health concern affecting both mostly developing countries and developed countries. In addition, foodborne diseases negatively impact the economy, trade, and industries of affected countries. For example, melamine has been detected in infant formula (milk powder) in China, leading to more than 290,000 infants suffering from severe health problems such as urinary tract stones [1]. Early and accurate detection of food safety is therefore very important for preventing, controlling, and mitigating the impact of potential outbreaks. Many analytic methods, including chromatography methods such as gas chromatography (GC) [2], high performance liquid chromatography (HPLC) [3], gas chromatography-mass spectrometer (GC-MS) [4], and liquid chromatography-mass spectrometer (LC-MS) [5], and immunological detection, such as enzyme linked immunosorbent assay (ELISA) [6] and lateral flow immunoassay [7], have been employed for food safety detection. Although those traditional methods are relatively sensitive and specific, they are expensive, laborious, and time-consuming and require well-trained personnel [8, 9], which make them incompatible for developing countries and areas are lacking equipped facilities and specialists. It is therefore urgent to develop rapid, accurate, sensitive, and online technologies for food safety detection.

Modern electrochemistry provides powerful analytical techniques for sensors, with the advantages of instrumental simplicity, low cost, and miniaturization, work on-site, and the ability to measure pollutants in complex matrices with minimal sample preparation [10]. Electrochemical sensors and methods are developed as suitable tools for different applications, including bioprocess control, agriculture, and military, and, in particular, for food quality control. Voltammetric techniques, such as cyclic voltammetry (CV) [10], linear sweep voltammetry (LSV) [11], differential pulse voltammetry (DPV) [12], and square wave voltammetry (SWV) [13], have been widely used in food analysis. Among these voltammetric techniques, DPV and SWV are commonly used, as low detection limits and multiplex analysis can be achieved with the two methods. These two techniques involve potential waveforms and their respective current response are shown in **Figure 1A**. The waveform of DPV consists of pulses of constant amplitude superimposed on a staircase waveform. This method has the highest sensitivity in electrochemistry because the charging current can be ignored against faradaic current, and their ratio is obtained as large. Moreover, SWV consists of symmetrical square-wave pulses superimposed on a staircase waveform.

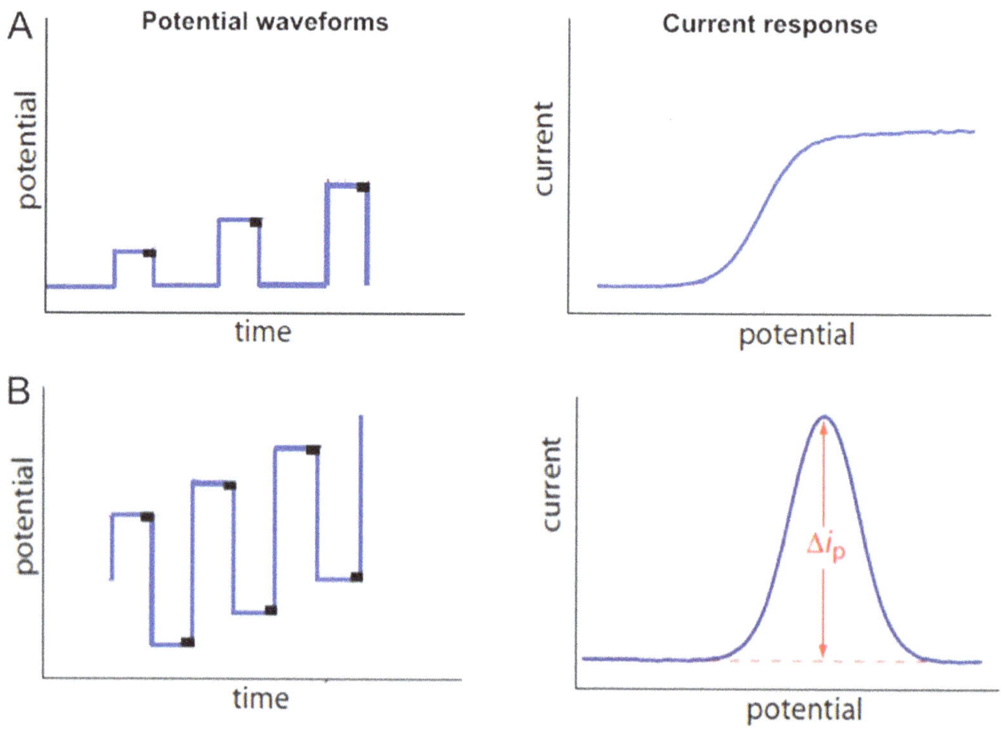

Figure 1. *Potential waveforms and their respective current response for (A) differential pulse voltammetry (DPV) and (B) square wave voltammetry (SWV).*

During each square wave cycle, the current is sampled twice, just before the end of each forward and each backward pulse followed by subtraction of the currents. The peak current heights (values) obtained by the two methods are directly proportional to the concentrations of the analyte. Amperometry is another important electrochemical analysis method in which the potential of the working electrode is constant and the resulting current from faradic processes occurring at the electrode is monitored with a function of time. In this method, the current is integrated over relatively longer time intervals, so it gives an improved signal to noise ratio [14].

Electrochemical sensors can be used as food safety monitoring tools in the assessment of biological/ecological quality or for the chemical monitoring of both inorganic and organic pollutants. In this chapter we provide an overview of electrochemical sensor systems for food safety applications, and in the following sections, we describe the various electrochemical sensors that have been developed for food safety detection.

Heavy metals

Heavy metals (HMs) are currently defined as metals with a specific gravity greater than 5 g cm^{-3}, which are considered as a serious source for polluting the biosphere throughout the world and causing many healthy and physiological diseases due to their prolonged half-life, non-biodegradability, and potential of accumulation in different parts of the human body [15, 16]. Heavy metals like cadmium, lead, arsenic, chromium, and mercury are considered as hazardous elements even at low concentrations [17–19]. Therefore, sensitive and selective determination of toxic heavy metals with cost-effective and convenient procedures is of paramount importance.

Due to the speed of detection, low cost, high sensitivity, and easy adaptability for in situ measurement [20], electrochemical sensors have attracted great interest in the detection of heavy metal ions for food safety.

For many years, anodic stripping voltammetry (ASV) at the mercury and its modified electrode was extensively applied to the determination of trace metal ions for the extensive cathodic potential range [21, 22]. However, the disposal of the mercury-containing device and the incorrect handling can lead to the formation of mercury vapors that are toxic and represent a significant health and environmental hazard [23]. Therefore, various mercury-free electrodes have been developed in the past few decades. For example, a nanostructured bismuth film electrode (nsBiFE) has been prepared for ASV detection of multiple heavy metals, in which the detection limits of 0.4 and 0.1 μg L^{-1} are obtained for Cd^{2+} and Pb^{2}, respectively [24]. Similar to bismuth, antimony nanoparticles have also been proven to be highly sensitive and reliable for tracing analysis of heavy metals [25]. To take into real application, more and more electrochemical sensors based on screen-printed carbon electrode (SPCE) have been fabricated for trace heavy metal detection in food safety as it is inexpensive, portable, and easy for mass production [26, 27].

Illegal additives

Addition of inedible substances and abuse of food additives are the prominent problems affecting food safety [28]. Typical illegal additives include melamine, clenbuterol, and Sudan I. These illegal actions may pose great threat to human health. For the detection of these chemicals, various nanomaterial-based biosensors have been developed. Various approaches aiming at analyzing specific chemical contaminants and illegal additives have been developed [29–31]. Li et al. developed a gold nanoparticles (AuNPs)-decorated reduced graphene oxide (RGO) modified electrode for detection of Sudan I in food samples including chili powder and ketchup sauce, demonstrating satisfactory sensitivity, selectivity, and recovery [11]. A sensitive and selective electrochemical sensor based on MIL-53@ XC-72 nanohybrid modified glassy carbon electrode (GCE) was also fabricated to determine melamine with a linear range from 0.04 to 10 μM and detection limit of 0.005 μM (S/N = 3) [32]. In addition, the sensor displayed excellent reproducibility, high stability, selectivity, and good recoveries for the determination of melamine in liquid milk. The synergistic effect of nitrogen-doped graphene (NGR) and nitrogen-doped carbon nanotubes (NCNTs) has also been investigated and applied to prepare an electrochemical sensor for simultaneous and sensitive determination of caffeine and vanillin [33]. Electrochemical sensors have also been developed for many other food additives, such as sunset yellow [34, 35].

Pesticide residues

Pesticides, including fungicides, herbicides, and insecticides, are widely used in most food production to control pests that would otherwise destroy or reduce food production [36]. In the area of agriculture, the usage of insecticides, herbicides, molluscicides, and fungicides has an increasing importance. However, many pesticides are toxic and can cause many health problems when consumed by animals and humans, such as bone marrow disorders, carcinogenicity, infertility, cytogenic effects, neurological diseases, and immunological and respiratory problems. Hence, pesticide residue detection is very important for food safety [37].

To date, many methods have been applied to determine pesticide residues in food samples. Electrochemical methods provide the elucidation of processes and mechanisms of redox reaction of pesticides and their residues [38]. They are sensitive, reliable, and fast. They can be easily miniaturized and integrated with other analytical methods [39, 40]. A magneto-actuated enzyme-free electrochemical sensor based on magnetic molecularly imprinted polymer was developed, and it showed outstanding analytical performance for the detection of methyl parathion in fish, with a limit of detection of as low as 1.22×10^{-6} mg L^{-1} and recovery values ranging from 89.4 to 94.7% [41]. Da Silva and coworkers [42] developed an acetylcholinesterase (AChE) biosensor for rapid detection of carbaryl in tomato samples by using electrode modified with reduced graphene oxide (rGO). The electrochemical response increased as the concentration of acetylthiocholine chloride increased, while the response decreased in the presence of AChE inhibitor OPs with a linear response to the inhibition of the thiocholine oxidation process for carbaryl concentrations from 10 to 50 nmol L^{-1} and 0.2 to 1.0 mol L^{-1}. Compared with AChE, organophosphorus hydrolase (OPH) enzymes catalyze the hydrolysis of organophosphorus pesticides (OPs) with a high turnover rate, can potentially be reused, and are, therefore, suitable for continuous monitoring of OPs [43, 44].

Veterinary drugs

Veterinary drugs mainly include antimicrobial drugs, antiparasitic drugs, and growth promoters, which are extensively used for treatment and prevention of diseases in animals, promotion of animal growth, and feed efficiency [45]. But the possible presence of veterinary drugs in animal-derived foods is one of the key issues for food safety, which arouses great public concern. So it is very important to develop quick and accurate methods to detect veterinary drug residues in animalderived food, and their quantity must be less than the maximum residue limits (MRL) defined in many countries on the basis of food safety [46].

Electrochemical sensors have drawn considerable attention in many fields such as food safety, disease diagnosis, and environmental monitoring [47, 48]. Lin et al. [49] developed a hybrid

CNT-modified electrode for simultaneous determination of toxic ractopamine and salbutamol in pork samples. Conzuelo et al. developed a novel strategy to construct disposable amperometric affinity biosensors by recombinant bacterial penicillin-binding protein (PBP) tagged by an N-terminal hexahistidine tail that was immobilized onto Co^{2+}-tetradentate nitrilotriacetic acid (NTA)-modified screen-printed carbon electrodes (SPCEs) for the specific detection and quantification of β-lactam antibiotic residues in milk, which was accomplished by means of a direct competitive assay using a tracer with horseradish peroxidase (HRP) for the enzymatic labeling [50]. The sensor showed limits of detection with the low part-per-billion level for the antibiotics tested in untreated milk samples and a good selectivity against other antibiotic residues frequently detected in milk and dairy products. In addition, Wang et al. proposed a simple, rapid, and highly sensitive homogeneous electrochemical strategy for the detection of ampicillin based on target-initiated T7 exonuclease-assisted signal amplification. This biosensor showed a low detection limit of 4.0 pM toward ampicillin with an excellent selectivity, which has been successfully applied to assay antibiotic in milk. Importantly, the sensor system could avoid the tedious and time-consuming steps of electrode modification, making the experimental processes much simpler and more convenient, which has great potential for the simple, easy, and convenient detection of antibiotic residues in food safety field [51].

Biological toxins

Mycotoxins are fungal secondary metabolites that have toxic effects on humans and animals. Generally, mycotoxins can be easily found in agriculture crops, dairy products, including milk and cheese, and alcohols [52]. Mycotoxins enter human or animal bodies through consumption of contaminated animals or industrial food products. Crops and food products that are highly susceptible to mycotoxin con-tamination include alcoholic beverages, wheat, corn, barley, sugarcane, cottonseed, peanuts, rice, sugar beets, sorghum, and hard cheese [53].

Many review articles have focused on mycotoxin detection using different transduction methods [54, 55]. However, only a few review articles have reported on the use of nanomaterials for the electrochemical (EC) sensing of mycotoxins [56]. The present review summarizes the recent developments of nanomaterial-based EC biosensors for mycotoxin detection. It describes the importance of mycotoxin detection and the current progress and necessity of POC analysis of food toxins [56]. Finally, it illustrates the role in mycotoxin detection of EC sensors based on carbon and graphene metal nanoparticles (NPs) combined with different recognition elements, such as aptamers, antibodies, and molecularly imprinted polymers (MIPs) [57, 58]. These sensors exhibited additional analytical merits such as a shortened analysis time with simplified analytical procedures and portability. As such, EC sensors are now acknowledged as promising options for the trace-level identification of mycotoxins in food processing and manufacturing industries.

Microbial pathogens

Microbial pathogens include bacteria, viruses, and protozoa, and failure to detect them can have severe impacts on public health and safety. In the food or water services industries, legislation developed by the appropriate associated regulatory bodies to monitor and control the presence of these microorganisms is vital. Rapid and cost-efficient detection methods, with high-through-put capacity, are essential to implement effective monitoring systems to protect human health [59]. In 2012, the Environmental Protection Agency (EPA) released new Recreational Water Quality Criteria recommendations for protecting human health in waters designated for primary contact recreation [60]. Guner et al. developed an electrochemical sensor for the detection of *E. coli* using a pencil graphite electrode that was modified with multiwalled CNT (MWCNT), chitosan, polypyrrole (PPy), and AuNPs. Anti-*E. coli* monoclonal antibody was immobilized on the hybrid bionanocomposite, and the detection range was from 3×10^1 to 3×10^7 CFU/mL of *E. coli* [61].

Gao et al. describe a novel electrochemical biosensor based on mouse monoclonal antibody immobilized on self-assembled monolayers (SAM)-modified gold (Au) electrodes for the detection of *Listeria monocytogenes* (LM) and the detection range is from 10^2 to 10^6 CFU/mL. More importantly, this biosensor could apply to detect LM in milk without sample pretreatment, which is a straightforward and reliable method for analysis of LM with a simple operation and sensitivity at a low cost [62]. SPCEs were modified with iron/gold core/ shell nanoparticles (Fe@Au) conjugated with anti-salmonella antibodies to develop an electrochemical biosensor for Salmonella detection. The biosensor was performed by square-wave anodic stripping voltammetry through the use of CdS nanocrystals and its calibration curve was established between 1×10^1 and 1×10^6 cells/mL with the detection limit of 13 cells/mL. The developed method showed that it is possible to determine the bacteria in milk at low concentrations and is suitable for the rapid (less than 1 h) and sensitive detection of *S. typhimurium* in real samples. Therefore, the developed methodology could contribute to the improvement of the quality control of food samples [63].

Summary

Food safety is undoubtedly one of the major global concerns. In this chapter, we summarize some representative electrochemical sensors toward food contaminants such as heavy metals, illegal additives, pesticide residues, veterinary drug residues, biological toxins, and foodborne pathogen. These electrochemical sensors for food safety detection continue to show many advantages including rapid response, field applicability, high sensitivity, high selectivity, and online analysis. Moreover, electrochemical sensors are much cheaper and easier to be miniaturized, which may play a key role on quality control in food processing, improving product quality and safety. However, the stability of the electrochemical sensors is still a challenging problem. Recently, we have developed an electrochemical instrument and a number of electrochemical sensors for the detection of heavy metal ions with excellent sensitivity and reproducibility. The instrument and sensors are being commercialized with satisfactory user feedback.

Author details

Lingwen Zeng*, Lei Peng, Dazhi Wu and Baoguo Yang

Institute of Environment and Safety, Wuhan Academy of Agricultural Sciences, Wuhan, China

*Address all correspondence to: zeng6@yahoo.com

References

[1] El-Nezami H, Tam PK, Chan Y, Lau AS, Leung FC, Chen SF. Impact of melamine-tainted milk on foetal kidneys and disease development later in life. Hong Kong Medical Journal.2013;**19**:S34e8

[2] Nolvachai Y, Kulsing C, Marriott PJ. Multidimensional gas chromatography in food analysis. TrAC Trends in Analytical Chemistry. 2017;**96**:124-137

[3] Armutcu C, Uzun L, Denizli A. Determination of Ochratoxin A traces in foodstuffs: Comparison of an automated on-line two-dimensional high-performance liquid chromatography and off-line immunoaffinity-high- performance liquid chromatography system. Journal of Chromatography. A. 2012;**1569**:139-148

[4] Wang Y, Liu SJ, Pu QK, Li YX, Wang XX, Jiang Y, et al. Rapid identification of *Staphylococcus aureus*, *Vibrio parahaemolyticus* and *Shigella sonnei* in foods by solid phase microextraction coupled with gas chromatography- mass spectrometry. Food Chemistry. 2018;**262**:7-13

[5] Malik AK, Blasco C, Picó Y. Liquid chromatography-mass spectrometry in food safety. Journal of Chromatography. A. 2010;**1217**:4018-4040

[6] Ma L, Nilghaz A, Choi JR, Liu X, Lu X. Rapid detection of clenbuterol in milk using microfluidic paper-based ELISA. Food Chemistry. 2018;**246**:437-441

[7] Raeisossadati MJ, Danesh NM, Borna F, Gholamzad M, Ramezani M, Abnous K, et al. Lateral flow based immunobiosensors for detection of food contaminants. Biosensors and Bioelectronics. 2016;**86**:235-246

[8] Zhou Y, Yang YJ, Deng X, Zhang GM, Zhang Y, Zhang CH, et al. Electrochemical sensor for determination of ractopamine based on aptamer/octadecanethiol Janus particles. Sensors and Actuators B: Chemical. 2018;**276**:204-210

[9] Thota R, Ganesh V. Selective and sensitive electrochemical detection of methyl parathion using chemically modified overhead projector sheets as flexible electrodes. Sensors and Actuators B. 2016;**227**:169-177

[10] Gayathri CH, Mayuri P, Sankaran K, Kumar AS. An electrochemical immunosensor for efficient detection of uropathogenic *E. coli* based on thionine dye immobilized chitosan/ functionalized-MWCNT modified electrode. Biosensors & Bioelectronics. 2016;**82**:71-77

[11] Li J, Feng H, Li J, Feng Y, Zhang Y, Jiang J, et al. Fabrication of gold nanoparticles-decorated reduced graphene oxide as a high performance electrochemical sensing platform for the detection of toxicant Sudan I. Electrochimica Acta. 2015;**167**:226-236

[12] Mishra RK, Hayat A, Catanante G, Istamboulie G, Marty JL. Sensitive quantitation of Ochratoxin A in cocoa beans using differential pulse voltammetry based aptasensor. Food Chemistry. 2016;**192**:799-804

[13] Silva NFD, Magalhães JMCS, Freire C, Matos CD. Electrochemical biosensors for salmonella: State of the art and challenges in food safety assessment. Biosensors and Bioelectronics. 2018;**99**:667-682

[14] Bard AJ, Faulkner LR. Electro- chemical Methods: Fundamentals and Applications. 2nd ed. New York: Wiley; 2001

[15] Gong T, Liu J, Liu X, Liu J, Xiang J, Wu Y. A sensitive and selective platform based on CdTe QDs in the presence of l-cysteine for detection of silver, mercury and copper ions in water and various drinks. Food Chemistry. 2016;**213**:306-312

[16] Lu YY, Liang XQ, Niyungeko C, Zhou JJ, Xu JM, Tian GM. A review of the identification and detection of heavy metal ions in the environment by voltammetry. Talanta. 2018;**178**:324-338

[17] Bansod BK, Kumar T, Thakur R, Rana S, Singh I. A review on various electrochemical techniques for heavy metal ions detection with different sensing platforms. Biosensors and Bioelectronics. 2017;**94**:443-455

[18] Gumpu MB, Sethuraman S, Krishnan UM, Rayappanabd JBB. A review on detection of heavy metal ions in water—An electrochemical approach. Sensors and Actuators B: Chemical. 2015;**213**:515-533

[19] Tsai WT, Nguyen MH, Lai JR, Nguyen HB, Lee MC, Tsengc FG. ppb-Level heavy metal ion detection by electrochemistry-assisted nanoPorous silicon (ECA-NPS) photonic sensors. Sensors and Actuators B: Chemical. 2018;**265**:75-83

[20] Afkhami A, Soltani-Felehgari F, Madrakian T, Ghaedi H, Rezaeivala M. Fabrication and application of a new modified electrochemical sensor using nanosilica and a newly synthesized Schiff base for simultaneous determination of Cd^{2+}, Cu^{2+} and Hg^{2+} ions in water and some foodstuff samples. Analytica Chimica Acta. 2013;**771**:21-30

[21] Wang J. Stripping Analysis Encyclopedia of Electrochemistry. Weinheim: Willey VCH; 2007

[22] Barek J, Fogg AG, Mick A, Zima J. Polarography and voltammetry at mercury electrodes. Critical Reviews in Analytical Chemistry. 2001;**31**:291-309

[23] Svancara I, Prior C, Hocevar SB, Wang J. A decade of bismuth electrodes in modern electroanalysis. Electroanalysis. 2010;**22**:1405-1420

[24] Zidarič T, Jovanovski V, Menart E, Zorko M, Kolar M, Veber M, et al. Multi-pulse galvanostatic preparation of nanostructured bismuth film electrode for trace metal detection. Sensors and Actuators B: Chemical. 2017;**245**:720-725

[25] Serrano N, Cristin JMDC, Esteban AM. Antimony-based electrodes for analytical determinations. TrAC Trends in Analytical Chemistry. 2016;**77**:203-213

[26] Yao Y, Wu H, Ping JF. Simultaneous determination of Cd (II) and Pb (II) ions in honey and milk samples using a single-walled carbon nanohorns modified screen-printed electrochemical sensor. Food Chemistry. 2019;**274**:8-15

[27] Jian JM, Fu LF, Ji JY, Lin LW, Guo XS, Ren TL. Electrochemically reduced graphene oxide/gold nanoparticles composite modified screen-printed carbon electrode for effective electrocatalytic analysis of nitrite in foods. Sensors and Actuators B: Chemical. 2018;**262**:125-136

[28] Martins FCOL, Sentanin MA, Souza DD. Analytical methods in food additives determination: Compounds with functional applications. Food Chemistry. 2019;**272**:732-750

[29] Zhang J, Na L, Jiang Y, Han D, Lou D, Jin L. A fluorescence quenching method for quantitative analysis of Ponceau 4R in beverage. Food Chemistry. 2017;**221**:803-808

[30] Yan W, Wang N, Zhang P, Zhang J, Wu S, Zhu Y. Simultaneous determination of sucralose and related compounds by high-performance liquid chromatography with evaporative light scattering detection. Food Chemistry. 2016;**204**:358-364

[31] Wang L, Li J, Zhang L. Determination of polyphosphates in fish andshrimp muscles by capillary electrophoresis with indirect UV detection after phosphatase inhibition using high pressure pretreatment. Food Chemistry. 2015;**185**:349-354

[32] Zhang WQ, Xu GR, Liu RQ, Chen J, Li XB, Zhang YD, et al. Novel MOFs@XC-72-Nafion nanohybrid modified glassy carbon electrode for the sensitive determination of melamine. Electrochimica Acta. 2016;**211**:689-696

[33] Jiang L, Ding Y, Jiang F, Li L, Mo F. Electrodeposited nitrogen- doped graphene/carbon nanotubes nanocomposite as enhancer for simultaneous and sensitive voltammetric determination of caffeine and vanillin. Analytica Chimica Acta. 2014;**833**:22-28

[34] Yin ZZ, Cheng SW, Xu LB, Liu HY, Huang K, Li L, et al. Highly sensitive and selective sensor for sunset yellow based on molecularly imprinted polydopamine-coated multi-walled carbon nanotubes. Biosensors and Bioelectronics. 2018;**100**:565-570

[35] Shah A, Malik MS, Zahid A, Iftikhar FJ, Anwar A, Akhter MS, et al. Carbamazepine coated silver nanoparticles for the simultaneous electrochemical sensing of specific food toxins. Electrochimica Acta. 2018;**274**:131-142

[36] Nsibande SA, Forbes PBC. Fluorescence detection of pesticides using quantum dot materials—A review. Analytica Chimica Acta. 2016;**945**:9-22

[37] London L, Nell V, Thompson ML, Myers JE. Effects of long-term organophosphate exposures on neurological symptoms, vibration sense and tremor amongst South African farm workers. Scandinavian Journal of Work, Environment & Health. 1998;**24**:18-29

[38] Chauhan N, Pundir CS. An amperometric acetylcholinesterase sensor based on Fe3O4 nanoparticle/ multi-walled carbon nanotube- modified ITO-coated glass plate for the detection of pesticides. Electrochimica Acta. 2012;**67**:79-86

[39] Grieshaber D, MacKenzie R, Voros J, Reimhult E. Electrochemical biosensors—Sensor principles and architectures. Sensors. 2008;**8**(3):1400-1458

[40] Rassaei L, Amiri M, Cirtiu CM, Sillanpaa M, Marken F, Sillanpaa M. Nanoparticles in electrochemical sensors for environmental monitoring. Trends in Analytical Chemistry. 2011;**30**:1704-1715

[41] Hassan AHA, Moura SL, Ali FHM, Moselhy WA, Sotomayor T, Sotomayor M d PT, et al. Electrochemical sensing of methyl parathion on magnetic molecularly imprinted polymer. Biosensors and Bioelectronics. 2018;**118**:181-187

[42] Da Silva MKL, Vanzela HC, Defavari LM, Cesarino I. Determination of carbamate pesticide in food using a biosensor based on reduced graphene oxide and acetylcholinesterase enzyme. Sensors and Actuators B: Chemical. 2018;**277**:555-561

[43] Stoytcheva M, Gochev V, Velkova Z. Electrochemical biosensors for direct determination of organophosphorus pesticides: A review. Current Analytical Chemistry. 2016;**12**:37-42

[44] Sahin A, Dooley K, Cropek DM, West AC, Banta S. A dual enzyme electrochemical assay for the detection of organophosphorus compounds using organophosphorus hydrolase and horseradish peroxidase. Sensors and Actuators B: Chemical. 2017;**158**:353-360

[45] Wu D, Du D, Lin YH. Recent progress on nanomaterial-based biosensors for veterinary drug residues in animal-derived food. TrAC Trends in Analytical Chemistry. 2016;**83**:95-101

[46] Lan LY, Yao Y, Ping JF, Ying YB. Recent advances in nanomaterial-based biosensors for antibiotics detection. Biosensors and Bioelectronics. 2017;**91**:504-514

[47] Kimmel DW, Blanc GL, Meschievitz ME, Cliffel DE. Electrochemical sensors and biosensors. Analytical Chemistry. 2012;**84**:685-707

[48] Zhu JL, Wen MQ, Wen W, Du D, Zhang XH, Wang SF, et al. Recent progress in biosensors based on organic- inorganic hybrid nanoflowers. Biosensors and Bioelectronics. 2018;**120**:175-187

[49] Lin KC, Hong CP, Chen SM. Simultaneous determination for toxic ractopamine and salbutamol in pork sample using hybrid carbon nanotubes. Sensors and Actuators B: Chemical. 2013;**177**:428-436

[50] Conzuelo F, Gamella M, Campuzano S, Ruiz PM, Torres ME, de las Rivas B, et al. Integrated amperometric affinity biosensors using Co^{2+}–tetradentate nitrilotriacetic acid modified disposable carbon electrodes: Application to the determination of β-lactam antibiotics. Analytical Chemistry. 2013;**85**:3246-3254

[51] Wang XZ, Dong SS, Gai PP, Duan R, Li F. Highly sensitive homogeneous electrochemical aptasensor for antibiotic residues detection based on dual recycling amplification strategy. Biosensors and Bioelectronics. 2016;**82**:49-54

[52] Schenzel J, Forrer HR, Vogelgsang S, Hungerbühler K, Bucheli TD. Mycotoxins in the environment: I. Production and emission from an agricultural test field. Environmental Science & Technology. 2012;**46**:13067-13075

[53] Marín S, Sancho GC, Sanchis V, Ramos AJ. The role of mycotoxins in the human exposome: Application of mycotoxin biomarkers in exposome- health studies. Food and Chemical Toxicology. 2018;**121**:504-518

[54] Chauhan R, Singh J, Sachdev T, Basu T, Malhotra BD. Recent advances in mycotoxins detection. Biosensors and Bioelectronics. 2016;**81**:532-545

[55] Anfossi L, Giovannoli C, Baggiani C. Mycotoxin detection. Current Opinion in Biotechnology. 2016;**37**:120-126

[56] Goud KY, Kailas SK, Kumar V, Tsang YF, Lee SE, Gobi KV, et al. Progress on nanostructured electrochemical sensors and their recognition elements for detection of mycotoxins: A review. Biosensors and Bioelectronics. 2018;**121**:205-222

[57] Li F, Yu Z, Han X, Lai RY. Electrochemical aptamer-based sensors for food and water analysis: A review. Analytica Chimica Acta. 2018. DOI: 10.1016/j.aca.2018.10.058

[58] Vidal JC, LlBonel AE, Susana H, Bertolín JR, Cubel C, Castilloa JR. Electrochemical affinity biosensors for detection of mycotoxins: A review. Biosensors and Bioelectronics. 2013;**49**:146-158

[59] Franz CMAP, den Besten HMW, Böhnlein C, Gareis M, Zwietering MH, Fusco V. Microbial food safety in the 21st century: Emerging challenges and foodborne pathogenic bacteria. Trends in Food Science & Technology. 2018;**81**:155-158

[60] United States Environmental Protection Agency. Office of Water Report 820-F-12-058. Fort Meade, MD: Environmental Science Center; 2012

[61] Güner A, Çevik E, Senel M, Alpsoy L. An electrochemical immunosensor for sensitive detection of Escherichia coli O157:H7 by using chitosan, MWCNT, polypyrrole with gold nanoparticles hybrid sensing platform. Food Chemistry. 2017;**229**:358-365

[62] Cheng CN, Peng Y, Bai JL, Zhang XY, Liu YY, Fan XJ, et al. Rapid detection of Listeria monocytogenes in milk by self-assembled electrochemical immunosensor. Sensors and Actuators B: Chemical. 2014;**190**:900-906

[63] Freitas M, Viswanathan S, Nouws H, Oliveira M, Delerue Matos C. Iron oxide/gold core/shell nanomagnetic probes and CdS biolabels for amplified electrochemical immunosensing of *Salmonella typhimurium*. Biosensors & Bioelectronics. 2014;**51**:195-200

7

Cardiovascular Disease and Nutrition

Javier Marhuenda, Débora Villaño, Begoña Cerdá and María Pilar Zafrilla

Abstract

Many studies have been published on the relationship between the risk of cardiovascular disease and various nutrients, foods, and eating patterns. Despite the well-accepted concept that diet has a significant influence on the development and prevention of cardiovascular disease, foods considered healthy or harmful have varied over the years. Cardiovascular diseases are one of the main causes of illness and death in Western countries, and cardiovascular drugs are the most commonly used medications. There are two types of factors involved in the development of cardiovascular disease. Some factor can be modified, like lifestyle, diet, environment, or smoking. Others such as genetic factors, gender, history, or age cannot be modified. In this chapter, some food, nutrients, and bioactive compounds that are susceptible to exert beneficial of harmful properties on cardiovascular disease are presented.

Keywords: nutrition, cardiovascular diseases, CVR, omega-3

Introduction

Diet and healthy lifestyle are the best tools to have good cardiovascular health. This relationship is so direct because the majority of cardiovascular diseases have their origin atherosclerotic plaque, hypertension, and obesity. These three cardiovascular risk factors are directly related to dietary habits and lifestyle. It is widely demonstrated from the scientific point of view that dietary habits influence cardiovascular health. There are diets such as the Dietary Approaches to Stop Hypertension (DASH) as the Mediterranean diet, which are clear examples of heart-healthy diets. However, there are discrepancies with regard to what are the components of a heart-healthy diet. There are foods that are considered healthy for the heart in all editions of food guides and recommendations, among which we can find fruits, vegetables, and whole grains, which have always been considered fundamental for health, and there are other foods that can currently be considered heart-healthy, since there are numerous studies that this is supported, such as virgin olive oil, pulses, fish, and nuts (especially nuts). This chapter focuses on the most recent food evidence (e.g., fruits and vegetables) and nutrients (such as fiber and omega-3) considered to be cardio-healthy today and as a counterpoint, the scientific clairvoyance that exists on those foods considered less heart-healthy because they are considered to increase cardiovascular risk (eggs, dairy products, meats, and salt).

Cardiovascular disease and its association with dietary patterns and nutrients

Meta-analysis related to dietary patterns and cardiovascular disease

Nowadays, most of the evidence supporting the beneficial and harmful effects of food and nutrients is based on observational epidemiological studies. The infor- mation of the present section aims to elucidate the current knowledge about dietary patterns and cardiovascular problems. The information is divided in food groups, in order to clarify as most as possible. Fruits and vegetables have traditionally been considered promoting health foods. This is due to the association between the greater consumption of these products and the reduction of the risk of suffering chronic diseases, such as cardio- vascular disease (CVD). Consequently, the current dietary guidelines recommend an increase in the consumption of fruits and vegetables up to five servings a day [1].

Current evidence is largely based on prospective cohort studies showing uniform associations between increased consumption of fruits and vegetables and reduced risk of both coronary artery disease (CAD) and stroke. However, these studies do not have the highest level of scientific evidence. In contrast, the number of controlled intervention trials (which provide a higher level of scientific evidence) in which the relationship between fruit and vegetable consumption and clinical endpoints has been investigated is unusual. However, the results of these studies show associations between increased consumption of fruits and vegetables and improvement of blood pressure and microvascular function. Meanwhile, associations with plasma lipid concentrations, risk of diabetes mellitus (DM), and body weight have not yet been definitely recognized [2].

The dietary habits of English population between 2001 and 2013 have been studied and reported in a recent study. It was observed that the consumption (seven daily servings of fruits and vegetables) reduces the specific risks of death from cancer and heart disease in 25 and 31%, respectively [3]. This report also showed that vegetables have a significantly greater beneficial health effect than fruits. It is important to emphasize that, whatever the starting point, the data indicate that the highest consumption of fruits and vegetables always provides a benefit. In addition, many confounding factors, such as poor access to fresh fruits and vegetables for people with preexisting health conditions or complicated lifestyles or those living in disadvantaged areas, affect the experimental approach used by these researchers. In conclusion, as reported by Berciano and Ordovás [2], the evidence indicating consumption of fruits and vegetables as dismissal of the risk of CVD is largely limited to observational epidemiology. Therefore, new intervention studies will be necessary to establish the existing real relationship.

Fruits and vegetables are very rich in both soluble and insoluble fibers, which structural and functional characteristics may vary greatly. Insoluble fibers, such as cellulose and lignin, are non-hydrolyzable and hardly undergo fermentation, while soluble fibers, such as pectin or inulin, are not hydrolyzed in the stomach but can be fermented by the gut microbiota. The main physiological effect associated with the consumption of insoluble fibers is the reduction of intestinal transit time which allows water retention, promotes an increase in fecal mass, and facilitates the movement of food through the intestine, due to mechanical stimulation of the intestinal walls. The distension caused also increases the feeling of fullness and can contribute to reducing caloric intake [4].

On the other hand, the main physicochemical properties of the soluble fibers that characterize their effects are viscosity, the ability to form gels, and fermentability. The increase in viscosity slows gastric emptying (which contributes to satiety) and increases transit time. This helps to produce the stabilization of the glucose and insulin response and reduces the absorption of dietary cholesterol [4].

Regarding CVD, the most important property of dietary fiber is fermentability that reduces the concentration of low-density lipoproteins (LDL) in the blood. The mechanism is mediated by short-chain fatty acids produced by colon bacteria. Apart from this effect, there are other important considerations related to the lymphocyte activation, the inhibition of cell proliferation and the anti-inflammatory effects and the bile acid binding activity exerted by the dietary fiber, which act as a kidnapper [5]. Despite knowing the different properties and effects on health that may have the various types and origins of fiber, most studies have provided insufficient data, which prevents an independent assessment of the associated risks of disease. However, total fiber intake is uniformly associated with a small reduction in the risk of CVD, coronary disease (CD), and stroke [6].

All existing reviews conclude that diets rich in fiber are significantly associated with lower risk of stroke, CVD, and CD. This inverse association reinforces what is indicated in the current guidelines, which recommend an increase in fiber consumption, although studies that have described results related to fractions of fiber are too scarce to establish specific recommendations on soluble/insoluble fiber and the types of origins of those fibers. Dose-response analyses have identified cutoff values that have not been validated and appear to show wide differences between different types of fiber. The broader study on this topic indicates that the existence of a threshold effect has not been verified and that the message to be retained must be rather than the greater the consumption of fiber, the greater the protection [2, 5, 6].

In the last years, coffee has been relegated to the background with the boom in tea consumption. Green tea is considered a healthy drink and consumed worldwide and has been attributed various beneficial effects to its regular intake, such as reducing the risk of suffering from diseases ranging from certain cancers to dementia and obesity. With regard to CVD, regular consumption of green tea has been associated with small reductions in CVD risk factors, such as LDL and blood pressure, which may have clinical relevance [7]. However, the number of studies reviewed is too low to be able to draw definitive conclusions, and there is a significant lack of long-term follow-up data and cardiovascular events to assess the long-term effects of green tea consumption.

Similar to green tea, wine and coffee are two beverages containing a wide variety of phytochemical substances that have been associated with a protective effect against heart disease. Although these compounds, mostly polyphenols, have been intensively studied over the past two decades, the main effects of wine (or alcoholic beverages in general) and coffee consumption continue to be attributed to ethanol and caffeine, respectively [8]. Recent reviews indicate that beer and especially red wine [7, 8] are associated with a greater reduction in the risk of CVD due to its high polyphenol content [9, 10]. The protective effects of coffee against CVD are not well established. In fact, a moderate consumption of coffee (two to four cups a day) has not shown any adverse effects in the long term [2]. However, it is well known that an excessive consumption of caffeine leads to hypertension, and in particular unfiltered coffee contributes to elevate the serum concentration of LDL, total cholesterol, and triglycerides [11]. It is important to note that the mentioned effects are subject to interpersonal differences, since there are many genetic polymorphisms that are known to affect different enzymes that are involved in their metabolism [2].

Regarding animal food, blue fish (like other many high-fat foods), such as olive oil, was on the list of "unhealthy" foods because of its high-fat content. However, from the earliest 1970s, omega-3 fats from blue fish were reported as beneficial to health and especially to health related to CVD [12]. However, there are still wide discrepancies regarding their effects on optimal doses, as well as their relationship with omega-6 fatty acids or other components of the diet. In fact, the results of the published randomized clinical trials (a total of 48 studies that included 36,913 individuals) have not shown a reduction in the risk of total mortality or the set of cardiovascular events in people who take supplementary omega-3 fats [2]. Consequently, despite the known effect of omega-3 fat on plasma triglyceride concentrations, there is no unequivocal evidence that omega-3 fats in the diet or supplements modify total mortality or the set of cardiovascular events. In fact, a recent study [13] raises certain doubts about the validity of the premises used to support the initial hypothesis on omega-3 and CVD [14].

Continuing with foods of animal origin, one of the most ancient are eggs, which were introduced in the diet prior to the appearance in the evolution of *Homo sapiens*. It is not surprising that eggs are an important source of nutrients such as proteins, unsaturated fats, fat-soluble vitamins, folate, choline, and minerals. The possible counterpoint derives from the fact that, on average, an egg contains 200 mg of cholesterol, one-third of the recommended daily amount. The rationale for this recommendation continues to be linked to the diet-heart hypothesis. In contrast, epidemiological evidence has consistently shown that it is unlikely that the consumption of one egg a day has any significant impact on the risk of CVD in healthy people.

Similarly, the relationship between egg consumption and the clinically relevant elevation of plasma cholesterol concentrations is too old. Newer studies revealed the actual hypothesis about egg consumption. One of the most recent studies is the HELENA study, showing that egg consumption was not associated with the lipid profile, adiposity, insulin resistance, blood pressure, good cardiorespiratory function, or the integrated CVD risk score [15]. In general, current evidence supports that egg consumption is not associated with risk of CVD, CD, or cardiac death in the general population and may even have a protective value against hemorrhagic stroke [16].

In contrast, egg consumption may be associated with an increase in the incidence of type 2 diabetes mellitus in the general population and the comorbidity of CVD in diabetic patients [17]. Consequently, it seems that the most recent results exonerate the eggs from their intended role of significant dietary factor of the CVD epidemic. In this regard, it is important to bear in mind that the absorption of cholesterol has great interindividual differences, and only a fifth of the population can respond with increases in plasma cholesterol to the presence of cholesterol in the diet [17]. Therefore, it is important to identify the genetic determinants of this variability.

Regarding meat, scientific literature has been focused on the relationship between diet meat, CVD, and total mortality, which have led to a situation less clear than in the case of egg consumption. What seems to be clear is the association between red meat consumption and total mortality related to CVD, as well as the risk of CVD, ischemic stroke, and type 2 diabetes mellitus.

However, this association can often be caused by the consumption of processed meats and not always by fresh red meat. In fact, it has been pointed out that the harmful effects observed by processed meat may be related to other components, such as sodium, nitrites, heme iron, and l-carnitine. For example, the effects of elevating blood pressure associated with the high sodium content of processed foods could explain the increased risk of people sensitive to salt. There is recent evidence reporting that trimethylamine, phosphatidylcholine, choline, and lcarnitine in processed and red meat can promote CVD [18]. The scientific literature indicates that the consumption of unprocessed red meat and processed red meat is not beneficial for cardiometabolic health. In fact, it can be observed that clinical and public health guidelines prioritize above all the reduction of consumption of processed meat.

Finally, other foods demonized in recent years are dairy products, in part due to their relatively high content of saturated fats and cholesterol. Consequently, after having occupied for decades a prominent place among recommended foods, dairy products also suffered the consequences of the "non-healthy anti-saturated fat fever." However, this group of foods had a relatively easy way out, and the dairy industry started to produce a whole range of low-fat products. As observed by Berciano and Ordovás [2], these products already have enough time on the market to evaluate them regarding the intrinsic benefits in terms of CVD compared to more traditional varieties.

The comparison between fatty and non-fatty dairy products is important because the relationship between CVD and saturated fats may not be as simple as initially thought. That fact can be due to multiple reasons.

First, not all fats would be the same and were, in origin, classified as good (unsaturated) and bad (saturated). However, actual knowledge seems to discuss that theory. In fact, it was appreciated that "healthy" fats as polyunsaturated fats omega-6 could not be as good as thought. Contrariwise, some of the "bad fats" could be healthy (the case of fats saturated from dairy foods) [19].

Second, the replacement of saturated fats in the diet with simple carbohydrates has led to an increase in obesity and health complications. Therefore, it is probable that some of the adverse effects associated with saturated fats in the past must be factors other than saturated fats. Thus, in recent times the relationship between dairy foods and the risk of CVD has been revisited on multiple occasions [19]. In an interesting study, Huth and Park [20] reviewed the published evidence on milk products with milk fat content and cardiovascular health. The results of this review indicate that most of the observational studies found no association between the consumption of dairy products and increased risk of CVD, CD, and stroke, regardless of the concentration of fat in the milk.

In general, it can be concluded that the consumption of dairy products provides protection against CVD or, at least, has no adverse effects. Consequently, the existing data support the concept that milk and low-fat milk products contribute to the prevention of hypertension and reduce the risk of stroke and, potentially, other CVD events. Another review revised the scientific literature related to observational studies on the relationship between the fat of dairy products and high-fat dairy foods, obesity, and cardiometabolic disease [21]. Of a total of 16 studies, in 68% there was an inverse association between the consumption of high-fat dairy products and the parameters of assessment of adiposity. In fact, studies conducted to examine the relationship between the consumption of high-fat dairy products and metabolic health has described an inverse association or no association [21]. Consequently, these results indicate that milk fat or high-fat dairy foods do not contribute to obesity or cardiometabolic risk and imply that the consumption of high-fat dairy products within the usual dietary patterns has an inverse association with the obesity risk.

Oxidative stress and antioxidants

It is commonly accepted by scientific community that oxidative stress is within the base of the etiology of cardiovascular diseases. However, the understanding of the role of reactive oxygen and nitrogen species (RONS) has evolved somewhat. They are not further seen in a whole negative perspective, but current knowledge supports that they are generated as part of normal metabolism, as well as a defense mechanism of cells from immune system to combat against infections; besides, they are implicated in intracellular signaling pathways [22]. Hence, low concentrations seem protective by triggering defense mechanisms that prevent cellular damage [23].

The levels of RONS are counteracted by cellular defenses in the form of antioxidants, to maintain an adequate balanced oxidative status. However, when an imbalance in the production/elimination of these reactive species occurs, a specific cellular function can be altered [24].

The excess of free radicals attacks macromolecules, mainly polyunsaturated fatty acids (PUFA) of cell membranes [25] that leads to cell death and conducts to different pathological conditions, as vascular diseases. Oxidation of PUFA generates fatty acid radicals, which adds oxygen to form fatty acid peroxyl radicals. These radicals can further oxidize PUFA molecules and initiate new chain reactions, producing lipid hydroperoxides that can produce more radical species [25].

Oxidative stress contributes markedly to endothelial dysfunction, with a reduced activity of nitric oxide (NO). NO induces vasodilation, inhibits platelet aggregation, prevents LDL oxidation, and decreases production of proinflammatory cytokines. Free radicals oxidize and inactivate NO impeding its protective action. Besides, vascular cells generate reactive species principally by NADPH oxidase pathway [26]. The increased NADPH oxidase activity and the decrease in antioxidant enzyme defenses and cysteine/cystine redox potential increase the risk of cardiovascular disease [22].

Free radicals induce the expression of adhesion molecules in vascular wall, as intercellular adhesion molecule 1 (ICAM-1), what activates the migration of monocytes and T cells to the vessel [27] and helps to their attachment to the endothelial surface. The oxidation of low-density lipoproteins (LDL) by free radicals is followed by their uptake by macrophages. Macrophage cells are converted into foam cells, accumulating in the wall and further activating cells from the immune system, perpetuating the damage. This is the hallmark of initiation of the process of atherosclerosis.

These oxidative changes can be prevented/ameliorated or mitigated by antioxidants. From a chemical point of view, antioxidants are molecules able to react with oxidative species, as free radicals, thus preventing oxidation of a third molecule. Based on their nature, antioxidants have been classified as enzymatic and nonenzymatic forms. Enzymes that break down and remove free radicals include superoxide dismutase (SOD), catalase (CAT), and glutathione peroxidase (GPx). SOD converts the superoxide radical O_2 into O_2 and H_2O_2 in the presence of metal ion cofactors as copper, zinc, or manganese. CAT converts H_2O_2 in H_2O and O_2, and GPx converts H_2O_2 to H_2O and fatty acid hydroperoxides to their corresponding alcohol forms. All of them show synergistic effect and play the major role in prevention of oxidative damage [25].

Low molecular weight antioxidants react due to one-electron reactions with free radicals and possess a chemical structure able to delocalize the one electron that resulted. They form relative stable radicals by delocalization of the unpaired electron within their structure. The term includes both endogenous (glutathione, uric acid, bilirubin) and exogenous antioxidants from dietary origin (ascorbic acid, α-tocopherol, carotenoids, and polyphenols, among others).

α-Tocopherol is the main antioxidant in lipid environment, as it scavenges lipid peroxides in cell membranes and lipid particles, including low-density lipoprotein (LDL), forming an α-tocopheroxyl radical. It intercepts lipid peroxyl radicals and terminates lipid peroxidation reactions [25].

Vitamin C has been considered the most important water-soluble antioxidant in extracellular environment. It scavenges various RONS and regenerates the α-tocopheroxyl radical back to tocopherol [28]. It forms ascorbyl radical, and two molecules react rapidly to produce one molecule of ascorbate and one molecule of dehydroascorbate.

Dietary polyphenols behave as scavenging antioxidants due to their chemical structure of benzo-γ-pyrene cycle. They are able to delocalize the unpaired electron formed after the reaction with free radicals, as they possess an ortho-dihydroxy structure in the B-ring and a [2, 3] double bond in conjugation, as well as the 4-hydroxyl function in C ring. Besides, they can chelate metal ions implicated in the generation of free radicals [29].

Epidemiological studies have shown that a regular intake of fruits and vegetables, rich in antioxidants, reduces the risk of degenerative diseases and cancer [30]. Animal models and in vitro studies performed with particular antioxidants have supported this point of view. There is a generalized and accepted idea that the excessive production of free radicals causes damage and that the scavenging of these radicals is health protective. Hence, a number of human clinical trials on different populations with antioxidant supplementation were performed some decades ago.

However, they showed non-antioxidant effects or even negative outcomes [31]. A meta-analysis of more than 300,000 individuals showed no prevention of cardiovascular disease after supplementation with vitamins E, C, and A and an increased risk of cancer in smokers with β-carotene supplementation [32]. Antioxidants have failed to prevent or delay the development of atherosclerosis [33, 34].

It must be pointed out that most in vitro and animal models used pharmacological doses of antioxidants in imposed oxidative stress conditions, far from the real physiological situation [35].

The contradictory results obtained in the human intervention studies prompted the investigators to undertake a better understanding toward the mechanisms of antioxidants to maintain a balanced redox status.

The classic perception of antioxidants as free radical scavengers has evolved to their action on cell signaling to stimulate enzymatic antioxidant protection. In fact, most free radicals and electrophile species are removed through enzymatic reactions using reducing power in the form of NADPH, GSH, and reduced thioredoxin [36]. Moreover, free radicals are extremely reactive within the cell, and the most effective protection mechanism is to prevent their formation, by enzyme-careactions, rather than trying to scavenge them once formed. Catalase dismutates H_2O_2 to H_2O and O_2, and peroxidase reduces hydroperoxides using GSH. The only possible biologically relevant antioxidant able to react with hydroxyperoxyl radicals is α-tocopherol [37]. Its subsequent radical formed, and the α-tocopheroxyl radical is reduced back by ascorbic acid [25].

Cells are able to adapt its redox potential increasing antioxidant enzymes, leading to transcription factors that act as redox sensors. Some antioxidants possess hormetic actions by upregulating the expression and activity of antioxidant defense enzymes, as well as by activating endothelial nitric oxide synthase (eNOS) that increases NO production and hence ameliorates vascular tone. The reaction of phytochemical antioxidants with free radicals gives oxidized products that are involved in signal transduction pathways. The last consequence is the activation of enzyme antioxidant activity and repair systems. Enzyme-catalyzed reactions occur at higher reaction rates than free radical scavenging by exogenous antioxidants.

One of the main pathways involved is nuclear factor erythroid 2-related factor 2 (Nrf2). Nrf2 is linked to the protein Keap 1 and remains inactive in the cytosol until Keap1 is oxidized. Nrf2 then translocates to nucleus where it activates ARE genes. The activation of the Nrf2 transcription factor and the antioxidant response element (ARE) to which Nrf2 binds conducts to the transcription of genes encoding phase II detoxification enzymes.

Reports about the activation of this signaling pathway by compounds within the diet are increasing recently. Dietary soy has shown to inhibit atherosclerotic lesion progression by a mechanism that involves this Nrf2 gene transcription. Other phytochemicals include curcumin from turmeric [38], diallyl sulfide from garlic [39], isothiocyanates as sulforaphane from broccoli [40], and polyphenols from apple [41].

These mechanistic studies have been performed with pure compounds, and it is conceivable that supplementation with antioxidants in concentrations that saturate this system can exert none or even harmful effects [24]. Hence, it is advisable to provide an adequate level of antioxidants by nutritional intake to regulate the antioxidant system in a physiological basis.

Bioactive compounds

"Bioactive compounds" are extranutritional constituents that typically occur in small quantities in foods. Epidemiological studies have demonstrated that nutritional habits, like those based on high consumption of foods rich in bioactive substances (natural products derived from plants, marine organisms, and animals), have been associated with a longer life expectancy and a significant decrease in the incidence and prevalence of several chronic diseases with inflammatory basis, such as CVD [42].

These bioactive compounds possess a wide range of biological activities including antitumor, anti-inflammatory, anticarcinogenic, antiviral, antimicrobial, antidiarrheal, antioxidant, and other activities [43].

Dietary supplementation with bioactive natural compounds demonstrated that lipid-lowering effects (cholesterol synthesis inhibitors, intestinal cholesterol absorption inhibitors, and LDL-C excretion stimulants) are currently supported by the international guidelines for CVD prevention and some international expert panels [44].

Omega-3

The functions of the fatty acids are diverse. In addition to their energetic value, they are also part of the phospholipids found in the membranes of the body's cells and determine in a greater or lesser extent the structure and functionality of the cell. Such functionality refers to aspects like fluidity and permeability, lipid peroxidation, etc. [45]. Experimental, epidemiological, and interventional studies have demonstrated the beneficial cardiovascular effects of eicosapentaenoic acid (EPA) and docosahexaenoic acid (DHA), which have anti-atherosclerotic, antithrombotic, antiarrhythmic, and anti-inflammatory effects.

Food contains omega-3 fatty acids in three main active forms: eicosapentaenoic acid (20: 5 omega 3, EPA), docosahexaenoic acid (22: 6 omega-3, DHA) and alphalinolenic acid (18: 3 omega-3, a-ALA). EPA and DHA forms can be found in fish oils, fish that mainly live in cold waters such as salmon, tuna, and sardines, among other varieties. EPA, DHA, and ALA are essential fatty acids, and they need to be ingested in the diet, since the body cannot synthesize them [46].

In a study, it was showed that the intake of EPA and DHA is inversely related to cardiovascular risk in a dose-dependent manner up to about 250 mg/day in healthy populations, and the intake of 1 g/day is associated with a marked protection from a sudden cardiac death [47]. The daily recommended intake of omega-3 fatty acids varies from 250 mg to 1 g of EPA and DHA.

Polyphenols

Polyphenols are bioactive compounds that can be found mostly in foods like fruits, cereals, vegetables, dry legumes, and chocolate and beverages such as coffee, tea, and wine. They are extensively used in the prevention and treatment of cardiovascular disease (CVD) providing protection against many chronic illnesses [48].

Polyphenols can regulate cellular lipid metabolism, vascular and endothelial function, hemostasis, as well as platelet function, which represent primary conditions for atherosclerotic plaque formation and development. The cardioprotective effects of polyphenols have been linked mainly to its antioxidant properties; however, recent findings attribute its anti-atherosclerotic potential to modulate simultaneous signaling and mechanistic pathways [42]. Recently, the PREDIMED study reported that dietary polyphenols intake such as extra-virgin olive oil and nuts were associated with improved CVD risk factors and decreased inflammatory biomarker levels in high-CVD-risk participants [49].

Moreover, polyphenols alter hepatic cholesterol absorption, triglyceride biosynthesis and lipoprotein secretion, the processing of lipoproteins in plasma, and inflammation [48]. A recent study showed that polyphenols intake decreased blood pressure (BP), increased plasma high-density lipoprotein (HDL) and decreased the inflammatory biomarkers of CVD, including vascular cell adhesion molecule 1 (VCAM-1), intercellular adhesion molecule 1 (ICAM-1), IL-6, TNF-α as well as MCP-1. Treatment with quercetin ameliorated the high-fat diet-induced MetS such as abdominal obesity, cardiovascular remodeling, and liver complications in rats by increasing the expression of Nrf2, HO-1, and carnitine palmitoyltransferase 1 (CPT1) and decreasing NF-κB [50].

Finally, it has been reported that the effects of polyphenols on human health depend on the amount consumed and on their bioavailability.

Phytosterols

Phytosterols are bioactive compounds found in foods of plant origin, which can be divided into plant sterols and plant stanols. Food sources of phytosterols include vegetable oils, mainly corn (909 mg/100 mL), sunflower (411 mg/100 mL), soybean (320 mg/100 mL), and olive (300 mg/100 mL); oleaginous fruits such as almonds (183 mg/100 g); cereals like wheat germ (344 mg/100 g) and wheat bran (200 mg/100 g); and in addition fruits and vegetables, such as passion fruit (44 mg/100 g), orange (24 mg/100 g), and cauliflower (40 mg/100 g) [51].

Clinical studies consistently indicate that the intake of phytosterols (2 g/day) is associated with a significant reduction (8–10%) in levels of low-density lipoprotein cholesterol (LDL-cholesterol). A typical Western diet contains approximately 300 mg of sterols and 30 mg of plant stanols, while vegetarian diets can achieve a higher content (300–500 mg/day). Phytosterols intake based on regular diets is considered too low to achieve their recommended daily intake -which are able to present therapeutic effects on LDL-cholesterol reduction-, (~2 g/day), and the consumption of foods enriched with phytosterols or, alternatively, the use of supplements of phytosterol are generally required [52].

In the last decades, purified plant sterols or stanols have been added to various food items to obtain functional foods with remarkable hypocholesterolemic activity. A daily intake of plant sterols or stanols of 1.6–2 g/day, incorporated in these foods, is able to reduce cholesterol absorption from the gut by about 30% and plasma LDL-cholesterol levels by 8–10% [53].

Most guidelines and consensus on the treatment of dyslipidemia and/or prevention of CVD recommend the intake of phytosterols in the amount of approximately 2 g/day with the goal of reducing LDL-cholesterol by approximately 10%, in association with lifestyle changes [54].

Hydroxytyrosol

Hydroxytyrosol, 2-(3,4-dihydroxyphenyl)-ethanol (OHTYR), is a phenolic compound present in the fruit and leaf of the olive (*Olea europaea* L.), which belongs to the family Oleaceae, comprising species distributed throughout the temperate regions of the world, and essentially localized in the Mediterranean basin. Another natural source of OHTYR is red wine [55]. In fact, daily intake of hydroxytyrosol in the Mediterranean area would be 2 mg (considering the maximum 50 mg/day). This amount would be insufficient to reach the recommended amount of 5 mg to develop the benefit of protection of LDL particles from oxidative damage [56].

Numerous human and animal studies have shown that olive polyphenols, particularly hydroxytyrosol, can improve blood cholesterol profiles and reduce the risk of potentially lethal thrombosis [57]. Hydroxytyrosol can be considered antithrombotic, since it significantly reduces platelet aggregation [58].

Various authors support the potential beneficial effects of hydroxytyrosol in atherogenesis through the reduction of LDL oxidation. In addition to hydroxytyrosol, oleuropein has also been shown to effectively inhibit LDL oxidation induced by copper sulfate [59].

Melatonin

Melatonin (N-acetyl-5-methoxytryptamine) is a neuroendocrine hormone, which is synthesized primarily by the pineal gland. The synthesis and secretion of melatonin are regulated by light intensity [60]. Melatonin-rich foods include various food components from both animal and plant origins such as chicken, lamb, pork, cow milk, strawberries, tomatoes, olives, grapes, wines, cereals, and cherries. Interestingly, melatonin concentrations are significantly higher in plants than in animals [61].

Importantly, recent research suggests that melatonin plays an important role in various cardiovascular diseases, including myocardial ischemia-reperfusion injury, atherosclerosis, hypertension, heart failure, drug-induced myocardial injury, pulmonary hypertension, vascular diseases, valvular heart diseases, and lipid metabolism.

Early experiments showed that treatment with melatonin can improve dyslipidemia. In patients with nonalcoholic fatty liver disease, treatment with melatonin (2 × 5 mg/day) for 14 months significantly reduced levels of triglycerides and LDL- cholesterol (LDL-C) compared with controls [62].

Yang et al. [63] demonstrated that melatonin reduces flow shear stress-induced bone marrow mesenchymal stem cell injury by acting on melatonin receptors and the adenosine monophosphate-activated protein kinase/acetyl-CoA carboxylase signaling pathway. These findings suggest that targeting melatonin relating signaling in tissue-engineered heart valves may be an effective strategy in treating valvular heart disease.

Melatonin may improve vascular dysfunction by affecting epigenetic regulation. In mice generated with assisted reproductive technologies, treatment with melatonin resulted in decreased arterial hypertension, which was thought to be due to its effects on normalizing nitric oxide levels by preventing impaired methylation of endothelial nitric oxide synthase [64].

Borghi and Cicero [65] confirmed the blood pressure (BP)-lowering effects of melatonin. It was shown that patients treated with melatonin (2–5mg/day for 7–90 days) had a decrease in nocturnal SBP as well as DBP. Additionally, it was demonstrated that the effect of melatonin on decreasing BP was most pronounced from 3:00 am to 8:00 am [66].

Pulmonary hypertension is a disease characterized by elevated pulmonary arterial pressure, which leads to right ventricular hypertrophy and failure. Various authors reported that treatment with melatonin alleviated right ventricular hypertrophy and dysfunction and also reduced interstitial fibrosis and plasma oxidative stress in a rat model of pulmonary hypertension [67].

As an inexpensive and well-tolerated drug, melatonin may be a new therapeutic option for cardiovascular disease [54].

Conclusions

There is a clear relationship between diet and cardiovascular health. A hearthealthy diet should contain fruits and vegetables, which are rich in fiber and bioactive compounds. Foods rich in omega-3 fatty acids such as nuts or blue fish should not be missing from this diet. There is no scientific evidence relating egg or daily products consumption with increased cardiovascular risk (CVR). In fact, dairy products protects against CVR. Finally, consumption of processed meats is related to increased CVR, due to its high salt content. In fact, dietary guidelines recommend the reduction consumption of these processed meats.

On the other hand, given that oxidative stress is the basis of CVD, a diet rich in antioxidants may be useful in prevention. Among the antioxidants we must highlight the α-tocopherols, vitamin C, and the polyphenols present in fruits and vegetables. However, supplementation has not been shown to have preventive effects on CVD.

Both omega-3, polyphenols, and phytosterols have been shown to decrease CVR factors and inflammatory markers in patients with elevated CVR.

Finally, we must highlight the hydroxytyrosol and melatonin, which are involved in the reduction of LDL oxidation and in the improvement of dyslipidemia, respectively.

Acknowledgements

The authors want to thanks the UCAM for supporting the present chapter.

Conflict of interest

The authors declare that they have no conflict of interest.

Author details

Javier Marhuenda, Débora Villaño, Begoña Cerdá and María Pilar Zafrilla* Bachelor in Pharmacy, Health Sciences Faculty, Catholic University of Murcia, Murcia, Spain

*Address all correspondence to: mpzafrilla@ucam.edu

References

[1] Alemán JA, Rentero MZ. Alimentación y riesgo cardiovascular. 2010

[2] Berciano S, Ordovás JM. Nutrición y salud cardiovascular. Revista Española de Cardiología. 2014;67(9):738-747

[3] Oyebode O, Gordon-Dseagu V, Walker A, Mindell JS. Fruit and vegetable consumption and all-cause, cancer and CVD mortality: Analysis of health survey for England data. Journal of Epidemiology and Community Health. 2014;68:856-862

[4] Pearce S, Ferguson N, Karl J, Arcidiacono S, Soares J, Racicot K, et al. Effects of dietary fiber by-product short-chain fatty acids on intestinal cell physiology and health. In: Abstracts of Papers of the American Chemical Society. AMER Chemical SOC 1155 16TH St, NW, Washington, DC 20036 USA. 2018

[5] Threapleton DE, Greenwood DC, Evans CEL, Cleghorn CL, Nykjaer C, Woodhead C, et al. Dietary fibre intake and risk of cardiovascular disease: Systematic review and meta-analysis. BMJ [Internet]. 2013;347. Available from: https://www.bmj.com/content/ bmj/347/bmj.f6879.full.pdf

[6] Chen G-C, Lv D-B, Pang Z, Dong J-Y, Liu Q-F. Dietary fiber intake and stroke risk: A meta-analysis of prospective cohort studies. European Journal of Clinical Nutrition. 2012;67:96

[7] Hartley L, Flowers N, Holmes J, Clarke A, Stranges S, Hooper L, et al. Green and black tea for the primary prevention of cardiovascular disease. Cochrane Database of Systematic Reviews. 2013;6:CD009934

[8] Ugai T, Matsuo K, Sawada N, Iwasaki M, Yamaji T, Shimazu T, et al. Coffee and green tea consumption and subsequent risk of acute myeloid leukemia and myelodysplastic syndromes in Japan. International Journal of Cancer. 2018;142(6):1130-1138

[9] Roth I, Casas R, Medina-Remón A, Lamuela-Raventós RM, Estruch R. Consumption of aged white wine modulates cardiovascular risk factors via circulating endothelial progenitor cells and inflammatory biomarkers. Clinical Nutrition. 2018

[10] Tverdal A, Magnus P, Selmer R, Thelle D. Consumption of alcohol and cardiovascular disease mortality: A 16 year follow-up of 115,592 Norwegian men and women aged 40-44 years. European Journal of Epidemiology. 2017;32(9):775-783

[11] Rebello SA, van Dam RM. Coffee consumption and cardiovascular health: Getting to the heart of the matter. Current Cardiology Reports. 2013;15(10):403

[12] Vergroesen AJ. Dietary fat and cardiovascular disease: Possible modes of action of linoleic acid. The Proceedings of the Nutrition Society. 1972;31(3):323-329

[13] Fodor JG, Helis E, Yazdekhasti N, Vohnout B. "Fishing" for the origins of the "Eskimos and heart disease" story: Facts or wishful thinking? The Canadian Journal of Cardiology. 2014;30(8):864-868

[14] Bang HO, Dyerberg J, Nielsen A. Plasma lipid and lipoprotein pattern in Greenlandic west-coast Eskimos. The Lancet. 1971;297(7710):1143-1146

[15] Soriano-Maldonado A, Cuenca- García M, Moreno LA, González-Gross M, Leclercq C, Androutsos O, et al. Ingesta de huevo y factores de riesgo cardiovascular en adolescentes; papel de la actividad física: Estudio HELENA. Nutrición Hospitalaria. 2013;28(3):868-877

[16] Nakamura Y, Okamura T, Kita Y, Okuda N, Kadota A, Miura K, et al. Re-evaluation of the associations of egg intake with serum total cholesterol and cause-specific and total mortality in Japanese women. European Journal of Clinical Nutrition. 2017;1

[17] Khawaja O, Singh H, Luni F, Kabour A, Ali SS, Taleb M, et al. Egg consumption and incidence of heart failure: A meta- analysis of prospective cohort studies. Frontiers in Nutrition. 2017;4:10

[18] Brown JM, Hazen SL. Meta- organismal nutrient metabolism as a basis of cardiovascular disease. Current Opinion in Lipidology. 2014;25(1):48

[19] Lawrence GD. Dietary fats and health: Dietary recommendations in the context of scientific evidence. Advances in Nutrition. 2013;4(3):294-302

[20] Huth PJ, Park KM. Influence of dairy product and milk fat consumption on cardiovascular disease risk: A review of the evidence. Advances in Nutrition. 2012;3(3):266-285

[21] Kratz M, Baars T, Guyenet S. The relationship between high-fat dairy consumption and obesity, cardiovascular, and metabolic disease. European Journal of Nutrition. 2013;52(1):1-24

[22] Mann GE, Bonacasa B, Ishii T, Siow RC. Targeting the redox sensitive Nrf2–Keap1 defense pathway in cardiovascular disease: Protection afforded by dietary isoflavones. Current Opinion in Pharmacology. 2009;9(2):139-145

[23] Sena LA, Chandel NS. Physiological roles of mitochondrial reactive oxygen species. Molecular Cell. 2012;48(2):158-167

[24] Sthijns MM, Weseler AR, Bast A, Haenen GR. Time in redox adaptation processes: From evolution to hormesis. International Journal of Molecular Sciences. 2016;17(10):1649

[25] Nimse SB, Pal D. Free radicals, natural antioxidants, and their reaction mechanisms. RSC Advances. 2015;5(35):27986-28006

[26] Förstermann U. Oxidative stress in vascular disease: Causes, defense mechanisms and potential therapies. Nature Reviews. Cardiology. 2008;5(6):338

[27] Krieglstein CF, Granger DN. Adhesion molecules and their role in vascular disease. American Journal of Hypertension. 2001;14(S3):44S-54S

[28] Huang J, May JM. Ascorbic acid spares α-tocopherol and prevents lipid peroxidation in cultured H4IIE liver cells. Molecular and Cellular Biochemistry. 2003;247(1-2):171-176

[29] Di Meo F, Lemaur V, Cornil J, Lazzaroni R, Duroux J-L, Olivier Y, et al. Free radical scavenging by natural polyphenols: Atom versus electron transfer. The Journal of Physical Chemistry. A. 2013;117(10):2082-2092

[30] Aune D, Giovannucci E, Boffetta P, Fadnes LT, Keum N, Norat T, et al. Fruit and vegetable intake and the risk of cardiovascular disease, total cancer and all-cause mortality—A systematic review and dose-response meta-analysis of prospective studies. International Journal of Epidemiology. 2017;46(3):1029-1056

[31] Bjelakovic G, Nikolova D, Gluud C. Antioxidant supplements and mortality. Current Opinion in Clinical Nutrition and Metabolic Care. 2014;17(1):40-44

[32] Fortmann SP, Burda BU, Senger CA, Lin JS, Whitlock EP. Vitamin and mineral supplements in the primary prevention of cardiovascular disease and cancer: An updated systematic evidence review for the US Preventive Services Task Force. Annals of Internal Medicine. 2013;159(12):824-834

[33] Yoshihara D, Fujiwara N, Suzuki K. Antioxidants: Benefits and risks for long-term health. Maturitas. 2010;67(2):103-107

[34] Ye Y, Li J, Yuan Z. Effect of antioxidant vitamin supplementation on cardiovascular outcomes: A meta- analysis of randomized controlled trials. PLoS One. 2013;8(2):e56803

[35] Ristow M. Unraveling the truth about antioxidants: Mitohormesis explains ROS-induced health benefits. Nature Medicine. 2014;20(7):709

[36] Forman HJ, Davies KJ, Ursini F. How do nutritional antioxidants really work: Nucleophilic tone and para-hormesis versus free radical scavenging in vivo. Free Radical Biology & Medicine. 2014;66:24-35

[37] Karbownik M, Lewinski A, Reiter RJ. Anticarcinogenic actions of melatonin which involve antioxidative processes: Comparison with other antioxidants. The International Journal of Biochemistry & Cell Biology. 2001;33(8):735-753

[38] Fattori V, Pinho-Ribeiro FA, Borghi SM, Alves-Filho JC, Cunha TM, Cunha FQ , et al. Curcumin inhibits superoxide anion-induced pain-like behavior and leukocyte recruitment by increasing Nrf2 expression and reducing NF-κB activation. Inflammation Research. 2015;64(12):993-1003

[39] Kim S, Lee H-G, Park S-A, Kundu JK, Keum Y-S, Cha Y-N, et al. Keap1 cysteine 288 as a potential target for diallyl trisulfide-induced Nrf2 activation. PLoS One. 2014;9(1):e85984

[40] Houghton CA, Fassett RG, Coombes JS. Sulforaphane and other nutrigenomic Nrf2 activators: Can the clinician's expectation be matched by the reality? Oxidative Medicine and Cellular Longevity. 2016;2016

[41] Sharma S, Rana S, Patial V, Gupta M, Bhushan S, Padwad YS. Antioxidant and hepatoprotective effect of polyphenols from apple pomace extract via apoptosis inhibition and Nrf2 activation in mice. Human & Experimental Toxicology. 2016;35(12):1264-1275

[42] Santhakumar AB, Battino M, Alvarez-Suarez JM. Dietary polyphenols: Structures, bioavailability and protective effects against atherosclerosis. Food and Chemical Toxicology. 2018;113:49-65

[43] Wang TH, Wang SY, Wang XD, Jiang HQ , Yang YQ , Wang Y, et al. Fisetin exerts antioxidant and neuroprotective effects in multiple mutant hSOD1 models of amyotrophic lateral sclerosis by activating ERK. Neuroscience. 2018;379:152-166

[44] Wastesson JW, Morin L, Tan EC, Johnell K. An update on the clinical consequences of polypharmacy in older adults: A narrative review. Expert Opinion on Drug Safety. 2018;17(12):1185-1196

[45] Piñeiro-Corrales G, Lago Rivero N, Culebras-Fernández JM. Papel de los ácidos grasos omega-3 en la prevención de enfermedades cardiovasculares. Nutrición Hospitalaria. 2013;28(1):1-5

[46] Castellanos L, Rodriguez M. El efecto de omega 3 en la salud humana y consideraciones en la ingesta. Revista Chilena de Nutricion. 2015;42(1):90-95

[47] Kirkhus B, Lamglait A, Eilertsen K-E, Falch E, Haider T, Vik H, et al. Effects of similar intakes of marine n-3 fatty acids from enriched food products and fish oil on cardiovascular risk markers in healthy human subjects. The British Journal of Nutrition. 2012;107(9):1339-1349

[48] Giglio RV, Patti AM, Cicero AF, Lippi G, Rizzo M, Toth PP, et al. Polyphenols: Potential use in the prevention and treatment of cardiovascular diseases. Current Pharmaceutical Design. 2018;24(2):239-258

[49] Medina-Remón A, Casas R, Tressserra-Rimbau A, Ros E, Martínez- González MA, Fitó M, et al. Polyphenol intake from a Mediterranean diet decreases inflammatory biomarkers related to atherosclerosis: A substudy of the PREDIMED trial. British Journal of Clinical Pharmacology. 2017;83(1):114-128

[50] Panchal SK, Poudyal H, Brown L. Quercetin ameliorates cardiovascular, hepatic, and metabolic changes in diet-induced metabolic syndrome in rats. The Journal of Nutrition. 2012;142(6):1026-1032

[51] Gupta A, Jacobson GA, Burgess JR, Jelinek HF, Nichols DS, Narkowicz CK, et al. Citrus bioflavonoids possess dipeptidyl peptidase-4 inhibition activity similar to gliptin antidiabetic medication. Biochemical and Biophysical Research Communications. 2018

[52] Cabral CE, Klein MRST. Phytosterols in the treatment of hypercholesterolemia and prevention of cardiovascular diseases. Arquivos Brasileiros de Cardiologia. 2017;109(5):475-482

[53] Marangoni F, Poli A. Phytosterols and cardiovascular health. Pharmacological Research. 2010;61(3):193-199

[54] Pirro M, Vetrani C, Bianchi C, Mannarino MR, Bernini F, Rivellese AA. Joint position statement on "Nutraceuticals for the treatment of hypercholesterolemia" of the Italian Society of Diabetology (SID) and of the Italian Society for the Study of Arteriosclerosis (SISA). Nutrition, Metabolism, and Cardiovascular Diseases. 2017;27(1):2-17

[55] Marhuenda J, Medina S, Martínez- Hernández P, Arina S, Zafrilla P, Mulero J, et al. Effect of the dietary intake of melatonin-and hydroxytyrosol-rich wines by healthy female volunteers on the systemic lipidomic-related oxylipins. Food & Function. 2017;8(10):3745-3757

[56] De La Torre R, Covas MI, Pujadas MA, Fitó M, Farré M. Is dopamine behind the health benefits of red wine? European Journal of Nutrition. 2006;45(5):307-310

[57] Vilaplana-Pérez C, Auñón D, García-Flores LA, Gil-Izquierdo A. Hydroxytyrosol and potential uses in cardiovascular diseases, cancer, and AIDS. Frontiers in Nutrition. 2014;1:18

[58] Dell'Agli M, Buscialà A, Bosisio E. Vascular effects of wine polyphenols. Cardiovascular Research. 2004;63(4):593-602

[59] Killeen MJ, Pontoniere P, Crea RH. An examination of its potential role in cardiovascular disease, inflammation, and longevity. Agro Food Industry Hi Tech. 2011;22:16-19

[60] Arendt J, Bojkowski C, Franey C, Wright J, Marks V. Immunoassay of 6-hydroxymelatonin sulfate in human plasma and urine: Abolition of the urinary 24-hour rhythm with atenolol. The Journal of Clinical Endocrinology and Metabolism. 1985;60(6):1166-1173

[61] Tan DX, Hardeland R, Manchester LC, Rosales-Corral S, Coto-Montes A, Boga JA, et al. Emergence of naturally occurring melatonin isomers and their proposed nomenclature. Journal of Pineal Research. 2012;53(2):113-121

[62] Celinski K, Konturek PC, Slomka M, Cichoz-Lach H, Brzozowski T, Konturek SJ, et al. Effects of treatment with melatonin and tryptophan on liver enzymes, parameters of fat metabolism and plasma levels of cytokines in patients with non-alcoholic fatty liver disease—14 months follow up. Journal of Physiology and Pharmacology.

2014;65(1):75-82

[63] Yang Y, Fan C, Deng C, Zhao L, Hu W, Di S, et al. Melatonin reverses flow shear stress-induced injury in bone marrow mesenchymal stem cells via activation of AMP-activated protein kinase signaling. Journal of Pineal Research. 2016;60(2):228-241

[64] Rexhaj E, Pireva A, Paoloni- Giacobino A, Allemann Y, Cerny D, Dessen P, et al. Prevention of vascular dysfunction and arterial hypertension in mice generated by assisted reproductive technologies by addition of melatonin to culture media. American Journal of Physiology-Heart and Circulatory Physiology. 2015;309(7):H1151-H1156

[65] Borghi C, Cicero AF. Nutraceuticals with a clinically detectable blood pressure-lowering effect: A review of available randomized clinical trials and their meta-analyses. British Journal of Clinical Pharmacology. 2017;83(1):163-171

[66] Gubin DG, Gubin GD, Gapon LI, Weinert D. Daily melatonin administration attenuates age- dependent disturbances of cardiovascular rhythms. Current Aging Science. 2016;9(1):5-13

[67] Torres F, González-Candia A, Montt C, Ebensperger G, Chubretovic M, Serón-Ferré M, et al. Melatonin reduces oxidative stress and improves vascular function in pulmonary hypertensive newborn sheep. Journal of Pineal Research. 2015;58(3):362-373

8

Microbial Contamination in Milk Quality and Health Risk of the Consumers of Raw Milk and Dairy Products

Valente Velázquez-Ordoñez, Benjamín Valladares-Carranza, Esvieta Tenorio-Borroto, Martín Talavera-Rojas, Jorge Antonio Varela-Guerrero, Jorge Acosta-Dibarrat, Florencia Puigvert, Lucia Grille, Álvaro González Revello and Lucia Pareja

Abstract

The dairy products industry is going toward safe milk and its products in the food market. Milk quality and food safety concern in the consumers' health and nutrition in public health surveillance prevent food-borne diseases, food poisoning, and zoonosis risk by raw milk and fresh dairy products. The aim of this work is focused on milk microbial contamination and its impacts on milk production and dairy industry with their implications in milk product quality, food-borne diseases from raw milk, and unpasteurized milk by food-borne pathogen microbial contamination and milk and dairy product spoilage. The microbial milk contamination source comes from herd hygiene and health status, mastitis prevalence, production environment, and milking parlor and milk conserving practices in dairy farm. Moreover, these facts are implicated in milk quality and milk spoilage and unsafe dairy products. The milk production system and the dairy plant operations keep track in pasteurized milk and fresh dairy products reviewing the traceability in field situational diagnosis report.

Keywords: cow milk production, food safety, food-borne disease, milk contamination, milk spoilage

Introduction

The objective of the dairy industry is to maintain productivity and competitiveness in a growing milk commerce, which is demanding a large volume of milk and a wide range of dairy products in the food market and the preferences of the final food consumer with remarkable differences according to patterns of consumer behavior by demographic categories, culture, and socioeconomic variations in the human population in the food market [1, 2]. The consumers prefer a safe and healthy milk product selection, with a great variety and availability in the market. This fact affects the health and nutrition consumer's information about the milk products made with raw milk [3, 4]. Milk is also an important source of bacterial infection for human health, when milk is consumed without pasteurization [5–7]. Milk is a basic food in the human diet with great value as a nutritious healthy food; in the first years of human life, milk and dairy products are an important nutritional fact in the diet of the adult population [8]. According to the sustainable production system, their main priorities are contributing to the regional social and economic development, land resource preservation, and animal welfare quality in dairy cattle husbandry maintaining a productive healthy cow herd to produce high milk quality [9]. The global responsibilities of the milk industry and big dairy farm and small holder producers are offering high-quality milk and safe dairy products in the commerce preventing food-borne diseases to spread in the population [10, 11].

The source of milk contamination

The milk market requires and offers safe and high-quality products, preventing a contamination source by good hygiene practices to reduce a possible exposure of food-borne pathogens and chemical milk residues. The mammary gland participates in the excretion of numerous xenobiotic substances from veterinary drug milk residues and contaminants originated from milk and other chemical residues to environmental pollutants on the grasslands, animal feedstuffs, and the field crops [12]. The presence of residual concentrations of milk contaminants and pathogens is an indicator of milk quality in cow dairy farms. In evaluating the raw milk bulk tank at the dairy farms, quick information about udder health status, environmental pathogens, milk chemical residues, and antibiotics is obtained [13–16]. The relationship among dairy cow production and milk safety and dairy product quality is considered in different subjects: raw and pasteurized milk contamination and microbial aspects of the quality of milk and dairy products, cow husbandry in animal welfare influence, feeding conditions, and herd hygiene practices and milk composition. Also the environmental pollutants, and chemicals from agriculture, pesticides residues, drug veterinary residues and management in dairy production. Those relationships that exist in milk production are auditable and selectively regulated to prevent milk contaminants. The contaminants agents are trackingand monitored at milk parlor, in refrigerated milk tank and the milk bulk tank on platform by the application of proper sampling methods required in the Control Analytical Methods for milk quality in Dairy Industry Management assurance the food safety [17]. Are affecting milk production and dairy products related to food safety and milk quality [18]. In the phenomenon of the climatic change, the zoonosis and food-borne diseases are priorities in the public health programs in many countries, ones of the surveillance task is the diseases transmitted by raw milk, and unpasteurized fresh dairy products [19, 20]. The aflatoxin M1 contamination levels in milk appear to be a serious health hazard derivate from hepatotoxic and carcinogen effects of aflatoxin M1, which show a high risk on milk food safety. The milk contamination risk is established through the forages, corn and concentrated feeds; those are contaminated by aflatoxin B1 (AFB1). There is an aim to watch over the limit exposure to aflatoxins in dairy by imposing regulatory limits [21]. The presence of biotics from grazing cows and conserved pastures and feeding grains, like aflatoxins AFB1 and AFM2, has been usually monitored in milk [22]. In dairy production, an important practice is oriented to reduce environment fungal contamination and the proper conserving methods of silages, forages, and grains for animal feed [23]. The controlled grazing land is a relevant characteristic of the milk produced at grazing, was its richness in beta-carotene, lutein, vitamin E and sesquiterpenes among winter seasonal period monitored farms. These conditions should have a great influence on the physicochemical milk profile of raw milk bulk tank at dairy farm, in comparison with the milk of the producers with herds fed with diets rich in concentrate, corn silage, and pasture [24]. The silage is a significant source of contamination of raw milk with spores compared with grass and maize silage. Preventive management of outgrowth of aerobic spores in silage by the application of acid lactic bacteria or chemical additives can improve the silage fermentation; it will contribute to reduce the total spore load of raw milk for dairy process [25]. The microbial contamination of milk could be produced from sources of bacteria and fungi are identified in grassland and other feedstuffs. The health herd status will be implicated in specific zoonosis produced by animal carriers of *Salmonella* spp., *Mycobacterium bovis, Mycobacterium avium* subsp. *paratuberculosis*, and Brucellosis and *Escherichia coli* 0157H7 are focused by sanitary conditions and the health risk [26, 27]. The health level status is an important issue in milk production; the maintenance of herd hygiene, disease control programs, and preventive management is oriented to reduce the prevalence of contagious diseases in dairy cattle [28]. The others sources of milk contamination may be present in the herd management, poor hygiene milk practices, mastitis, infectious pathogens in infected cows and the presence of environmental pathogens by poor animal hygiene [7]. The good hygiene practices in the herd cow is an important fact for to reduce contamination from production environment, feces, slurry, soil and mud those are microbial sources for the udder contamination. The poor hygiene practices could occurs microbial milk contamination, pathogens dissemination, and udder contamination may be occurred at milking time between cows, hands of milkier man and milk machine from others [29]. The microbial analysis of raw milk are influenced by microorganisms present in the teat canal and the surface of teat skin [30]. The bad hygiene practices and poor cleanness procedure equipment, the surrounding air in the milk parlor, as well as other environmental factors including housing conditions, water supply, and during feeding have an important effect on the milk contamination [31, 32]. Other microbial contamination of milk possibility may occur during the long milk storage, under low insufficient temperature [33]. Usually contaminated environments are a potential source of food-borne pathogens and spoilage bacteria present in raw milk bulk tank in the dairy farm, which are affecting the milk quality and emerging public health risk [34–36]. The cow herd should be monitored for preventing possible food-borne pathogens and food intoxications, which is a preventive strategy for health risks and to diminish the poor dairy product quality. The variation of the milk components of bulk milk among herds, could give an approach of the grassland interaction among the dairy cows, the environmental pollutants, and the environment health status have a potential public health risk [37]. In dairy farms the milk tank study is widely used for monitoring the herd udder health status as an indicator of quality for milk producers used by the dairy industry [38]. Through a microbiological study, it is possible to know the possible bacterial contamination source for modifying hygiene practices and to recall critical bacterial contamination in milk traceability for preventing the milk spoilage on the quality of the pasteurized milk and dairy products, affecting the consumer's acceptability.

When milk food-borne disease outbreaks occur in the human population, there are other many reasons to trace back and investigate; fresh cheeses are elaborated with non-pasteurized milk or elaborated without proper hygiene conditions using pasteurized and unpasteurized milk [3, 28, 39]. Outbreaks of milk food-borne diseases (**Table 1**) have been associated with diseases due to infected foods and contaminated dairy products after pasteurization [40]. Another consideration of food-borne pathogens in raw milk into dairy food processing plants can persist in biofilms, with subsequent contamination of processed milk products. Inadequate milk pasteurization allows survival of food-borne pathogens in milk and dairy products [41, 42]. The health educational program for the human population should be oriented to reduce the risk of exposure for food borne diseases by the information in the end of the food chain, by adequate handling of milk and dairy products at home for prevention of the risk of food-borne diseases thought the consumption of non-pasteurized raw milk and dairy products prepared with unsafe hygiene practices in dairy food process [42–44].

Table 1. *Food-borne pathogens and food poisoning in milk production source.*

Mammary gland health status	Cow herd health status	Production environment	Production land water source
S. aureus *Streptococcus agalactiae* *Streptococcus* spp. *Streptococcus pyogenes* *Streptococcus zooepidemicus* (B-hemolytic *Streptococcus* Lancefield C group) *Corynebacterium ulcerans*	*Mycobacterium bovis* *Mycobacterium avium* subsp. *paratuberculosis* *Brucella* ssp. *S. aureus* MRSA-LA *Salmonella typhimurium* phage type 561 (STM DT7)	*Listeria monocytogenes* *Salmonella ssp.* *E. coli O 157:H7* *E. coli (STEC)* *E. coli (EHEC)* *Yersinia enterocolitica* *Enterobacter sakazakii* *Campylobacter jejuni* *Enterococcus faecalis* *Citrobacter freundii* *Bacillus cereus* +*Cryptosporidium parvum* *Coxiella burnetii** *Toxoplasma gondii**	Hepatitis A virus* *Leptospira* spp.* +*Bacillus licheniformis* +*Bacillus subtilis* +*Pseudomonas aeruginosa* +*Clostridium disporicum* *Aspergillus* spp. Aflatoxin M1 Mycotoxin B1

*Occasionally
+Involved in enteric diseases

Udder health and the milk quality

The infectious bovine mastitis in milk production is considered a disease with high economic impact reducing milk yield and the industrial dairy process and food safety. *S. aureus* and *Streptococcus agalactiae* are the most prevalent contagious pathogens in bovine mastitis from dairy herds around the world. The intramammary infection in dairy cows is relationship with infections by contagious pathogens and environmental pathogens as coliforms bacteria and *Streptococcus uberis* mostly are occurring in the dry period and the lactation in clinical cases regularly [45]. In the dairy herd with low prevalence of subclinical mastitis, the milk losses could be estimated between 3 and 5 % of the milk yield production, comparing to a herd average within milk somatic cell counts about 200,000 cells/mL [46]. The change in milk yield and composition depends of the severity and duration of the mammary gland infection and somatic cells counts.

In an uninfected mammary gland that contains <100,000 somatic cells/ mL, >200,000/mL, somatic cells counts suggest an incipient mammary gland inflammatory response [47, 48]. The bovine mastitis in dairy herds affects milk composition and somatic cells counts, serum protein, and proteolytic enzymes. Other undesirable milk mastitis conditions are bacterial toxins and abnormal proteins derived from inflammatory tissular response, which influence milk flavor and taste as well as milk product stability in the dairy process [46]. A wide variety of environmental pathogen exposure routes have been documented during the last decade; at present new pathogens and transmission routes are emerging. The main food-borne disease outbreaks comes from notified from the consumption of milk food products. The accidental ingestion of fresh dairy products contaminated with *E. coli* and other food-borne pathogens were originated from the soil or water provokes mainly enteric diseases. The knowledge regarding to biotic and abiotic factors involved in the survival or enhance of the agents, and their potential dissemination in the environment, and exposure routes of the main food borne pathogens, are considered now in the investigation of the public health risks from dairy farms [49]. In the prevention and control strategies applied to mastitis in dairy herds, can be included in the program by a situational diagnosis previous provide information about of herd somatic cell counts, microbial agents and mastitis in different clinical stages. This wide study is done to provide strategic information of herd hygiene status, milking hygiene practices, and milk machines' regular maintenance for proper functioning. The monitoring of somatic cell counts from the milk tank, and the lactating dairy cows, and dry cow period. To bring information about of the mammary gland health status in the surveillance program [50–52]. Antibiotic milk residues, are commonly associated with mastitis treatment in lactating cows; non observe the legal restriction and milk discard period in medicated cows; in those cases are expected more mastitis incidence of the cows, with lower milk somatic cells counts herd-year SCC, with mean values of >500,000 somatic cells/mL, are indicating an increases of mastitis cases in the cow population during the lactation period. It will have potential detection of antibiotic residues in the tank milk; these situations illustrate the importance of the maintenance of udder health and milk hygiene practices and cow selection genetic programs [45, 53]. Preand post-milking disinfectant routines help to reduce dramatically the infection, while udder hygiene in the milking routine directly dismisses mastitis cow pathogen transmission [50]. The prudent antibiotic use in cow herd medication schemes will help efficacy in clinical mastitis cases and dry cow infections. In contrast an increase in the incidence of mastitis in lactating cows will increase the potential risk for antibiotic residues of milk and antibiotic bacterial resistance in herd [54].

The development of antibiotic resistance in bacterial pathogens from dairy herds, is considered an emerging public health risk as many countries derived from dairy herds and the development of antibiotic resistance in bacterial pathogens [55]. *S. aureus* resistant strains (ORSA/MRSA), which are subject of surveillance programs of bacterial antibiotic resistance in human health [56, 57]. The use of antibiotics in animal food is incriminated as to be partly responsible for emergence of antibioticresistant bacteria with an importance in human medicine. The methicillin-resistant *S. aureus* (MRSA) strain was identified in animal companion and small dairy herds. The MRSA in humans is wildly studied in nosocomial infections and home care patients [58, 59]. The regulations of antibiotic and veterinary drug administration surveillance in animal food should be observed by agriculture department authorities [60]. The bacterial growth inhibitor test is to be performed by different conventional methods, such as the agar diffusion test with *Bacillus stearothermophilus* variety *calidolactis*, sensitive to β-lactamic antibiotics. The test is less effective in the detection of spiramycin, sulfonamide, or chloramphenicol milk residues. When the test of inhibitors of bacterial growth is testing with *Streptococcus thermophilus, Bacillus subtilis, Bacillus megaterium, Bacillus* cereus, and *Micrococcus luteus*, the sensitivity of the test for antibiotic macrolides and sulfonamides will increase slightly [61].

Food-borne pathogens from milk

The surveillance of food-borne disease in primary purpose in the herd is to characterize potential pathogens which are recovered from animal, milk tank, milk pipelines, and milking equipment, including the man milkers and the production environments. The monitoring programs have been designed to determine the milk production process' critical points, the health herd level, and control of animal risk for food-borne pathogens; a survey is oriented to cut the chain of disease and exposure routes to humans preventing milk and dairy product contamination [62, 63]. The surveillance of food-borne diseases usually is difficult to research an area for population monitoring. An outbreak survey of human gastrointestinal disease could be an epidemiological indicator of food-borne disease, which may be originated from drinking unpasteurized milk; *Salmonella* species can be found in ice cream and fresh cheeses as well as *Brucella melitensis* in non-pasteurized milk and homemade dairy products mostly goat cheese [42, 64]. The main zoonotic pathogens identified in raw milk were *Brucella* ssp., mainly *Brucella melitensis, Listeria monocytogenes, Salmonella* ssp., *Mycobacterium bovis, Yersinia enterocolitica, Streptococcus pyogenes*, and *Streptococcus agalactiae,* and *Escherichia coli* O157:H7 and *Enterobacter sakazakii* are recently reported [5, 65]. New emerging pathogens causing milk food-borne diseases are considered: hepatitis A virus, *Mycobacterium avium* subsp. *paratuberculosis, Streptococcus zooepidemicus* (B-hemolytic *Streptococcus* Lancefield C group), *Campylobacter jejuni, Citrobacter freundii, Corynebacterium ulcerans*, and *Cryptosporidium parvum* [66]. The food-borne pathogens predominantly have been involved in human disease and have originated often in many food animals as well as animal in active carrier states such as in *Salmonella* species, *E. coli* O157:H7, *Campylobacter* species, *Yersinia enterocolitica, Listeria* species, *Aeromonas hydrophila, Leptospira interrogans*, and *Mycobacterium* species. In contrast, *Coxiella burnetii, Cryptosporidium parvum*, and *Toxoplasma gondii* may be infrequent [67]. The Campylobacter infections are expected seasonally as many cases are reported to public health services [4]. Food-borne outbreaks are incriminated occurring with contaminated fresh milk and dairy products provoking acute infections and food intoxications, occurring in family's at small villages, in declared official cases confirmed with consumption of homemade fresh dairy products elaborated with non-pasteurized milk [66, 68]. The outbreaks of food-borne disease could occur after milk pasteurization and manipulating dairy products. Outbreak cases were investigated and tested by laboratory microbial probe tests for rapid detection of microbial contamination and toxins produced by *Salmonella* species, *Listeria* species, and *S. aureus* enterotoxins [39, 67]. The enzyme-linked assays for microbial and toxins and the DNA probe test are very useful for screening food samples before processing and traceability in food conserving microbial testing [49, 68]. The dairy cattle are also known reservoirs for *Salmonella* species; the animal carrier is often asymptomatic and difficult to identify because *Salmonella* prevalence is fluctuating in the seasonal period from fecal samples, tank milk, filters milk, and water. Other areas in the farm were also positives in samples from production environments like high-animal-traffic areas [34]. The dairy cow farms suspected to *Salmonella typhimurium* phage type 561 (STM DT7 international typing scheme), are strongly investigated in environment and microbiological carrier cows prompt agent detection, for triggering control measures and herd hygiene for to cut off contamination level in dairy products [69]. The *Klebsiella* species, *Enterobacter* ssp., and *Salmonella* ssp. might be present in raw milk depending of hygienic practices in the herd [1]. *Yersinia enterocolitica* O: 8 outbreaks resulted from post-pasteurization contamination. In other cases no deficiencies in pasteurization procedures or equipment were detected. *Y. enterocolitica* O: 8 were isolated from raw-milk sample and a fecal sample, and from a fecal sample and is a such as milk bottles rinsing with untreated water prior to filling milk [70]. *E. coli* infection may occur among small residents of a community, closely related to a possible common source of infection. The epidemiologic evidence of the *E.coli* infection is evidence are supported from raw milk is the cause of infections by the number of ill persons that drank raw milk. The O157:H7 is isolated from raw milk samples and environmental samples [71]. The *E. coli's* ability to persist in cattle production environments contributes to the contamination and recontamination cycle of dairy cattle as well as human infection. *Escherichia coli* (STEC) are the most important emergent food-borne pathogens. Shiga toxinproducing STEC are common as colonizers in the intestine of healthy cattle and easily spread into the environment by fecal shedding by the surface application of farm effluent on soil. The bacteria can be transmitted to humans through food, such as ground beef inadequately cooked or unpasteurized milk. The prevalence of Shiga-like toxin produced by *E. coli* (STEC) in raw milk cheeses, including soft, hard, unripened, and blue mold cheeses, was mainly related to effective control strategies and must be considered on cattle farms in order to limit entry of STEC strains into the production environment [72]. The prevalence of Shiga-like toxin produced by *E. coli* (STEC) in raw milk cheeses was mainly related to serotypes O6, O174, O175, O176, O109, O76, and O162 and in minor frequency O22 serogroup [44]. Enterohemorrhagic *E. coli* (EHEC), EHEC O26: H-, has emerged as a significant cause of hemolytic-uremic syndrome in human (HUS). The source of the vehicle of contamination with EHEC O26 is not often identified; fecal samples were taken from cows of the farm that produced the incriminating milk. *E. coli* O26 infection illustrates the hazards associated with the consumption of raw milk [73, 74]. *Brucella* spp. is identified in ewes' milk cheese as an important human infection source, and it has been an important public health risk. The isolation of *Brucella* species on raw milk, goats' cheese, and ewes' cheese has been reported; *B. melitensis* was isolated from cheese samples [63]. *Bacillus* spp. contamination of raw milk from the environment of production might be originated from different sources, air, milking equipment, feed, soil, and feces, and grass differences in feeding and housing strategies of cows may influence the microbial quality of milk. *Bacillus licheniformis, Bacillus pumilus, Bacillus circulans* and *Bacillus. subtilis* and strain types of the species belonging to the *Bacillus cereus* group. Higher numbers of thermotolerant sporulated organisms in milk were found from conventional dairy farms compared to organic farms [75]. Contamination of milk by bacterial spores occurred during grazing season, the spore content of milk by *Bacillus cereus* psychotropic, affects post-pasteurized milk by spore total number; this was attributed to the nipple teat contamination with soil due by low evaporation of soil water and dirty farm access this was attributed to the nipple contamination with wet soil, due by low evaporation of soil water and farm access dirty [76]. The assurance of microbial quality in dairy product, requires monitoring and identifying bacteria associated with food safety concerns in raw milk and traditional cheeses in local industry, semi hard cheese could preserve microbial contamination for a few months; *Staphylococcus sciuri, Staphylococcus epidermidis, Staphylococcus saprophyticus, Staphylococcus aureus* was not detected in old cheese. *Staphylococcus agnetis, S. chromogenes, S. devriesei, Staphylococcus equorum, S. haemolyticus, Staphylococcus lentus, S. sciuri, Staphylococcus vitulinus* and *S. xylosus.* The probability of finding *S. chromogenes* and *S. agnetis* on the teat and inguinal region increased with age [77].

Raw and pasteurized milk microbial contamination

In human population raw milk and dairy products are often tangled up in food-borne disease outbreaks; occasionally pasteurized milk may be contaminated and lead to bacteria spoilage of milk and dairy product storage during the dairy processing with a potential health risk for the consumers [5]. The microbiological quality of dairy products reflects good hygienic practices during the dairy milking process; raw milk contamination may occur in diseased or infected cows with environmental bacteria [1]. In raw milk samples collected from the milk-producing areas tested for *L. monocytogenes* and *Salmonella* spp., the presence and enumeration of mesophilic aerobes and total coliforms is an indicator of *E. coli* contamination and poor microbiological quality of dairy products and causes interference with the native microbiota and other important pathogens [52]. The bacteria acid lactic species (BAL) identified mainly as *Lactococcus lactis* subsp. *lactis* and *Enterococcus faecium* were considered as antagonistic bacteria for the enteric pathogens [36]. The microbial contamination, affects fresh dairy products quality raw milk elaborated. This condition might constitute a potential risk in milk food-borne diseases and public health and dairy food quality [77]. The presence of highly heat-resistant spores of *Bacillus sporothermodurans* in ultrahigh temperature or sterilized milk has emerged as an important item in the dairy industry. The predominant bacterial species isolated at the dairy farm comes from the water, feedstuffs, and milking equipment, in this aspect Bacillus licheniformis and Bacillus pallidus acts as entry points for highly heat-resistant spores into the raw milk and the contamination risk level aerobic spore-forming bacteria that could lead to spoilage of milk and dairy products [30]. The milk products are contaminated by *Pseudomonas* spp. in the systems processing milk; it has direct effects on the product shelf life in the dairy industrial plants. The spoilage of milk components has produced by *Pseudomonas* fluorescens, and *Pseudomonas putida* in raw and pasteurized milk provoked by different enzyme systems of the bacteria comes from of protease, lecithinase, and lipase activities. The bacterial contamination source was a derivate from production herd environment and the hygienic farm measures [78, 79]. The hygiene in the production environment in the dairy farm is a very important fact to prevent food-borne diseases and food quality [18]. The incidence of food-borne infections in human population is increasing in the recent years. Oftenlly the expose was occurred in private homes and food markets, were prevail the microbial risk contamination in the cases related to the prepared food dairy products, raw milk consumption and eggs, from others food products [80]. Bovine colostrum in human food is considered an excellent source of bioactive proteins, to improve gastrointestinal health and enhance body condition. The consumers are demanding safe and high-quality milk products. There is no influence of herd size and localization in the bacteriological colostrum quality. In milk quality, the animal hygiene and herd health status is considered a goal to warranty the milk as free of *Salmonella* ssp., *S. aureus*, coagulase negative staphylococci, *Streptococcus agalactiae* and streptococci non-agalactiae and coliforms and non-coliforms [36]. In the milk industry, spore-forming bacteria can survive food-processing thermal treatments particularly *Bacillus* and *Clostridium* species to determine the shelf life of a variety of heat-treated milk products, mainly if the level of post-process contamination is low. The management approach of the food production chain, based on raw materials, ingredients and environmental sources, influences the quality of the final product. The strategy on the farm to reduce contamination by foodborne pathogens is to establish hygienic practices on the farm in various components of the milk production chain. Contamination by *Clostridium tyrobutyricum* was consistently found in milk related to farm administration rather than food contamination. Because rottenly *Clostridium disporicum*, identified as an important member of clostridia populations transferred to milk, as a bacteria present in soil, forage, grass silage, maize silage, dry hay. These clostridia may contribute to raw milk contamination by the environmental bacteria as present in soil, forage, grass silage, maize silage, and dry hay [81, 82]. Other virulence factors identified in isolation were assayed: biofilm formation and adhesion to mammalian cells and antibiotic resistance. The genes encoding for virulence factors were present in *Enterococcus faecalis* more than in *Enterococcus faecalis and Enterococcus faecium*. The enterococci were also implicated in vancomycin-resistant strains and the severe multiresistant human nosocomial infection. The recovery of bacteriocinogenic *Enterococcus faecium* isolated with no virulence traits suggests a potential use for biotechnological applications in food animal production [83]. The fecal contamination of the milking equipment is also responsible for the raw milk contamination. Lactobacilli were identified in cows' teats, raw milk, the milking machine, and the milking parlor on one farm. The lactobacilli present in the feces were predominantly *Lactobacillus mucosae* and *Lactobacillus brevis*. The majority of enterococcal isolates from cow feces were identified as *Aerococcus viridans* [36]. *Bacillus cereus* spores are implicated in the herd with environmental microbial contamination; a large number of spores were present in free stalls and bedding material, especially with sawdust beds. A positive relationship was observed between raw milk and the number of spores determined in the feed and feces [84]. *Bacillus licheniformis* and *Bacillus cereus* contamination was present in raw milk, pasteurized milk, and yogurt during dairy processing of dairy milk products as well as other different strains in raw milk and yogurt. The evidence of dairy environmental contamination was attributed to *Bacillus* strains during the technological processing of milk [85]. The enterotoxigenic *Bacillus cereus* and their enterotoxins could be detected in milk products from retail shops. *Bacillus cereus* was isolated from milk products. Enterotoxigenic *B. cereus* hemolytic was identified from milk and milk products and *B. cereus* non-hemolytic enterotoxins just like in milk [86]. The evaluation of the hygienic quality of raw milk is meant to be possible based on the presence of fecal contamination evaluated in raw milk indicated by the coliforms bacteria, and Bifidobacteria species (*Bifidobacterium pseudolongum* subsp. *globosum*), identified isolates compared with bifidobacteria isolated from dung of the cows and the contaminated raw milk samples. The raw milk samples harbored *Bifidobacterium pseudolongum* subsp. *globosum* [87].

Microbiological quality of milk and dairy products: spoilage bacteria

Milk and dairy product quality is the consequence of all activities developed during the production process, from the farms to the transformation in the dairy industry [88, 89]. Cow's milk contains the nutritional requirements necessary for the growth of the calf, since it is a source rich in lipids, proteins, amino acids, vitamins, and minerals, which added to its high activity of water (aw) and makes it an excellent matrix for the growth of a large number of spoilage microorganisms (**Table 2**) and pathogens for humans [90, 91]. Not so long ago, it was believed that the milk contained in the mammary gland was sterile and that the microorganisms isolated had their origin from external contamination. Nevertheless, this idea has been questioned due to the development of more sensitive molecular methods which suggests that there is colonization of a wide variety of microorganisms in the healthy mammary gland [92].

Table 2. *Principal causes and defects in milk and dairy products caused by spoilage microorganisms.*

Kind of defect	Cause	Related microorganism	Reference
Pasteurized, sterilized, and UHT milk			
Precipitation when milk added to hot beverage (bitty cream)	Activity of phospholipases and proteinases and fat destabilization	*Bacillus* spp.	[130]
Gelation	Thermoresistant proteinases	Psychrotrophic bacteria (Gram-negative and Gram-positive): *Pseudomonas* spp. (10^6–10^8 cfu mL^{-1})	[131, 132]
Shorter shelf life	Proteolytic and lipolytic activities	*Bacillus cereus* spp. (10^6 cfu mL^{-1})	[130, 133]
Undesirable flavor: unclean, fruity, bitter, rancid, yeasty	High concentration of free fatty acids due to activity of thermostable lipases; protein hydrolysis due to activity of heat stabile proteinases	*Pseudomonas fragi* *P. fluorescens*	[130]
Increase of free fatty acids and casein hydrolyses, destabilizing the casein micelles (acid coagulation of milk)	Proteolytic and lipolytic activities	*Bacillus* spp.	[133]; [134]; [120]
Milk spoiling	Biofilm formation	Consortium of species	[135]
Powder milk			
Shorter shelf life, rancidity, and bitterness	Bacterial proteinases and lipases and increase of free fatty acid	*Bacillus* spp.	[111]
Cheese			

Destabilization of the natural plasmin system of milk. Affect the quality of cheese, flavor and texture development, and reduce the yield of the curd	Activity of lipases and proteinases remain in curd that ongoing hydrological changes during ripening; cause spoilage of milk and dairy product.	Psychrotrophic spp. (>10^3 cfu mL^{-1})	[114, 136, 137]
Change coagulation time and quality of curd (fragile and less compact)	Higher concentration of free amino acids (bacterial proteinases) which stimulates starter culture which growth.		
Undesirables flavor: rancid taste in hard cheeses (ripening)	Longer coagulation time: higher concentration of free fatty acids (bacterial lipases) which inhibits starter culture growth	*Bacillus* spp. (≥10^6 cfu mL^{-1})	[133, 138]
	Lipases: free fatty acids increase		
Bitterness and off-flavors			[130]
Fermented milks			
Changes of texture and flavor: more firm gel and higher viscosity, more pronounced syneresis		Psychrotrophic	[139]
Lipolytic changes (free fatty acid): atypical flavor as bitter, rancid, unclean, and fruity			[140]
Reduced shelf life Rancidity and off-flavor Fruity, bitterness, soapy	High concentration of lipases and proteinases in milk (cream) High concentration of free fatty acids (C4-C6; C110-C12)	Psychrotrophic *Pseudomonas* spp. *Bacillus* spp. *Pseudomonas fragi* *P. fluorescens*	[141, 142]

The microbial composition of milk is influenced by several different parameters such as, in the case of raw milk, the microorganisms present in the teat canal, on the surface of teat skin, in the surrounding air, and in feed as well as other environmental factors including housing conditions, the quality of the water supply, and equipment hygiene [93–95]. Moreover, the insufficient cold capacity and long storage times can also increase the bacterial count owing to the bacterial growth during milk storage [96]. Therefore, it is not always easy to determine the cause of a high bacterial count in raw milk; there are several parameters that can give an insight of the source of contamination [97].

Bulk milk analysis is used by dairy industry, veterinarians, and milk producers as an indicator of quality [98]. Through a microbiological profile, it is possible to prevent and modify the possible contamination points. For this reason, the bacterial count of bulk milk is a useful tool for monitoring the environment hygiene, translating high values as negative effects on the quality of the pasteurized milk and milk products, reducing the shelf life and its sensory characteristics [99]. Regarding these indicators, the standard plate count (SPC) in milk represents those bacteria that grow between 30 and 35°C under aerobic conditions and is conformed mainly by bacteria coming from teat skin, feces, milker's hands, equipment, soil, water, etc. [100]. Their importance is given by the fact that they reflect not only the hygienic quality of the raw milk but also the way in which the product was handled. The higher values of SPC indicate raw milk not suitable for consumption, poor handling practices in its elaboration, and an increased risk of the presence of pathogenic microorganisms. Additionally, this parameter reflects the efficiency of cleaning procedures and storage temperatures as well as the hygiene of the udders during milking [100]. With regard to dairy products, this parameter acquires remarkable importance particularly in the elaboration of cheeses, recommending low counts in order to minimize the alteration of the composition of the milk and the final yield obtained [101]. According to the regulations of the European Union, the dairy farms remittent to processing plants of these products must have bacterial counts below 100,000 cfu/mL [102].

In relation to the factors of variation in SPC, there are several studies supporting that the seasonal effect is of great significance in the production of quality milk in terms of hygiene [103]. A work in raw milk from Canada [104] determined that high bacterial counts in summer and spring are related to higher room temperatures that favor the rapid bacterial multiplication. The whole routine of milking, from the presealed and post-sealed to the implementation and maintenance of practices of cleaning and disinfection of dairy equipment, has a great influence in the improvement of milk quality, although for counts below 50,000 cfu/mL, the major factor is hygiene [105].

On the other hand, the rapid cooling of milk and the maintenance of its coldness for prolonged periods stimulate the growth of psychrotrophic bacteria, modifying the native microbiota in favor of Gram-negative ones in approximately more than 90% of the total population [99, 106]. *Psychrotrophic* microorganisms are defined as mesophilic microorganisms which are adapted to grow at refrigeration temperature (7°C or lower), although their optimum temperature of multiplication is higher. They can be widely distributed in the environment: soil, water, and being part of the normal microbiota of animals and man [107]. Numerous psychrotrophic microorganisms have been isolated from raw milk: *Pseudomonas* (*Ps.*), *Enterobacter*, *Flavobacterium*, *Klebsiella*, *Aeromonas*, *Acinetobacter*, *Alcaligenes*, and *Achromobacter* have been reported as the most representative genera [108], while the most frequently isolated species are *Ps. fluorescens*, *Ps. fragi*, *Ps. aeruginosa*, and *Ps. putrefaciens* [109]. In terms of quality, psychotropic bacteria have become a problem of special importance for the dairy industry, being recognized as one of the main agents causing deterioration ending in significant economic losses for the sector [110]. In general, psychrotrophs are capable of producing extracellular or intracellular enzymes (proteases, lipases, and phospholipases), many of which are heat-resistant, which means that they are capable of maintaining their activity after heat treatment (pasteurization or more severe treatment) and also generating big adverse changes in the quality of dairy products [111]. This deterioration in milk quality translates as changes in flavor, undesirable coagulation of proteins, and an increase in the concentration of free fatty acids and amino acids [110].

With regard to other aspects of quality, such as the suitability of milk for the production of dairy products, psychrotrophs have a significant negative effect on yields and in the reduction of their shelf life [112]. When coming from the environment, psychrotrophs are also considered indicators of the hygienic quality of milk [108]. In some countries its count is used as a complement to the bacterial count to determine the quality of the milk and is of special interest when the milk will be subjected to certain technological processes. For example, the regulatory limits for hygienic quality in the Czech Republic are set at ≤100,000 cfu/mL of bacterial count and ≤50,000 cfu/mL of psychrotrophs [113]. Furthermore, in the case where milk is used in technological processes, the requirements increase using the limits set by the EU of <30,000 cfu/mL for bacterial counts and <5000 cfu/mL for psychrotrophs [102]. In Scotland, an average of 130.000 cfu/mL psychrotrophs in silos of dairy industries from which 70.2% were *Pseudomonas* was found [114].

In terms of food safety, the pasteurizing milk was established as a necessary step for the consumption of fluid milk and other dairy products [115, 116]. In spite of that, this procedure applied in dairy industries for the elimination of pathogenic microorganisms does not completely inactivate all microorganisms, even in the most severe thermal treatments. For instance, some bacteria like thermoduric bacteria resist milk pasteurization. Also, the spores highly resistant to heat can survive the ultrahigh temperature (UHT) process and even to the processes of spray-drying persisting in pasteurized powders [116, 117]. For these reasons, the Food and Drug Administration (FDA) in the USA declared the thermoduric, thermophilic, psychrotrophic, and spore-forming bacteria as the microorganisms with the highest risk of spoilage in dairy products [118]. The thermoduric count is used as an indicator of sanitization of equipment in the industry and establishments [99], being the ideal ranges those between 100 and 200 cfu/mL [119]. Of this group, *Bacillus cereus* is the most commonly found in milk and dairy products [120], and their spores are characterized by having the ability to survive the thermal processing used in the industry [121]. In addition, some species can multiply at refrigeration temperatures, which is why it is also considered a psychotropic microorganism [122]. *Bacillus* spp. produces extracellular proteases and lipases and phospholipases (lecithinase) resistant to thermal treatments, comparable with the enzymes produced by *Pseudomonas* [123]. The combination of these characteristics in a microbial species indicates a great deteriorating potential [124]. Raw milk contamination by spores of *B. cereus* has been reported as the main cause of the presence of these groups of microorganisms in processed milks [125]. The spores of thermoduric microorganisms can be found in processed products, such as pasteurized milk and stored cream, decreasing their shelf life [91, 126]. To ensure the shelf life of the pasteurized milk, it is necessary to comply with a maximum spore limit of *B. cereus* of 3 log spores/mL [127]. In dehydrated products, they have a main importance because these products are more prone to thermoduric deterioration because of having a long useful life [116].

Therefore, psychrotrophs and thermodurics are of great importance in the quality of the milk that will be industrialized, mainly due to its effects on the composition. The lipolytic and proteolytic enzymes that they produce cause deterioration during the storage of milk and dairy products [107]. Moreover, studies suggest that these proteases found in raw milk are produced by psychrotrophic bacteria, especially of the genus *Pseudomonas* [128]. In this regard, a study conducted in fresh milk observed a production of extracellular proteases of psychrotrophs, which cause an increase in plasmin activity, hydrolyzing casein and decreasing its levels (count above

10^7 cfu/mL); this increase in plasmin activity could affect the quality of cheeses or other dairy products [129]. In the case of thermodurics, it has been reported that *B. cereus* can also release proteases that degrade casein by damaging the milk. The κ-casein is the protein fraction which is more affected by hydrolysis; after 7 days of storage at 20°C, all κ-casein is converted to para-κ-casein, while β-casein is reduced by 70%. Furthermore, as part of the deterioration caused by this microorganism in milk, it has been observed that it releases peptides of low molecular weight causing undesirable flavors [120].

In summary, milk and milk products provide favorable conditions for the growth of various microorganisms. These include groups capable of growing at refrigeration temperatures, withstanding heat treatments and producing heat-resistant enzymes, which are responsible for the deterioration and reduction of the shelf life of milk and by-products. The effectiveness in the control of these microorganisms is a critical challenge for the dairy industry, and its relevance has been discussed in this chapter.

Conclusions

The paper remarks the importance among the milk production and food safety, closely related in the assurance of the milk quality and the prevention of milk spoilage. The dairy industry management programs as for food safety, the milk quality and the dairy products. Preventing the microbial and chemical contamination. The food-borne diseases in public health programs are a priority in the surveillance of milk food-borne diseases by the monitoring of food-borne pathogens and the microbial contamination in milk products. Actually dairy farms are compromised to reduce the milk contamination source from udder and the dairy cow herd health status and the production environment, by hygiene practices in the cow herd management and good milk conserving in the raw milk bulk tank. The food hygiene protocols are fundament for to reduce the microbial contamination of the raw milk and pasteurized milk, regarding the health risk by the microbial pathogens in the food borne diseases and bacterial spoilage, source of deteriorating dairy products and milk. The microbial quality of foods is required for the traceability in dairy products industry. Consumers education programs and practices of good handling of foods, could be reduce the exposure to food borne pathogens and the consumption of unsafe food products. The traceability of milk and dairy products, from the production-distribution chain food and the consumption is a good policy for to the assurance the quality and to reduce the public health risks.

Acknowledgements

We appreciate the selfless and participatory collaboration of the authors in the preparation and communication of the book chapter.

Conflict of interest

The authors declare that there is no conflict of interest in the participation and collaboration in the elaboration of this work and its divulgation.

Author details

Valente Velázquez-Ordoñez[1]*, Benjamín Valladares-Carranza[1],

Esvieta Tenorio-Borroto[1], Martín Talavera-Rojas[1], Jorge Antonio Varela-Guerrero[1], Jorge Acosta-Dibarrat[1], Florencia Puigvert[3], Lucia Grille[3], Álvaro González Revello[2] and Lucia Pareja[4]

1. Facultad de Medicina Veterinaria y Zootecnia, Centro de Investigación y Estudios Avanzados en Salud Animal, Universidad Autónoma del Estado de México (CIESA-FMVZ-UAEM), Toluca, Mexico

2 Departamento de Ciencia y Tecnología de la Leche, Facultad de Veterinaria, Universidad de la Republica, Montevideo, Uruguay

3 Departamento de Ciencia y Tecnología de la Leche, Facultad de Veterinaria, Universidad de la Republica, CENUR-Litoral Norte, Paysandú, Uruguay

4 Facultad de Química, Universidad de la Republica, Estación Experimental Dr. Mario A. Cassinoni, Paysandú, Uruguay

*Address all correspondence to: vvo@uaemex.mx

References

[1] Kongo JM, Gomes AP, Malcata FX. Monitoring and identification of bacteria associated with safety concerns in the manufacture of São Jorge, a Portuguese traditional cheese from raw cow's milk. Journal of Food Protection. 2008;**71**(5):986-992

[2] Patilk SR, Cates SA, Morales R. Consumer food safety knowledge, practices, and demographic differences: Findings from a meta- analysis. Journal of Food Protection. 2005;**68**(9):1884-1994

[3] Johnson EA. Microbiological safety of cheese made from heat-treated milk. I. Executive summary, introduction and history. Journal of Food Protection. 1990;**53**:441

[4] Murinda SE, Nguyen LT, Nam HM, Almeida RA, Headrick SJ, Oliver SP. Detection of sorbitol-negative and sorbitol-positive Shiga toxin-producing *Escherichia coli*, *Listeria monocytogenes*, *Campylobacter jejuni*, and *Salmonella* spp. in dairy farm environmental samples. Foodborne Pathogoly Disease. 2004;**1**(2):97-104. DOI: 10.1089/153531404772914446

[5] Frank JF. Milk and dairy products. In: Doyle PM, Beuchant LR, Monteville TJ, editors. Food Microbiology: Fundamentals and Frontiers. 2nd ed. Washington, DC: ASM Press; 2001. p. 111

[6] Entis P. Food Safety: Old Habits New Perspectives. Washington, DC: ASM Press; 2007

[7] Oliver SP, Boor KJ, Murphy SC, Murinda SE. Food safety hazards associated with consumption of raw milk. Foodborne Pathogens and Disease. 2009;**6**(7):793-806. DOI: 10.1089/ fpd.2009.0302

[8] FAO. In: Muehlhoff E, Bennett A, McMahon D. Milk and Dairy Products in Human Nutrition. Rome, Italy: Food and Agriculture Organization of the United Nations (FAO); 2013. E-ISBN 978-92-5-107864-8 (PDF). Available from: http://www.fao.org/ docrep/018/ i3396e/i3396e.pdf

[9] FAO y FIL. Guía de buenas prácticas en explotaciones lecheras. Roma, Italia: Organización de las Naciones Unidas para la Alimentación y la Agricultura (FAO) y Federación Internacional de la Leche (FIL). Directrices FAO: Producción y Sanidad Animal No. 8; 2012. ISBN 978-92-5-306957-6

[10] Msalya G. Contamination levels and identification of bacteria in milk sampled from three regions of Tanzania: Evidence from literature and laboratory analyses. Hindawi Veterinary Medicine International. 2017; Article ID 9096149, 10 p. DOI: 10.1155/2017/9096149

[11] In: Velázquez-Ordoñez V, Castañeda-Vázquez H, Wolter W, Švarc Gajic J, Bedolla-Cedeño C, Guerra-Liera JE, editors. Producción y Calidad de la Leche. México, DF: Editorial Juan Pablos Editor; 2015. ISBN 978-607-711-310-2

[12] Velázquez-Ordoñez V, Valladares- Carranza B, Gutiérrez-Castillo del CA, Talavera-Rojas M, Pescador-salas N, Valdés-ramos R. Milk production and safety food. In: Svarc-Gajic, editor. Nutritional Insigthts and Food Safety. New York, NY: Nova-Publishers, Inc.; 2011. pp. 334-357

[13] Simsek O, Gültekin R, Oksüz O, Kurultay S. The effect of environmental pollution on the heavy metal content of raw milk. Die Nahrung. 2000;**44**(5):360-363

[14] Bean NH, Goulding Joy S, Lao C, Angulo FJ. Surveillance for foodborne- disease outbreaks in the United States, 1988-1992. MMWR. 1996;**45**(SS-5):1-66

[15] Murinda SE, Nguyen LT, Ivey SJ, Gillespie BE, Almeida RA, Draughon FA, et al. Molecular characterization of Salmonella spp. isolated from bulk tank milk and cull dairy cow fecal samples. Journal of Food Protection. 2002;**65**:1100-1105

[16] CLSI. Performance Standards for Antimicrobial Disk and Dilution Susceptibility Tests for Bacteria Isolated from Animals; Approved Standard. 3rd ed. Wayne, PA: Clinical Laboratory Institute (CLSI). Document M31-A3; 2008. p. 99

[17] Bauman CA, Barkema HW, Dubuc J, Keefe GP, Kelton DF. Canadian National Dairy Study: Herd-level milk quality. Journal of Dairy Science. 2018;**101**(3):2679-2691. DOI: 10.3168/ jds.2017-13336

[18] Callaway TR, Oliver SP. On-farm strategies to reduce foodborne pathogen contamination. Foodborne Pathogenesis Disease. 2009;**6**(7):753. DOI: 10.1089/ fpd.2009.9996

[19] FAO. Climate Change: Implications for Food Safety. Roma, Italia: Organización de las Naciones Unidas para la Alimentación y la Agricultura (FAO); 2008. Available from: http:// www.fao.org/ag/agn/agns/files/ HLC1_ Climate_Change_and_Food_Safety.pdf [Consultado 24 de diciembre de 2018]

[20] Velázquez-Ordoñez V, Valladares- Carranza B, Castañeda-Vázquez H, Gutiérrez-Castillo A d C, Alonso-Fresan MU. Efecto del cambio climático en la producción de leche y riesgos a la salud pública asociados a las enfermedades transmitidas por alimentos. In: Loredo P, Castellanos Editores S, editors. Crisis alimentaria y la salud en México. Mexico, DF, SA de CV; 2016. pp. 309-330. ISBN 968-5573-42-3

[21] Roussi V, Govaris A, Varagouli A, Botsoglou NA. Occurrence of aflatoxin M(1) in raw and market milk commercialized in Greece. Food Additives and Contaminants. 2002;**19**(9):863-868

[22] Tajik H, Rohani SM, Moradi M. Detection of aflatoxin M1 in raw and commercial pasteurized milk in Urmia, Iran. Pakistan Journal of Biological Sciences. 2007;**10**(22):4103-4107

[23] Sugiyama K, Hiraoka HV, Sugita- Konishi Y. Aflatoxin M1 contamination in raw bulk tank milk and the presence of aflatoxin B1 in corn supplied to dairy cattle in Japan. Shokuhin Eiseigaku Zasshi. 2008;**49**(5):352-355

[24] Agabriel C, Cornu A, Journal C, Sibra C, Grolier P, Martin B. Tanker milk variability according to farm feeding practices: Vitamins A and E, carotenoids, color, and terpenoids. Journal of Dairy Science. 2007;**90**(10):4884-4896. DOI: 10.3358/ shokueishi.49.352

[25] Te Giffel MC, Wagendorp A, Herrewegh A, Driehuis F. Bacterial spores in silage and raw milk. Antonie Van Leeuwenhoek. 2002;**81**(1-4):625-630

[26] OIE. Código Sanitario para los Animales Terrestres. Paris, Francia: Organización Mundial de Sanidad Animal (OIE); 2006. ISBN 92-9044-679-X

[27] Murinda SE, Nguyen LT, Ivey SJ, Gillespie BE, Almeida RA, Oliver SP. Prevalence and molecular characterization of Escherichia coli O157:H7 in bulk tank milk and fecal samples from cull dairy cows: A 12-month survey of dairy farms in East Tennessee. Journal of Food Protection. 2002;**65**:752-759

[28] Nauta MJ. Modular process risk model (MPRM). In: Schaffner WD, editor. A Structured Approach to Food Chain Exposure Assessment: Microbial Risk Analysis of Foods. Washington, DC: ASM Press; 2008. p. 99

[29] Gillespie BE, Headrick SI, Boonyayatra S, Oliver SP. Prevalence and persistence of coagulase-negative Staphylococcus species in three dairy research herds. Veterinary Microbiology. 2009;**134**(1-2):65-72. DOI: 10.1128/ JCM.02239-16

[30] Adkins PRF, Dufour S, Spain JN, Calcutt MJ, Reilly TJ, Stewart GC, et al. Cross-sectional study to identify staphylococcal species isolated from teat and inguinal skin of different-aged dairy heifers. Journal of Dairy Science. 2018;**101**(4):3213-3225. DOI: 10.3168/ jds.2017-13974

[31] Fox LK, Norell RJ. *Staphylococcus aureus* colonization of teat skin as affected by postmilking teat treatment when exposed to cold and windy conditions. Journal of Dairy Science. 1994;**77**(8):2281-2288. DOI: 10.3168/jds. S0022-0302(94)77171-X

[32] Pangloli P, Dje Y, Ahmed O, Doane CA, Oliver SP, Draughon FA. Seasonal incidence and molecular characterization of Salmonella from dairy cows, calves, and farm environment. Foodborne Pathogens and Disease. 2008;**5**(1):87-96. DOI: 10.1089/ fpd.2008.0048

[33] Lin H, Shavezipur M, Yousef A, Maleky F. Prediction of growth of *Pseudomonas fluorescens* in milk during storage under fluctuating temperature. Journal of Dairy Science. 2016;**99**(3):1822-1830. DOI: 10.3168/ jds.2015-10179

[34] Van Kessel JS, Karns JS, Wolfgang DR, Hovingh E, Jayarao BM, Van Tassell CP, et al. Environmental sampling to predict fecal prevalence of Salmonella in an intensively monitored dairy herd. Journal of Food Protection. 2008;**71**(10):1967-1973

[35] Viljoen BC. The interaction between yeasts and bacteria in dairy environments. International Journal of Food Microbiology. 2001;**69**(1-2):37-44

[36] Kagkli DM, Vancanneyt M, Hill C, Vandamme P, Cogan TM. Enterococcus and Lactobacillus contamination of raw milk in a farm dairy environment. International Journal of Food Microbiology. 2007;**114**(2):243-251. DOI: 10.1016/S0168-1605(01)00570-0

[37] Parkpian P, Leong ST, Laortanakul P, Thunthaisong N. Regional monitoring of lead and cadmium contamination in a tropical grazing land site, Thailand. Environmental Monitoring and Assessment. 2003;**85**(2):157-173

[38] Velthuis AG, van Asseldonk MA. Process audits versus product quality monitoring of bulk milk. Journal of Dairy Science. 2011;**94**(1):235-249. DOI: 10.3168/jds.2010-3528

[39] Srinivasan V, Sawant AA, Gillespie BE, Headrick SJ, Ceasaris L, Oliver SP. Prevalence of enterotoxin and toxic shock syndrome toxin genes in Staphylococcus aureus isolated from milk of cows with mastitis. Foodborne Pathogens and Disease. 2006;**3**(3): 274-283. DOI: 10.1089/fpd.2006.3.274

[40] Straley BA, Donaldson SC, Hedge NV, Sawant AA, Srinivasan V, Oliver SP, et al. Public health significance of antimicrobial-resistant gram-negative bacteria in raw bulk tank milk. Foodborne Pathogens and Disease. 2006;**3**(3):222-223. DOI: 10.1089/ fpd.2006.3.222

[41] Jørgensen HJ, Mørk T, Rørvik LM. The occurrence of *Staphylococcus aureus* on a farm with small-scale production of raw milk cheese. Journal of Dairy Science. 2005;**88**(11):3810-3817. DOI: 10.3168/ jds.S0022-0302(05)73066-6

[42] Cremonesi P, Perez G, Pisoni G, Moroni P, Morandi S, Luzzana M, et al. Detection of enterotoxigenic *Staphylococcus aureus* isolates in from raw milk cheeses in France. Letters in Applied Microbiology. 2005;**41**(3):235-241. DOI: 10.1111/j.1472-765X.2005.01756.x

[43] Tsegmed U, Normanno G, Pringle M, Krovacek K. Occurrence of enterotoxic *Staphylococcus aureus* in raw milk from yaks and cattle in Mongolia. Journal of Food Protection. 2007;**70**(7):1726-1729

[44] Vernozy-Rozand C, Montet MP, Berardin M, Bavai C, Beutin L. Isolation and characterization of Shiga toxin-producing *Escherichia coli* strains from raw milk cheeses in France. Letters in Applied Microbiology. 2005;**41**(3):235-241. DOI: 10.1111/j.1472-765X.2005.01756.x

[45] Velázquez-Ordoñez V, Vázquez CHJC, Pescador SN, Saltijeral OJ. Niveles de células somáticas en leche y resistencia a la mastitis. Producción Animal. 2005;**207**:15-23

[46] Oliver SP, Calvinho LF. Influence of inflammation on mammary gland metabolism and milk composition. Journal of Animal Science. 1995;**73**:18-33

[47] Damm M, Holm C, Blaabjerg M, Bro MN, Schwarz D. Differential somatic cell count—A novel method for routine mastitis screening in the frame of Dairy Herd Improvement testing programs. Journal of Dairy Science. 2017;**100**(6):4926-4940. DOI: 10.3168/ jds.2016-12409

[48] Frössling J, Ohlson A, Hallén- Sandgren C. Incidence and duration of increased somatic cell count in Swedish dairy cows and associations with milking system type. Journal of Dairy Science. 2017;**100**(9):7368-7378. DOI: 10.3168/jds.2016-12333

[49] Srinivasan V, Gillespie BE, Lewis MJ, Nguyen LT, Headrick SI, Schukken YH, et al. Phenotypic and genotypic antimicrobial resistance patterns of *Escherichia coli* isolated from dairy cows with mastitis. Veterinary Microbiology. 2007;**124**(3-4):319-328. DOI: 10.1016/j. vetmic.2007.04.040

[50] Oliver SP, Lewis MJ, Gillespie BE, Ivey SJ, Coleman LH, Almeida RA, et al. Evaluation of a postmilking teat disinfectant containing a phenolic combination for the prevention of mastitis in lactating dairy cows. Journal of Food Protection. 1999;**62**(11):1354-1357

[51] Rea MC, Cogan TM, Tobin S. Incidence of pathogenic bacteria in raw milk in Ireland. The Journal of Applied Bacteriology. 1992;**73**(4):331-336

[52] Nero LA, de Mattos MR, Barros M d A, Ortolani MB, Beloti V, Franco BD. Listeria monocytogenes and Salmonella spp. in raw milk produced in Brazil: Occurrence and interference of indigenous microbiota in their isolation and development. Zoonoses and Public Health. 2008;**55**(6):299-305. DOI: 10.1111/j.1863-2378.2008.01130.x

[53] Ruegg PL, Tabone TJ. The relationship between antibiotic residue violations and somatic cell counts in Wisconsin dairy herds. Journal of Dairy Science. 2000;**83**:2805-2809. DOI: 10.3168/jds.S0022-0302(00)75178-2

[54] Tan X, Jiang YW, Huang YJ, Hu SH. Persistence of gentamicin residues in milk after the intramammary treatment of lactating cows for mastitis. Journal of Zhejiang University. Science. B. 2009;**10**(4):280-284. DOI: 10.1631/jzus. B0820198

[55] Chao G, Zhou X, Jiao X, Quian X, Xu L. Prevalence and antimicrobial resistance of food borne pathogens isolated from food products in China. Foodborne Pathogens and Disease. 2007;**5**(3):277-284. DOI: 10.1089/ fpd.2007.0088

[56] Velázquez-Ordoñez V, Lagunas BS, Gutiérrez GB, Talavera RM, Alonso FU, Saltijeral OJ. *Staphylococcus aureus* methicillin resistant strain(MRSA) mínimum inhibitory enrofloxacin concentration in *Staphylococcus aureus* isolations obtained from cows with subclinical mastitis in family dairy farms. In: Krynsky A, Wrzesien R, editors. Proceedings XIIth International Congress ISAH 2005. Warsaw, Poland: International Society for Animal Hygiene, Faculty of Animal Science, Agricultural University; 2005. pp. 338-341

[57] Trakulsonboon S, Danchaivijitr S, Rongrun-Granugruang Y, Dhiraputra C, Susaegrant W, Ito T, et al. First report of methicillin-resistant *Staphylococcus aureus* with reduced susceptibility to vancomycin in Thailand. Journal of Clinical Microbiology. 2001;**32**(2):591-595. DOI: 10.1128/ JCM.39.2.591-595.2001

[58] Cercenado E, Ruiz de Gopegui E. Community-acquired methicillin- resistant *Staphylococcus aureus*. Enfermedades Infecciosas y Microbiología Clínica. 2008;**13**:19-13

[59] López-Vázquez M, Martínez- Castañeda JS, Talavera-Rojas M, Valdez-Alarcón JJ, Velázquez-Ordóñez V. Detection of mecA, mecI and mecR1 genes in methicillin-resistant *Staphylococcus aureus* strains of bovine origin isolated from Family Dairy Farms, Mexico. Archivos de Medicina Veterinaria. 2015;**47**:245-249

[60] Committee on drug use in food animals, Panel of animal health, Food safety, and Public Health, Board on Agriculture, National Research Council. In: National Academy of Sciences, editor. The Use of Drugs in Food Animals: Benefits and Risks. Washington, DC: National Academic Press; 1999. p. 63

[61] Bruhn JC, Ginn RE, Messer JW, Mikolajcik EM. Detection of antibiotic residues in milk and dairy products. In: Richarson GM, editor. Standard Methods for the Examination of Dairy Products. Washington, DC: American Public Health Association; 1985. pp. 265-287

[62] Oliver SP, Mitchell BA. Prevalence of mastitis pathogens in herds participating in a mastitis control program. Journal of Dairy Science. 1984;**67**:2436-2440. DOI: 10.3168/jds. S0022-0302(84)81592-1

[63] Kasimoğlu A. Determination of Brucella ssp in raw milk and turkish white cheese in Kirikkale. Deutsche Tierärztliche Wochenschrift. 2002;**109**(7):324-326

[64] Hoob BC, Roberts D. Food Poisoning and Food Hygiene. 6th ed. London, UK: Edward Arnolds Publishers Limited; 1990

[65] Lal M, Kaur H, Gupta LK, Sood NK. Isolation of Yersinia enterocolitica from raw milk and pork in Ludhiana. Indian Journal of Pathology and Microbiology. 2005;**48**(2):286-287

[66] Skovgaard N. New trends in emerging pathogens. International Journal of Food Microbiology. 2007;**120**(3):217-224. DOI: 10.1016/j. ijfoodmicro.2007.07.046

[67] Doyle MP, Beuchant L, Monteville TJ. Food Microbiology: Fundamentals and Frontiers. 2nd ed. Washington, DC: ASM Press; 2001

[68] Rohrbach BW, Draughon FA, Davidson PM, Oliver SP. Prevalence of *Listeria monocytogenes*, *Campylobacter jejuni*, *Yersinia enterocolitica*, and Salmonella in bulk tank milk: Risk factors and risk of human exposure. Journal of Food Protection. 1992;**55**:93-97

[69] Dewey-Mattia D, Manikonda K, Hall AJ, Wise ME, Crowe SJ. Surveillance for foodborne-disease outbreaks in the United States, 2009-2015. MMWR Surveillance Summaries. 2018;**67**(10):1-11. DOI: 10.15585/mmwr.ss6710a1

[70] Van Duynhoven YT, Isken LD, Borgen K, Besselse M, Soethoudt K, Haitsma O, et al. A prolonged outbreak of Salmonella Typhimurium infection related to an uncommon vehicle: Hard cheese made from raw milk. Epidemiology and Infection. 2009;**19**:1-10

[71] Ackers ML, Schoenfeld S, Markman J, Smith MG, Nicholson MA, De Witt W, et al. An outbreak of Yersinia enterocolitica O:8 infections associated with pasteurized milk. The Journal of Infectious Diseases. 2000;**181**(5): 1834-1837. DOI: 10.1089/fpd.2006.3.274

[72] Denny J, Bhat M, Eckmann K. Outbreak of *Escherichia coli* O157:H7 associated with raw milk consumption in the Pacific Northwest. Foodborne Pathogens and Disease. 2008;**5**(3): 321-328. DOI: 10.1089/fpd.2007.0072

[73] Fremaux B, Prigent-Combaret C, Vernozy-Rozand C. Long-term survival of Shiga toxin-producing *Escherichia coli* in cattle effluents and environment: An updated review. Veterinary Microbiology. 2008;**132**(1-2):1-18. DOI: 10.1016/j.vetmic.2008.05.015

[74] Paneto BR, Schocken-Iturrino RP, Macedo C, Santo E, Marin JM. Occurrence of toxigenic *Escherichia coli* in raw milk cheese in Brazil. Arquivo Brasileiro de Medicina Veterinária e Zootecnia. 2007;**59**(2):508-512

[75] Allerberger F, Friedrich AW, Grif K, Dierich MP, Dornbusch HJ, Mache CJ, et al. Hemolytic-uremic syndrome associated with enterohemorrhagic *Escherichia coli* O26:H infection and consumption of unpasteurized cow's milk. International Journal of Infectious Diseases. 2003;**7**(1):42-45

[76] Coorevits A, De Jonghe V, Vandroemme J, Reekmans R, Heyrman J, Messens W, et al. Comparative analysis of the diversity of aerobic spore-forming bacteria in raw milk from organic and conventional dairy farms. Systematic and Applied Microbiology. 2008;**31**(2):126-140. DOI: 10.1016/j.syapm.2008.03.002

[77] Christiansson A, Bertilsson J, Svensson B. Bacillus cereus spores in raw milk: Factors affecting the contamination of milk during the grazing period. Journal of Dairy Science. 1999;**82**(2):305-314. DOI: 10.3168/jds.S0022-0302(99)75237-9

[78] Scheldeman P, Pil A, Herman L, De Vos P, Heyndrickx M. Incidence and diversity of potentially highly heat-resistant spores isolated at dairy farms. Applied and Environmental Microbiology. 2005;**71**(3):1480-1494. DOI: 10.1128/AEM.71.3.1480-1494.2005

[79] Dogan B, Boor KJ. Genetic diversity and spoilage potentials among Pseudomonas spp. isolated from fluid milk products and dairy processing plants. Applied and Environmental Microbiology. 2003;**69**(1):130-138. DOI: 10.1128/AEM.69.1.130-138.2003

[80] Guan RF, Liu DH, Ye XQ , Yang K. Use of fluorometry for determination of skim milk powder adulteration in fresh milk. Journal of Zhejiang University. Science. B. 2005;**6**(11):1101-1106. DOI: 10.1128/AEM.69.1.130-138.2003

[81] Baumann A, Sadkowska- Todys M. Foodborne infections and intoxications in Poland in 2006. Przegląd Epidemiologiczny. 2008;**62**(2):275-286

[82] Julien MC, Dion P, Lafrenière C, Antoun H, Drouin P. Sources of clostridia in raw milk on farms. Applied and Environmental Microbiology. 2008;**74**(20):6348-6357. DOI: 10.1128/ AEM.00913-08

[83] Gomes BC, Esteves CT, Palazzo IC, Darini AL, Felis GE, Sechi LA, et al. Prevalence and characterization of Enterococcus spp. isolated from Brazilian foods. Food Microbiology. 2008;**25**(5):668-675. DOI: 10.1016/j. fm.2008.03.008

[84] Magnusson M, Christiansson A, Svensson B. Bacillus cereus spores during housing of dairy cows: Factors affecting contamination of raw milk. Journal of Dairy Science. 2007;**90**(6):2745-2754. DOI: 10.3168/jds.2006-754

[85] Banykó J, Vyletelová M. Determining the source of *Bacillus cereus* and *Bacillus licheniformis* isolated from raw milk, pasteurized milk and yoghurt. Letters in Applied Microbiology. 2009;**48**(3):318-323. DOI: 10.1111/j.1472-765X.2008.02526.x

[86] Ombui JN, Nduhiu JG. Prevalence of enterotoxigenic *Bacillus cereus* and its enterotoxins in milk and milk products in and around Nairobi. East African Medical Journal. 2005;**82**(6):280-284

[87] Beerens H, Hass Brac de la Perriere B, Gavini F. Evaluation of the hygienic quality of raw milk based on the presence of bifidobacteria: The cow as a source of faecal contamination. International Journal of Food Microbiology. 2000;**54**(3):163-169

[88] Joint FAO/WHO Codex Alimentarius Commission, Food and Agriculture Organization of the United Nations. Animal Food Production. Rome: Food and Agricultural Organization; 2008. 192 p

[89] Vilar MJ, Rodríguez-Otero JL, Sanjuán ML, Diéguez FJ, Varela M, Yus E. Implementation of HACCP to control the influence of milking equipment and cooling tank on the milk quality. Trends in Food Science & Technology. 2012;**23**:4-12. DOI: 10.1016/j.tifs.2011. 08.002

[90] Haug A, Hostmark A, Harstad O. Bovine milk in human nutrition—A review. Lipids in Health and Disease. 2007;**6**:25. DOI: 10.1186/1476-511X-6-25

[91] Hill B, Smythe B, Lindsay D, Shepherd J. Microbiology of raw milk in New Zealand. International Journal of Food Microbiology. 2012;**157**:305-308. DOI: 10.1016/j.ijfoodmicro.2012.03.031

[92] Addis MF, Tanca A, Uzzau S, Oikonomou G, Bicalho RC, Moroni P. The bovine milk microbiota: Insights and perspectives from-omics studies. Molecular BioSystems. 2016;**12**: 2359-2372. DOI: 10.1039/C6MB00217J

[93] Verdier-Metz I, Michel V, Delbès C, Montel MC. Do milking practices influence the bacterial diversity of raw milk? Food Microbiology. 2009;**26**: 305-310. DOI: 10.1016/j.fm.2008.12.005

[94] Vacheyrou M, Normand AC, Guyot P, Cassagne C, Piarroux R, Bouton Y. Cultivable microbial communities in raw cow milk and potential transfers from stables of sixteen French farms. International Journal of Food Microbiology. 2011;**146**:253-262. DOI: 10.1016/j.ijfoodmicro.2011.02.033

[95] Braem G, De Vliegher S, Verbist B, Heyndrickx M, Leroy F, De Vuyst L. Culture-independent exploration of the teat apex microbiota of dairy cows reveals a wide bacterial species diversity. Veterinary Microbiology. 2012;**157**: 383-390. DOI: 10.1016/j.vetmic.2011. 12.031

[96] Elmoslemany AM, Keefe GP, Dohoo IR, Jayarao BM. Risk factors for bacteriological quality of bulk tank milk in Prince Edward Island dairy herds. Part 1: Overall risk factors. Journal of Dairy Science. 2009;**92**:2634-2643. DOI: 10.3168/jds.2008-1812

[97] Murphy SC, Boor KJ. Trouble- shooting sources and causes of high bacteria counts in raw milk. Dairy, Food and Environmental Sanitation. 2000;**20**:606-611

[98] Gillespie BE, Lewis MJ, Boonyayatra S, Maxwell ML, Saxton A, Oliver SP, et al. Short communication: Evaluation of bulk tank milk microbiological quality of nine dairy farms in Tennessee. Journal of Dairy Science. 2012;**95**: 4275-4279. DOI: 10.3168/jds.2011-4881

[99] Barbano DM, Ma Y, Santos MV. Influence of raw milk quality on fluid milk shelf life. Journal of Dairy Science. 2006;**89**:E15-E19. DOI: 10.3168/jds. S0022-0302(06)72360-8

[100] American Public Health Association (APHA), Downes FP, Ito K. Compendium of Methods for the Microbiological Examination of Foods. 4th ed. Washington, DC: American Public Health Association; 2001. 676 p

[101] Innocente N, Biasutti M. Automatic milking systems in the Protected Designation of Origin Montasio cheese production chain: Effects on milk and cheese quality. Journal of Dairy Science. 2013;**96**:740-751. DOI: 10.3168/ jds.2012-5512

[102] European Union. Regulation (EC) N° 853/2004 of the European Parliament and of the Council of 29 April 2004, laying down specific hygiene rules for food of animal origin [Internet]. 2004. Available from: https://eur-lex.europa.eu/LexUriServ/ LexUriServ.do?uri=OJ:L:2004:139: 0055:0205:EN:PDFPDF [Accessed: 2018-12-15]

[103] Cziszter L, Acatinc S, Neciu FC, Ionel R, Ilie DE, Costin LI, et al. The influence of season on the cow milk quantity, quality and hygiene. Scientific Papers: Animal Science and Biotechnologies. 2012;**45**:305-312

[104] Elmoslemany AM, Keefe GP, Dohoo IR, Wichtel JJ, Stryhn H, Dingwell RT. The association between bulk tank milk analysis for raw milk quality and on-farm management practices. Preventive Veterinary Medicine. 2010;**95**:32-40. DOI: 10.1016/j.prevetmed.2010.03.007

[105] Zucali M, Bava L, Tamburini A, Brasca M, Vanoni L, Sandrucci A. Effects of season, milking routine and cow cleanliness on bacterial and somatic cell counts of bulk tank milk. Journal of Dairy Research. 2011;**78**:436-441. DOI: 10.1017/ S0022029911000598

[106] Martins ML, Pinto CLO, Rocha RB, de Araújo EF, Vanetti MCD. Genetic diversity of Gram-negative, proteolytic, psychrotrophic bacteria isolated from refrigerated raw milk. International Journal of Food Microbiology. 2006;**111**:144-148. DOI: 10.1016/j. ijfoodmicro.2006.06.020

[107] Jay JM. Microbiología Moderna de los Alimentos. 5th ed. Acribia: Zaragoza; 2009. 788 p

[108] Hayes MC, Ralyea RD, Murphy SC, Carey NR, Scarlett JM, Boor KJ. Identification and characterization of elevated microbial counts in bulk tank raw milk. Journal of Dairy Science. 2001;**84**:292-298. DOI: 10.3168/jds. S0022-0302(01)74479-7

[109] Signorini M, Sequeira G, Bonazza J, Dalla Santina R, Otero J, Rosmini M. Variación estacional en los principales indicadores de higiene de leche cruda de un tambo de la cuenca central. FAVE Sección Ciencias Veterinarias. 2003;**2**:97-110. DOI: 10.14409/favecv.v2i2.1391

[110] Samarzija D, Zamberlin S, Pogacic T. Psychrotrophic bacteria and milk and dairy products quality. Mljekarstvo. 2012;**62**:77-95

[111] Chen L, Daniel RM, Coolbear T. Detection and impact of protease and lipase activities in milk and milk powders. International Dairy Journal. 2003;**13**:255-275. DOI: 10.1016/S0958-6946(02)00171-1

[112] Cousin MA. Presence and activity of psychrotrophic microorganisms in milk and dairy products: A review. Journal of Food Protection. 1982;**45**: 172-207. DOI: 10.4315/0362-028X-45.2.172

[113] Cempírková R. Psychrotrophic vs. total bacterial counts in bulk milk samples. Veterinarni Medicina-Praha. 2002;**47**:227-233

[114] Mcphee J, Griffiths M. Psychrotrophic bacteria Pseudomonas spp. In: John WF, editor. Encyclopedia of Dairy Sciences. 2nd ed. San Diego: Academic Press; 2011. pp. 379-383

[115] Gleeson D, O'Connell A, Jordan K. Review of potential sources and control of thermoduric bacteria in bulk- tank milk. Irish Journal of Agricultural and Food Research. 2013;**52**:217-227

[116] Buehner KP, Anand S, Djira GD, Garcia A. Prevalence of thermoduric bacteria and spores on 10 Midwest dairy farms. Journal of Dairy Science. 2014;**97**:6777-6784. DOI: 10.3168/ jds.2014-8342

[117] Thomas A, Prasad V. Thermoduric bacteria in milk—A review. International Journal of Science and Research. 2012;**3**:2438-2442

[118] Hull R, Toyne S, Haynes I, Lehmann F. Thermoduric bacteria: A re-emerging problem in cheesemaking. Australian Journal of Dairy Technology. 1992;**47**:91-95

[119] Jayarao BM, Pillai SR, Sawant AA, Wolfgang DR, Hegde NV. Guidelines for monitoring bulk tank milk somatic cell and bacterial counts. Journal of Dairy Science. 2004;**87**:3561-3573. DOI: 10.3168/jds.S0022-0302(04)73493-1

[120] Janštová B, Dračková M, Vorlová A. Effect of Bacillus cereus enzymes on the milk quality following ultra high temperature processing. Acta Veterinaria Brno. 2006;**75**:601-609. DOI: 10.2754/avb200675040601

[121] Cronin UP, Wilkinson MG. Bacillus cereus endospores exhibit a heterogeneous response to heat treatment and low-temperature storage. Food Microbiology. 2008;**25**:235-243. DOI: 10.1016/j.fm.2007.11.004

[122] Zhou G, Zheng D, Dou L, Cai Q , Yuan Z. Occurrence of psychrotolerant *Bacillus cereus* group strains in ice creams. International Journal of Food Microbiology. 2010;**137**:143-146. DOI: 10.1016/j.ijfoodmicro.2009.12.005

[123] Meer RR, Baker J, Bodyfelt FW, Griffiths MW. Psychrotrophic Bacillus spp. in fluid milk products: A review. Journal of Food Protection. 1991;**54**:969-979. DOI: 10.4315/0362-028X-54.12.969

[124] Matta H, Punj V. Isolation and identification of lipolytic, psychrotrophic, spore forming bacteria from raw milk. International Journal of Dairy Technology. 1999;**52**:59-62. DOI: 10.1111/j.1471-0307.1999.tb02072.x

[125] Svensson B, Eneroth ÅSA, Brendehaug J, Molin G, Christiansson A. Involvement of a pasteurizer in the contamination of milk by *Bacillus cereus* in a commercial dairy plant. Journal of Dairy Research. 2000;**67**:455-460. DOI: 10.1017/ S0022029900004313

[126] Griffiths M. *Bacillus cereus* in liquid milk and other milk products. Bulletin of International Dairy Federation. 1992;**275**:36-39

[127] Walstra P. Ciencia de la leche y tecnología de los productos lácteos. Zaragoza: Acribia; 2001. 730 p

[128] Gebrte-Egziabher A, Humbert E, Blankenagel G. Hydrolysis of milk proteins by microbial enzymes. Journal of Food Protection. 1980;**43**:709-712. DOI: 10.4315/0362-028X-43.9.709

[129] Fajardo-Lira C, Oria M, Hayes KD, Nielsen SS. Effect of psychrotrophic bacteria and of an isolated protease from *Pseudomonas fluorescens* M3/6 on the plasmin system of fresh milk. Journal of Dairy Science. 2000;**83**:2190-2199. DOI: 10.3168/jds. S0022-0302(00)75102-2

[130] Samaržija D, Zamberlin Š, Pogačić T. Psychrotrophic bacteria and milk and dairy products quality. Mljekarstvo. 2001;**62**:77-95. DOI: 10.1016/ S0924-2244(97)01006-6

[131] Datta N, Deeth HC. Diagnosing the cause of proteolysis in UHT milk. LWT-Food Science and Technology. 2003;**36**:173-182. DOI: 10.1016/ S0023-6438(02)00214-1

[132] Nörnberg MFBL, Friedrich RSC, Weiss RDN, Tondo EC, Brandelli A. Proteolytic activity among psychrotrophic bacteria isolated from refrigerated raw milk. International Journals Dairy Technology. 2010;**63**:41-46. DOI: 10.1111/j.1471-0307.2009.00542.x

[133] Rukure G, Bester BH. Survival and growth of bacillus cereus during gouda cheese manufacturing. Food Control. 2001;**12**:31-36. DOI: 10.1016/ S0956-7135(00)00016-5

[134] Janštová B, Lukášová J, Dračková M, Vorlová L. Influence of Bacillus spp. enzymes on ultra high temperature- treated milk proteins. Acta Veterinaria Brno. 2004;**73**:393-400. DOI: 10.2754/ avb200473030393

[135] Perin LM, Moraes PM, Nero LA. Interference of storage temperatures in the development of mesophilic, psychrotrophic, lipolytic and proteolytic microbiota of milk R. Semina: Ciências Agrárias. 2012;**33**:333-342. DOI: 10.1590/1808-1657000102013

[136] Cousin MA, Marth EH. Changes in milk proteins caused by psychrotrophic bacteria. Milkwissenschaft. 1977;**32**(377):341. Available from: https://eurekamag.com/ research/000/310/000310950.php

[137] Mankai M, Boulares M, Moussa OB, Karoui R, Hassouna M. The effect of refrigerated storage of raw milk on the physicochemical and microbiological quality of Tunisian semihard gouda-type cheese during ripening. International Journals Dairy Technology. 2012;**65**:250-259. DOI: 10.1017/S0022029900032957

[138] Corsetti A, Rossi J, Gobbetti M. Interactions between yeasts and bacteria in the smear surface-ripened cheeses. International Journal of Food Microbiology. 2001;**69**:1-10. DOI: 10.1016/S0168-1605(01)00567-0

[139] Gassem MA, Frank JF. Physical properties of yogurt made from milk treated with proteolytic enzymes. Journal of Dairy Science. 1991;**74**:1503-1511. DOI: 10.3168/jds. S0022-0302(91)78310-0

[140] Sørhaug T, Stepaniak L. Psychrotrophs and their enzymes in milk and dairy products: Quality aspects. Trends in Food Science and Technology. 1997;**8**:35-41. DOI: 10.1016/ S0924-2244(97)01006-6

[141] Stead D. Microbial lipases: Their characteristic, role in food spoilage and industrial uses. Journal of Dairy Research. 1986;**53**:481-505. DOI: 10.1017/ S0022029900025103

[142] JD MP, Griffiths MW. In: Roginski H, Fuquay WJ, Fox FP, editors.

Pseudomonas spp. Encyclopedia of Dairy Sciences. Vol. 4. Academic Press; 2002. pp. 2340-2350

9

Nutritional Quality and Effect on Disease Prevention of Vegetables

João Silva Dias

Abstract

Vegetables have remarkable nutritional and health benefits. There are good reasons to include vegetables in human diet since they are enriched in bioactive compounds and by this reason they may help reduce the risk of some diseases. In this chapter, the nutrition quality and the effect on disease prevention of vegetables were analyzed. Each vegetable family and each vegetable contain a unique combination of bioactive compounds. The health benefit of vegetables should not be linked to one type of vegetable. Some experimental research evidences that vegetables exert antioxidative, anticarcinogenic, antidiabetic, and cardiovascular disease lowering effects are presented. The mechanism by which vegetable bioactive compounds decrease the risk of some of these diseases is complex and sometimes unknown.

Keywords: vegetables, health benefits, healthier life, nutrition, ANDI, bioactive compounds, antioxidants, dietary fiber, vitamins, minerals, phytochemicals

Introduction

Vegetables are important for nutritional balanced diets since they supply bioactive compounds such as dietary fiber, vitamins, minerals, and phytochemicals [1–3]. They are also associated with disease prevention by improvement of gastrointestinal health, good vision, and reduced risk of chronic and degenerative diseases such as cardiovascular diseases, certain cancers, diabetes, rheumatoid arthritis, and obesity [3–8]. In recent years consumers began to be more aware of the relation of eating patterns with nutrition and human disease prevention, and there is a general agreement among scientists, nutritionists, and dieticians that the promotion of a greater consumption of vegetables will improve nutrition quality and will bring health benefits.

The mechanisms by which vegetable consumption prevents diseases have not yet been fully understood [2, 3]. However, scientists, nutritionists, and dieticians believe that the bioactive compounds such as dietary fiber, vitamins, minerals, and phytochemical contents are responsible for mitigating some human diseases. All these different compounds may contribute to the overall health benefit. So, the health benefit of vegetables should not be linked to only one bioactive compound or one type of vegetable, but rather with a balanced diet that includes more than one type of vegetable [1–3].

Some vegetable phytochemicals (glucosinolates, thiosulfates, polyphenols, bioactive peptides, etc.) have positive effects on health. They are strong antioxidants, and they reduce the risk of chronic diseases by protecting against free radical damage, by modifying metabolic activation and detoxification of carcinogens, or even by influencing mechanisms that alter the course of tumor cells [1–3]. Phytochemicals are the key to better health as well as disease prevention.

All vegetables are sources of important vitamins (C, A, B1, B6, B9, E) and minerals and consequently have nutritional and health benefits [2, 3].

Dietary fiber is a major constituent of vegetables. Dietary fiber and other bioactive molecule contents have been usually addressed separately in nutritional studies. However, vegetable dietary fiber transports, through the human gut, a significant amount of phytochemicals, vitamins, and minerals linked to the fiber matrix [9, 10]. Therefore, associated phytochemicals, vitamins, and minerals of the whole aliment may contribute to the overall health benefit usually attributed to the dietary fiber of vegetables [2, 3].

The objective of this paper is to explore the nutritional quality and effect on disease prevention of vegetables.

Nutritional quality of vegetables

Vegetables

From more than 1000 plants that are used as vegetables, Kays and Dias [11, 12], based on a world survey, report that at least 402 vegetables are cultivated and commercialized worldwide. They represent 69 families and 230 genera. From these great diversity, leafy and stalk vegetable group comprised 53% of the total, followed by fruit and flower vegetable group (15%) and belowground (root, bulb, and tuber) vegetable group (17%). Many of these vegetable crops have more than one part used. Leafy and stalk vegetable group include lettuce, chicory, coles (head cabbages, kales, tronchudas, collards, Brussels sprouts, etc.), Chinese cabbage, pak-choi, turnip greens, mustards, rocket, watercress, Swiss chard, spinach, purslane, New Zealand spinach, celery, asparagus, rhubarb, fennel, chives, parsley, coriander, etc.

Fruit and flower vegetable group include tomato, pepper, eggplant, watermelon, melon, cucumber, squash, pumpkin, zucchini, bitter gourd, peas, beans, lentils, okra, sweet maize, cauliflower, broccoli, kailan, broccoletti, artichoke, etc.

Root, bulb, and tuber vegetable group include carrot, garden beet, turnip, radish, rutabaga, parsnip, sweet potato, cassava, celeriac, onion, garlic, shallot, leek, Welsh onion, potato, etc.

Vegetables and human nutrition

Until few years ago, it was believed that the key for human nutrition and health was only 14 vitamins and 16 essential minerals. Recently, with the great developments in chemistry, it was found that, in addition to these vitamins and minerals, vegetables contain thousands of beneficial phytochemicals. As mentioned some vegetable's phytochemicals are robust antioxidants and are believed to reduce the risk of some chronic and degenerative diseases [2–4].

With the exclusion of the organosulfur compounds (OSCs) glucosinolates and thiosulfates (which are distinct phytochemicals of Brassicaceae and Alliaceae families, respectively), the phytochemical, vitamin, and mineral contents of many vegetables lie principally in dietary fiber, polyphenols (carotenoids, flavonoids), vitamin C, folate, calcium, and selenium [2, 3]. The principal dissimilarity is that each vegetable family incorporates a distinct amalgam and amount of these bioactive compounds, which differentiate them from other vegetables [2, 13].

Vegetables of the Apiaceae family (carrot, parsnip, celery, celeriac, fennel, parsley, coriander, etc.) are rich in flavonoids, carotenoids, vitamin C, and vitamin E. For example, celery and parsley are among the best vegetable sources for the flavonoid apigenin and vitamin E [2, 14], and carrots have a unique combination of three flavonoids: kaempferol, quercetin, and luteolin [15–17].

Vegetables of the Asteraceae or Compositae family (lettuce, endive and escarole chicories, stem lettuce, globe artichoke, etc.) are rich in flavonoids, tocopherols, and conjugated quercetin. Crozier et al. [18] observed sizeable variations in flavonol content within lettuce cultivars. The outer leaves of "Lollo Rosso," a red cultivar, contained 911 µg/g fresh weight of quercetin, in contrast with the common head lettuce that contained only 11 µg/g. And, the levels in iceberg lettuce were even lower than in the head lettuce. The red color of "Lollo Rosso" lettuce is due to high levels of anthocyanins, which like quercetin are products of the phenylpropanoid pathway. As one end product of the pathway has been elevated, it may well be that other related compounds, including the flavonols, are also found in higher concentrations. Roman lettuce is richer in lutein than head lettuces; and leafy and roman lettuces are richer in quercetin [3, 13].

The Chenopodiaceae family vegetables (Swiss chard, spinach, garden beet, quinoa, etc.) are among those that are rich in oxalates [19, 20] but also excellent sources of dietary fiber, vitamins, calcium, manganese, flavonoids, and carotenoids. When oxalates become too concentrated in body fluids, they can crystallize and cause health problems such as kidney calcium oxalate stones.

The Cucurbitaceae family vegetables (e.g., squash, pumpkin, cucumber, melon, bitter gourd, etc.) are rich in carotenoids, and tocopherols, and vitamin C [21]. Burger et al. [22] in a survey of 350 melon accessions observed a 50-fold variation in ascorbic acid content, ranging from 0.7 to 35.3 mg/100 g fresh weight. Ascorbic acid and β-carotene content ranged from 7.0 to 32.0 mg/100 g and 4.7 to 62.2 µg/100 g, respectively, in sweet melons [23].

The vegetables of the Leguminosae or Fabaceae family (all the legumes, e.g., pea, bean, soybean, lentils, chickpea, etc.), mature and immature seeds, are great sources of dietary fiber, resistant starch, protein, isoflavonoids [24], calcium, and iron. Mallillin et al. [25] studied the total, soluble, and insoluble fiber and fermentability characteristics of 10 legume mature seeds (mung bean, soybean, peanut, pole sitao, cowpea, chickpea, green pea, lima bean, kidney bean, and pigeon pea). They concluded that the dietary fiber content in these ten legumes ranged from 20.9 to 46.9 g/100 g and that the best sources after in vitro fermentation using human fecal inoculum-stimulating conditions in the human colon (as mmol/g/ fiber isolate of acetate, propionate, and butyrate produced after fiber fermentation) were pole sitao and mung bean (acetate), kidney bean and pigeon pea (propionate), and peanut and cowpea (butyrate). High-flavonol legumes include sugar snap peas and mange tout, which were found to contain 98 and 145 µg quercetin/g, respectively [2]. As mentioned some legumes are also rich in iron. Trinidad et al. [26] studied the mineral availability in vitro of iron, zinc, and calcium in 10 local legumes (cowpeas, mung beans, pole sitao, chickpeas, green peas, groundnuts, pigeon peas, kidney beans, lima beans, and soybeans). They found that the highest iron availability among these legumes was for lima beans and mung bean, while for zinc and calcium, the highest availability was for kidney beans and pigeon peas. Groundnuts have the lowest iron, zinc, and calcium availability. They concluded that mineral availability of iron, zinc, and calcium from legumes differs and may be attributed to their mineral content, mineral-mineral interaction, and their phytic and tannic acid content. Mung bean either eaten as whole pod grains or grown to produce bean sprouts is an important source of iron for women and children throughout South Asia [1, 27].

Vegetables of the Brassicaceae or Cruciferae family, which include kales, collards, cabbages, Brussels sprouts, cauliflower, broccoli, kailan, pak-choi, Chinese cabbage, turnip, broccoletti, swede, watercress, radish, horseradish, rocket, mustards, etc., are high sources of glucosinolates, as well as vitamin C, carotenoids, folates, and calcium, and can accumulate selenium. Comparative studies of glucosinolate profiles within each Cruciferae, and among accessions and plant parts, indicate significant quantitative and qualitative differences [28–39]. Kushad et al. [34] observed in 65 broccoli cultivars that glucoraphanin was the predominant glucosinolate and that there was more than 27-fold difference between the highest concentration in "Brigadier" and the lowest in "EV6–1." Hansen et al. [40] also observed in 21 red cabbage and 6 white cabbage cultivars, a considerable variation in the concentration of glucosinolates. Red cabbages were found to contain significantly higher concentrations of glucoraphanin compared to white ones. There were also significant differences within the red cabbages examined: "Rodima" had the highest level of glucoraphanin (7.4 mg/g), whereas "Primero" has the lowest (0.6 mg/g). The white cabbages presented significantly higher levels of glucoiberin than the red ones: white cabbage "Bartolo" had the highest concentration of glucoiberin (7.4 mg/g), whereas "Candela" has the lowest (1.7 mg/g), and red cabbages ranged from 3 to 0.3 mg/g. The red cabbages were also found to contain significantly higher levels of gluconasturtiin than white: "Amager Garo" had the highest level of gluconasturtiin (1 mg/g), whereas "Primero" had the lowest (0.1 mg/g).

In turnip and rutabagas, similar differences between accessions were also observed [30]. Fahey et al. [41] evaluated glucosinolate content of broccoli sprouts and found that they contain nearly 20- to 50-fold higher glucosinolate concentrations than tissue from mature plants. In broccoli heads, the predominant glucosinolates are glucoraphanin, glucobrassicin, progoitrin, and gluconasturtiin [32, 34, 36, 38, 42, 43]. In cabbage, Brussels sprouts, cauliflower, kale, tronchuda, and collard, the most significant glucosinolates are sinigrin, progoitrin, and glucobrassicin [29, 32, 34, 39, 40, 44]. In turnip and rutabagas, the major glucosinolates are glucoerucin, glucoraphanin, and glucobrassicin [30, 33]. In radish, the most significant glucosinolates are glucoerucin, glucoraphanin, and glucobrassicin [31, 35]. Each of these Cruciferae also contains smaller amounts of other glucosinolates.

Cao et al. [45] observed that in Brassicaceae vegetables vitamin C is the most abundant vitamin in coles (cabbage, broccoli, cauliflower, Brussels sprouts, tronchuda, and kale) and that kale rated as the second highest vitamin content and the second highest among 22 vegetables. They are also excellent sources of folate. Brussels sprouts and broccoli rank among the highest vegetable sources for folate [46, 47]. Most of the Cruciferae are also good sources of calcium. Kales, tronchudas, and collards contain the highest content in fiber and calcium when compared to other Brassicaceae. Vegetables of the Cruciferae family are able to accumulate selenium when grown on selenium-enriched soils. Banuelos and Meek [48] stated that broccoli-grown soils with high-selenium levels accumulated sevenfold more selenium than cabbage, collards, and Swiss chard.

Vegetables of the Alliaceae family (e.g., onions, garlic, shallots, leek, Welsh onion, chives, etc.) are rich in thiosulfates, flavonoids, calcium, potassium, manganese, and chromium and can accumulate selenium. The types and composition of thiosulfates differ from *Allium* [49]. Kalra et al. [50] reported that garlic fresh bulbs contain 33 thiosulfates. The major thiosulfates in the cytoplasm of *Allium* species are S-allyl-cysteine sulfoxide (alliin), S-methyl-cysteine sulfoxide (methiin), and γ-glutamyl-L-cysteine [51]. Other minor thiosulfates include S-propenyl-cysteine sulfoxide (isoalliin) and S-ethyl-cysteine (ethiin) [52]. None of the thiosulfates found in *Allium* have been detected in other vegetables, except S-methyl-cysteine sulfoxide (methiin) which was detected in some Cruciferae [53]. The most important thiosulfates detected in onion bulbs are isoalliin (49%), methiin (34%), propiin (6%), ethiin (5%), and alliin (5%) and in garlic alliin (92%) and methiin (8%) and trace amounts of ethiin, propiin, and isoalliin [51, 53–55].

The second most important group of bioactive compounds in *Allium* is flavonoids. Miean and Mohamed [56] mentioned that onion leaves had the highest total flavonoid content among 62 different vegetables. About 55% of this total of flavonoids is quercetin, 31% kaempferol, and 14% luteolin. Two flavonoids are found in onion bulbs: anthocyanins in red onions and flavonols like quercetin (more than 95%) and kaempferol in most yellow onion varieties [57]. White onion cultivars have significantly less quercetin than the red ones [2, 3, 58]. In garlic cloves, 72% of the total flavonoids is myricetin, 23% apigenin, and 5% quercetin [56]. In chive, garlic chive, and leek, the predominant flavonoid is kaempferol [58].

Onion and garlic are excellent sources of calcium, potassium, and manganese providing up to 10% of the human daily requirements. Most of the onions and garlics contain very low concentrations of selenium but can accumulate selenium when grown on selenium-enriched soils. Ip and Lisk [59] reported that garlic fertilized with a high selenium and low sulfur fertilizer accumulated between 110 and 150 ppm selenium, while onion accumulated up to 28 ppm. Onions also contain chromium [2]. Two hundred grams of onions contain up to 20% of the daily requirements in chromium. Onions are a rich source of dietary fibers and especially of inulin, a polyfructosan, that has prebiotic properties [2, 3]. Vegetables of the Solanaceae family that includes tomato, potato, sweet and hot peppers, eggplant, etc. are very diverse, in their contribution to bioactive compounds.

Tomato is the second most produced and consumed vegetable in the world after potato. Tomato has a unique nutritional and phytochemical profile. Carotenoids are the major bioactive compounds in tomato with 60–64% lycopene, 10–12% phytoene, 7–9% neurosporene, and 10–15% carotenes [60]. Red varieties of tomato contain more lycopene (on average 90 mg/kg) than yellow ones (5 mg/kg) [61].

The average daily intake of lycopene in human diet is about 25 mg/day. Processed tomatoes (juice, sauce, paste, and ketchup) contain higher lycopene (2- to 40-fold) than fresh tomatoes [60, 62, 63]. Lycopene is a very potent antioxidant [64, 65].

Tomato contains also significant amounts of α-, β-, γ-, and δ-carotene (0.6–2.0 mg/kg) which make it for consumers a top contributor of provitamin A and vitamin A [66, 67]. Tomatoes are also an excellent source of vitamin C [68]. Tomato contains small amounts of lutein, α-, β-, and γ-tocopherols and conjugated flavonoids (quercetin and kaempferol) [66, 69–71]. About 98% of these flavonoids are present in the peel [72]. Cherry tomato cultivars have higher flavonoid contents than beef ones, and field-grown tomatoes have higher flavonoid contents than greenhouse-grown ones [18, 72]. Tomatoes are also an excellent source of potassium.

Potato is usually only associated as a source of carbohydrates. But it is also an excellent source of essential amino acids (such as lysine) and other bioactive compounds [2]. In addition to superior quality proteins, potato tubers also have significant amounts of vitamins and minerals, as well as phytochemicals (phenolics, phytoalexins, etc.), and protease inhibitors [73, 74]. There are yellow-, red-, and purple-fleshed potato cultivars with high content of phytochemicals; nevertheless, some cultivars are known to have lower [2]. Other bioactive antioxidants presented in potato tubers include α-tocopherol, lutein, β-carotene, folates, and selenium [73, 74].

Peppers are excellent sources of vitamins C, K, carotenoids, and flavonoids [75]. They provide also a respectable amount of dietary fiber. Peppers contain in average 1–2 g/kg of vitamin C, which is equivalent to 200–300% of the recommended daily allowance [76]. Their content of provitamin A carotenoids (α- and β-carotene) depends in the cultivar. Some cultivars of hot pepper have 12 mg/kg total carotenoids, while others have trace amounts [76, 77]. In pepper, the major conjugated flavonoids are quercetin and luteolin. Their content varies among cultivars ranging from not detectable to 800 mg/kg [78]. Red bell peppers have significantly higher levels of bioactive compounds than green ones. Red bell peppers also contain lycopene [74].

In hot peppers or chilies, the major phytochemicals are capsaicinoids [2, 74]. More than 20 capsaicinoids, belonging to capsaicin and dihydrocapsaicin groups, have been identified. Capsaicin contributes about 70% for the pungent/hot fire flavor in chili peppers, while dihydrocapsaicin represents 30% [79]. Significant variations in capsaicinoids are found between and within peppers, ranging from about 220 ppm in *Capsicum annum* (sweet pepper) to 20,000 ppm in Capsicum chinense (hot pepper) [80]. Fresh chili peppers have high levels of vitamins and minerals. Just 100 g of hot peppers, red or green, provides 240% of vitamin C, 39% of vitamin B6-complex group, 32% of vitamin A, 13% of iron, 14% of copper, and 7% of potassium of the recommended daily allowance [81]. Chili peppers contain a good amount of manganese and magnesium [2].

Eggplant besides vitamins (C, K, B6-complex group, folate, and niacin) and minerals (magnesium, copper, manganese, molybdenum, potassium) also contains important phytochemicals like flavonoids, such as nasunin, and phenolic compounds, such caffeic and chlorogenic acid [2, 74]. Nasunin is the major phytochemical in purple eggplant cultivars. Nasunin is part of the antho- cyanin purple pigment found in the skin of eggplant [82–84]. Matsuzoe et al. [85] examined the profile of anthocyanins in several eggplants and found that nasunin represents between 70 and 90% of the total anthocyanins in the skin. Nasunin is an antioxidant that effectively scavenges reactive oxygen species, such as hydrogen peroxide, hydroxyl, and superoxide, as well as inhibits the formation of hydroxyl radicals, probably by chelating ferrous ions in the Fenton reaction [82, 84]. The predominant phenolic compound found in all cultivars of eggplant tested by Matsuzoe et al. [85] is chlorogenic acid, which is one of the most potent free radical scavengers found in plant tissues. Benefits attributed to chlorogenic acid include antimutagenic (anticancer), antimicrobial, and anti-low-density lipoproteins and antiviral activities. In addition to chlorogenic acid, Whitaker and Stommel [86] found 13 other phenolic acids present in seven eggplant cultivars. "Black Magic" was found by these authors to have nearly three times the amount of antioxidant phenolics as the other eggplant cultivars studied. Eggplant fruits also contain several other antioxidants including flavonoids myricetin and kaempferol as well as carotenoids lycopene, lutein, and α-carotene [56, 87]. Eggplant is richer in nicotine than any other edible vegetable and contains measurable amounts of oxalates [2, 74]. Due to oxalates individuals with already existing and untreated kidney or gallbladder problems may avoid eating eggplant [74, 88].

Looking generally for the nutrition quality of vegetables groups we can say. In the leafy and stalk vegetables, they are fiber sources, rich in important minerals such as calcium, magnesium, and iron and vitamins C and A and riboflavin. In this group, young fresh leaves contain more vitamin C than mature plants. The thinner and greener leaves are more nutritious respecting vitamins and minerals but less nutritious respecting dietary fiber. The green outer leaves of the head or pseudo-head leafy vegetables such as cabbage, lettuce, and endive chicory are usually richer in calcium, magnesium, iron, and vitamins than the inner leaves. Stalk vegetables like tronchuda cabbage, pak-choi, celery, and asparagus are rich in dietary fiber.

In the fruit and belowground organ vegetables, the skin and inside color reflect different bioactive compounds/pigment present. Anthocyanins (flavonoid) give vegetable leaves, belowground organs, and fruits their purple and purple-red color appearance, such as in red anthocyanin lettuce and endive chicory, red cabbage, Swiss chard, rhubarb, etc. (leafy and stalk vegetables); garden beet, purple carrot, red onion, purple- and purple-red-skinned potato, purple sweet potato, etc. (below ground vegetables); and purple eggplant, purple tomato, purple pepper, purple and black broccoli, purple corn, etc. (fruit and flowering vegetables). The most abundant carotenoids in vegetables are α-carotene, β-carotene, and lycopene (carotenes) and lutein, zeaxanthin, and β-cryptoxanthin (xanthophylls) [2, 74, 89]. The most common carotenes are β-carotene and lycopene. β-Carotene (as well as α-carotene) can be found in orange and yellow skin fruits, belowground organs, and leafy vegetables [2, 74]. As a rule of thumb, the greater the intensity of the orange color, the more β-carotene the vegetable contains [2, 74]. Lycopene can be found in red fruits (e.g., tomato), red belowground organs (e.g., red carrot), and red leafy vegetables. Lutein is the most abundant xanthophyll [2, 74]. Xanthophylls are responsible for the yellow color of vegetables.

ANDI and nutritional quality of vegetables

Aggregate Nutrient Density Index (ANDI) is a scoring system based on nutrient content, rated on a 1–1000 scale that was established by Fuhrman [90]. This index are scores attributed to a variety of vegetables (and other foods) based on how many nutrients they deliver to our body in each calorie consumed. It was calculated by evaluating the content of dietary fiber, vitamins, minerals, phytochemicals, antioxidant capacities, etc. It is an index that estimates the nutritional quality of vegetables. **Table 1** presents the highest ANDI scores in leafy vegetables.

Three main vegetable families are shown in this table: Brassicaceae (kale, collard greens, mustard greens, turnip greens, watercress, pak-choi, Chinese cabbage, Brussels sprouts, rocket, cabbage and broccoletti), Chenopodiaceae (Swiss chard and spinach), and Asteraceae (green leaf lettuce, chicory, and romaine lettuce). The highest ANDI scores of non-leafy vegetables are presented in **Table 2.**

Table 2 also shows other Brassicaceae like radish, turnip, kohlrabi, cauliflower, and rutabaga. Different vegetables from various families are also shown as well as differences among the peppers, where orange pepper is better than the red and red better than the green pepper.

Leafy vegetables thus have the highest ANDI scores compared to other vegetables. They are rich in dietary fiber, carotenoids, vitamin C, vitamin E, flavonoids, calcium, magnesium, etc. All the leafy vegetables are good sources of magnesium because they have chlorophyll.

The leafy vegetables with high ANDI scores are Brassicaceae. They have dietary fiber, are a rich source of glucosinolates and other bioactive nutrients, and have a very high content in calcium and β-carotene. They are excellent sources of lutein and can also accumulate selenium.

Table 1. *List of identified leafy vegetables with the highest ANDI scores.*

Vegetable	ANDI	Vegetable	ANDI
1.Kale	1000	9.Chinese cabbage	714
2.Collard greens	1000	10.Brussels sprouts	672
3.Mustard greens	1000	11.Rocket	604
4.Swiss chard	1000	12.Lettuce (green leaf)	585
5.Turnip greens	1000	13.Chicory	516
6.Watercress	1000	14.Romaine lettuce	510
7.Pak-choi	865	15.Cabbage	481
8.Spinach	739	16.Broccoletti	455

Table 2. *List of identified non-leafy vegetables with the highest ANDI scores.*

Vegetable	ANDI	Vegetable	ANDI
1.Radish	502	7.Cauliflower	315
2.Turnip	473	8.Rutabaga	296
3.Carrots	458	9.Bell pepper (red)	265
4.Winter squash "Acorn"	444	10.Bell pepper (green)	258
5.Bell pepper (yellow/orange)	371	11.Artichoke	244
6.Kohlrabi	352	12.Asparagus	234

Another important family is Chenopodiaceae. A recent research has shown that Swiss chard leaves contain at least distinct polyphenol antioxidants [91] comprising the flavonoids kaempferol and syringic acid [91–93]. Swiss chard and garden beet leaves have a unique source of the bioactive antioxidants named betalains [2, 74]. Nine betacyanin pigments were identified in the reddish-purple stems and veins of the leaves of Swiss chard and beet [94]. In the Swiss chard's yellowish stems and veins, 19 betaxanthin pigments were identified, including histamine-betaxanthin, alanine- betaxanthin, tyramine-betaxanthin, and 3-methoxytyramine-betaxanthin [94].

In Asteraceae, lettuces and chicories are the main vegetables used in raw salads. Leaf and romaine lettuces have higher ANDI scores (585 and 510, respectively) than iceberg lettuce. Besides, the nutritive value of leaf and romaine lettuce is higher than head lettuces (butter and batavia types). They have more dietary fiber, minerals, vitamins, and phytochemicals. Raw vegetables are the healthiest food we can eat since some phytochemicals are only available if we eat the vegetables raw [95].

In the non-leafy vegetables, we have after radish and turnip (both Brassicaceae) the carrots. They are high in fiber and nutrient rich. Carrots have different colors. Orange carrots have α- and β-carotene (vitamin A-rich carotenoids), and purple carrots are rich in anthocyanins (flavonoids) and low in carotenoids [96, 97]. Winter squash "Acorn" has a high β-carotene content. Kohlrabi, cauliflower, and rutabaga are also Brassicaceae, and so they are good sources of vitamins, minerals, and healthy glucosinolates. Kohlrabi (stem) and rutabaga (roots) besides having high vitamin C and antioxidant content due to glucosinolates are good alternative to potatoes since they are not starchy as potato and can be eaten raw and when sliced they do not produce discoloration. The nutritional value of the outer leaves of cauliflower is much higher than the flower buds. Artichoke is rich in fiber and a good source of minerals, namely, calcium, potassium, and phosphorus. It contains also many bioactive compounds such as glycosides and phenolics, mainly caffeicinic acid [98]. Asparagus besides rich in fiber is a very rich source of folic acid.

Effect on disease prevention of vegetables

Effect on cancers

The International Agency for Research on Cancer (IARC) estimates that the percentage of cancers due to unbalanced diets with low vegetable intake and low consumption of complex carbohydrates and dietary fiber ranges from 5 to 12% for all cancers and 20–30% for upper gastrointestinal tract cancers [2, 3]. The World Health Organization (WHO) states that about 14% of worldwide deaths are attributable to gastrointestinal cancers due to inadequate vegetable and fruit consumption [99]. The American Cancer Society observed that more than two-thirds of cancer deaths in the United States are avoidable and reported that one-third of cancer deaths can be prevented by a proper diet rich in vegetables [100, 101].

Numerous epidemiological studies conducted in the United States and in developed countries, which include results from tests on adenomatous polyps (the precursors to colorectal cancer), concluded that high vegetable intake decreases the risk of colorectal cancer [26, 102–106]. Witte et al. [107] observed significantly lower incidence of colorectal polyps in men and women ages between 50 and 74 years old who consumed higher rates of vegetables, namely, crucifers, garlic, and tofu. It is also interesting also that this research concluded that vegetables have more beneficial effects against colorectal polyps than fruits or fiber from grains. In another research with 41,837 women aged between 55 and 69 years old, Steinmetz et al. [106] found a 20–40% reduction in risk of colon cancer in populations with higher vegetable consumption. Other studies have also estimated lower risk of colon cancer, ranging from three- to eightfold due to high vegetable and fruit intake [26, 108–110]. Increasing the consumption of vegetables reduces the risk of cancer since the antioxidants in vegetables prevent the oxidative damage of the cells in the body [111, 112]

Leafy vegetables have protective effects against cancers, especially gastrointestinal carcinomas, mainly due to dietary fiber, but also to phytochemicals, vitamins (C, E, K, and A), and minerals they contain [113]. Tewani et al. [114] state that spinach shows protective effects against gastrointestinal cancer by reducing oxidative stress thanks to vitamins (C and E), carotenes (mainly β-carotene), lutein, and flavonoids (mainly flavones) it contains.

Cruciferous vegetables rich in glucosinolates have been shown to protect against lung cancer, prostate cancer, breast cancer, and chemically induced cancers [115–119]. The evidence concerning the anticarcinogenic effect of glucosinolates of cruciferous vegetables were from in vivo studies, mainly with broccoli, using animal models and human volunteers [116, 118–124].

Intact glucosinolates have no biological activity against cancer. However, their breakdown products have been shown to stimulate mixed-function oxidases involved in detoxification of carcinogens, reducing the risk of certain cancers [28, 125, 126]. Not all glucosinolate breakdown products have anticancer activity [127]. The glucosinolates glucoraphanin, glucoiberin, glucobrassicin, and gluconasturtiin are involved in the anticarcinogenic activity, and glucoraphanin is known to bolster the defenses of cells against carcinogens through an upregulation of enzymes of carcinogen defense.

Epidemiological data show that a diet rich in cruciferous vegetables can reduce the risk from several cancers by an intake of at least 10 g per day [115, 116, 118]. Epidemiological studies have suggested that diets rich in broccoli may reduce the risk of prostate cancer, and consumption of one or more portions of broccoli per week can reduce the incidence and the progression from localized to aggressive forms of prostate cancer [118, 119]. There is also strong evidence that isothiocyanates (an important group of breakdown products of glucosinolates) from cruciferous vegetables prevent bladder cancer, namely, transitional cell carcinoma of the urinary bladder [128].

Consumption of *Allium* vegetables has been also found to retard growth of several types of cancers. A number of epidemiological studies show inverse correlations between the consumption of *Allium* vegetables, mainly onions and garlics, and the reduced incidence of cancers.

There is a strong link between the consumption of onions and the reduced incidence of stomach and intestine cancers [129, 130]. Control studies reveal that consumption of one to seven portions of onions per week reduces the risks of colon, ovary, larynx, and mouth cancers [131].

Mortality due to prostate cancer also appears to be reduced by a diet making a large consumption of onions [132]. Onion extracts prevent tumors by inhibiting the mutation process [133] and reducing the proliferation of cancer cells [134].

Epidemiological researches show the correlation between moderate garlic intake and a low esophageal and stomach tract cancer incidence [131, 135, 136]. Garlic extracts prevent tumor initiation by inhibiting the activation of pro-carcinogens and by stimulating their elimination [137, 138]. A regular consumption of garlic has been associated also with the reduction in the incidence of preneoplastic lesions occurring in the gastric mucosa of individuals infected by *Helicobacter pylori* [139]. Other studies analyzing the preventive effect of garlic have evidenced their suppressive potential on the development and progression of colorectal adenomas [110, 140]. A reduced cancer risk by regular consumption of garlic has been widely documented also for colorectal and prostate cancers [131, 136, 141, 142]. The impact of a diet rich in *Allium* vegetables in antiprostate cancer is higher in men presenting localized rather than advanced forms [142].

The impact of a regular intake of *Allium* vegetables on the incidence of cancers affecting the breast, endometrium, and lungs has been studied in a limited number of investigations [143–145]. The risk of breast cancer was shown to decrease as consumption of *Allium* increased [143]. Onion extracts have apoptosis-inducing effects in epithelial MDA-MB-231 cells that cause breast cancer [146].

In tomato several investigations have shown an inverse relationship between plasma/serum lycopene concentrations and the risk of some cancers [147–153]. Reports on 13 cancer types were identified in literature, of which breast, colorectal, gastric-gastrointestinal, and prostate cancers. For breast, colorectal, and gastric cancers, the existing data support a potential protective association between tomato and lycopene intake and cancer risk. People consuming diets rich in tomato/lycopene and tomato-based products were found to be less likely to develop stomach and rectal cancers than those who consume lesser amounts [154]. Among the cancers investigated, prostate cancer is the most widely researched. Tomato and lycopene intake is preventive against prostate cancer [13, 155]. Hadley et al. [156] in an epidemiological study found that consuming tomato and tomato products was associated with a lower incidence of prostate cancer [156]. A prostate cancer risk reduction of nearly 35% was observed when the test subjects consumed 10 or more servings of tomato per week [157]; and the effect was much stronger for patients with more aggressive and advanced stages of cancer [157].

Other Solanaceae associated with cancer prevention are chili peppers and eggplant. Chili peppers are tough to prevent cancer cells from growing, developing, and spreading due to it capsaicin content [158]. A study of Nagase et al. [159] showed that eggplant extract inhibited human fibrosarcoma HT-180 cell invasiveness.

Consumption of legumes like soybean, chickpea, and lentil rich in isoflavonoids daidzein, genistein and glycitein have been suggested to have multiple beneficial effects in a number of diseases, including certain types of cancer [160, 161]. Ziegler et al. [162] observed that Asian-American women who consumed a diet rich in soy had low risk of breast cancer incidence. Later studies of soy-rich diets confirmed that the main anti-breast cancer ingredient is genistein [163–165]. Dong et al. [166] in a meta-analysis of prospective studies pointed out that soybean isoflavonoid intake is associated with a significantly reduced risk of breast cancer incidence in Asian populations, but not in Western populations. Epidemiological indications jointly with clinical data from animal and in vitro studies highly supported a positive correlation between soybean isoflavonoid consumption and protection toward prostate cancers [164, 167]. Besides breast and prostate cancer, soy isoflavonoids also exhibit inhibitory effects on ovarian cancer, leukemia, and lung cancer [168].

Anticarcinogenic effect of carrot juice extracts on myeloid and lymphoid leukemia cell lines was investigated by Zaini et al. [169]. Carrot juice extracts owned the ability to "kill" leukemia cells and inhibit their progression. Those researchers believed that β-carotene and falcarinol present in the carrot juice extract may have been responsible for this positive effect. As a complement of this study, Larsen et al. [170] examined the impact of carrot and falcarinol feeding toward the development of azoxymethane-induced colon preneoplastic lesions in the rat colon. The results of this study demonstrated that diets with carrot and falcarinol have the potential to delay the development of large aberrant crypt foci and colon tumors on rats. Purup et al. [171] observed also that carrot extracts which contain falcarinol and related aliphatic C17-polyacetylenes (falcarindiol and falcarindiol 3-acetate) had significant inhibitory effect on intestinal cancer cell proliferation. Pisani et al. [172] in a case–control study show that smokers who eat carrots more than once a week have a smaller risk of lung cancer.

Effect on cardiovascular diseases

Vegetables offer protection against cardiovascular diseases since they are free of saturated fat, trans fat, and cholesterol and rich in bioactive compounds such as dietary fibers, OSCs, flavonoids, carotenoids, phytoestrogens, monoterpenes, and sterols. Unbalanced diets with low vegetable intake have been estimated to cause about 31% of ischemic heart disease and 11% of stroke worldwide [3]. A healthy diet with high vegetable consumption has been associated with lower risk of cardiovascular disease in humans [173, 174]. Liu et al. [175] test the influence of vegetable intake on the incidence of cardiovascular disease among 15,220 male physicians without a history of heart disease or stroke. The results of this investigation show that the participators who consumed more than two servings of vegetables per day had 25% less cardiovascular disease than those who consumed less than one serving. Based on this and other researches, the American Heart Association (AHA) has concluded that a diet high in vegetables and fruits may reduce the risk of cardiovascular disease in humans [176].

Prevention of cardiovascular diseases has been attributed to regular garlic consumption. Epidemiological studies demonstrate that there is an inverse correlation between garlic consumption and incidence of cardiovascular diseases [3, 74]. Yeh and Liu [177] show that garlic extracts and their OSCs have cholesterol and lipid-lowering effects by inhibiting monooxygenase and HMG-CoA reductase, two key enzymes involved in cholesterol and fatty acid synthesis. Moriguchi et al. [178] reported that garlic extracts have fibrinolytic effect by inhibiting lipid peroxidation and hemolysis of erythrocytes. Chang et al. [179] in their studies reported also the antiplatelet effect of sodium 2-propenyl thiosulfate from garlic, by inhibiting cyclooxygenase enzyme activity.

Similar to garlic, onions also contain a number of OSCs and flavonoids, such as quercetin, that can reduce the risks for cardiovascular diseases by increasing antioxidant capacity [3, 74, 180]. Hubbard et al. [181] in a pilot study in humans showed that the consumption of the equivalent of three onions in a soup was sufficient to significantly reduce the blood platelet aggregation. Platelet aggregation is an important risk for the development of coronary thrombosis and atherosclerosis. Briggs et al. [182] observed that by cutting raw onions S-alkenyl-L-cysteine sulfoxides are converted by enzyme alliinase into thiosulfinates and copaenes and these compounds inhibit platelet aggregation. Ried et al. [183] report also that onion and garlic had a blood pressure lowering effect by inhibiting angiotensin-converting enzyme activity and inducing intracellular nitric oxide and hydrogen sulfide production.

The consumption of leafy vegetables, due to bioactive compounds, increases antioxidant capacity and protects against oxidative stress which play an important role in the pathogenesis of cardiovascular diseases. Another reason is their low sodium and high calcium and magnesium content [3, 74]. Furthermore, that consumption also reduces blood pressure, inhibits platelet aggregation, and improves endothelial dysfunction due to their rich inorganic nitrate content [184]. In diets where the consumption of leafy vegetables is high, the rate of cardiovascular diseases is lower compared with diets with less consumption [3, 74, 185]. Rastogi et al. [186] observed that individuals with consumption of more than three portions of leafy vegetables a day have an incidence of about 60% less of ischemic heart disease than those consuming less than one portion. Saluk et al. [187] report that anthocyanin extracted from red cabbage has a protective effect on blood platelets.

In broccoli, indole-3-carbinol and sulforaphane, which are hydrolysis breakdown products of glucosinolate glucoraphanin, are thought to be the major bioactive compounds protective against cardiovascular diseases [188, 189]. Jeffery and Araya [189] report that indole-3-carbinol and sulforaphane besides protecting against ischemic damage of the heart also protect against inflammation by inhibiting cytokine production [189]. Murashima et al. [190] reported in a study, with multiple biomarkers for metabolism and oxidative stress, that broccoli sprouts decrease levels of total cholesterol and low-density lipoprotein cholesterol and increase levels of high-density lipoprotein cholesterol.

Jorge et al. [191] show in their studies that eggplant is effective in the treatment of high blood cholesterol. Guimarães et al. [192] showed a significant decrease in blood levels of total cholesterol and low-density lipoprotein cholesterol in human volunteers who were fed with eggplant powder. Kwon et al. [193] presented eggplant phenolics as inhibitors of key enzymes relevant for type 2 diabetes and hypertension.

Legumes are also protective against cardiovascular diseases due to their high saponin and soluble fiber content [2, 3, 74]. Soluble fiber delays gastric emptying, slows glucose absorption, and lowers serum cholesterol levels [194]. In several epidemiologic studies, a positive correlation between increased legume consumption and reduced mortality due to cardiovascular disease was observed [195, 196]. Consumption of legumes reduces the levels of total cholesterol and low-density lipoprotein cholesterol by inhibiting the absorption of bile acid from intestines and by promoting the formation of propionic acid and other short-chain fatty acids that inhibit the synthesis of cholesterol [197].

Nicolle et al. [198] suggest that carrot intake may exert a protective effect against cardiovascular disease and that this protective effect may be due to the synergistic action of dietary fiber and antioxidant polyphenols in carrot. Gramenzi et al. [199] state that the consumption of carrots is associated with smaller risk of acute myocardial infarction in women. Gilani et al. [200] examined in rats the antihypertensive effect of DC-2 and DC-3, two coumarin glycosides from carrot. Their results showed that these glycoside compounds caused a decrease in arterial blood pressure in the rats. Further in vitro studies by the same researchers demonstrate that the decreased blood pressure observed may be due to the calcium channel blocking action of coumarin glycosides DC-2 and DC-3 from carrots.

Effect on diabetes

Dias and Imai [95] highlight the nutritional and health benefits of different vegetables and their dietary fiber, vitamin C, vitamin E, carotenoids, flavonoids, thiosulfates, magnesium, selenium, zinc, and chromium contents, to prevent and reverse diabetes. Besides they also analyzed when we should eat the vegetables, and mainly the effect of eating vegetables before carbohydrates on postprandial blood glucose levels, and glycemic control. Data of these authors shows that eating vegetables before carbohydrates is effective to reduce postprandial hyperglycemia in type 2 diabetes patients, as well as in healthy people. So, vegetables should be eaten before carbohydrates at every meal [95].

Carter et al. [201] in a systematic review and meta-analysis found that greater leafy vegetable consumption was colligated with 14% decrease in risk of type 2 diabetes. Another previous research reported that each daily serving of leafy green vegetables generates a 9% decrease in risk of type 2 diabetes [202]. Khan et al. [203] saw that oral feeding of regular rats for 60 days with a mustard (Brassica juncea) diet (10% w/w) led to significant hypoglycemic effect. This result was associated to the positive stimulation of glycogen synthetase and to the suppression of glycogen phosphorylase and some other gluconeogenic enzymes. As mentioned Swiss chard leaves contain syringic acid that have blood sugar-regulating properties [91–93]. Syringic acid was demonstrated to inhibit the activity of α-glucosidase enzyme. When α-glucosidase gets inhibited, fewer carbohydrates are converted to sugars, and blood sugar is able to remain more steady [204]. Garden beet leaves have the same properties, since beet and Swiss chard are both from the Chenopodiaceae family [3, 74]. Yoshikawa et al. [205] in an oral glucose tolerance test (OGTT) conducted in rats, that measures the body's ability to metabolize glucose [206], observed that several glycosides isolated from the root extract of beet increase glucose tolerance. Gu et al. [207] report that purslane had hypoglycemic effects in a study comparing the hypoglycemic and antioxidant activities of the fresh and dried purslane in insulin-resistant HepG2 cells and streptozotocin-induced diabetic mice. In another study in adult patients with type 2 diabetes, it was found that consumption of purslane extract significantly reduced HbA1c levels and postprandial blood glucose [208].

Alliaceae vegetables are necessary ingredients of a diabetes prevention diet. Garlic lowers blood sugar levels in diabetic patients [209], and administration of S-methyl cysteine sulfoxide isolated from onion restrained blood glucose and showed significant hypoglycemic effect in rats [2, 74]. El-Demerdash et al. [210] in a biochemical study on the hypoglycemic effects of onion and garlic in alloxaninduced diabetic rats report that these vegetables had a hypoglycemic effect. Other investigations evaluating the hypoglycemic, antioxidant, and hepatoprotective potentials of onion show that onion consumption increased the levels of enzymes superoxide dismutase, catalase, and glutathione peroxidase [211] and reduce insulin resistance [212]. Onions and other Alliaceae also contain chromium that is linked to diabetes prevention by enhancing insulin receptor kinases [213]. Clinical surveys on diabetic patients showed that chromium can decrease fasting glucose, ameliorate glucose tolerance, and bring down insulin levels. Swamy et al. [209] observed that 200 g of some cultivars of onions contain chromium up to 20% of the daily requirements.

Nutritionists and dieticians commonly recommend diabetic eating carrots in moderation because they say that carrots contain more sugar than other vegetables. Although carrots are not a negative vegetable for the diabetic since they have fiberrich fractions that transports a significant amount of polyphenols and carotenoids linked to the fiber matrix, they are relatively low in calories and the glycemic load is only 3 [97]. Glycemic effect of carrots when eaten raw is lessened further as the body does not absorb all of the calories in raw aliments [3, 74]. Chau et al. [214] comparing the characteristics, functional properties, and in vitro hypoglycemic effects of various carrot-insoluble fiber-rich fractions confirmed the great relationship between dietary fiber intake and lower risk of type 2 diabetes since those authors concluded, from their study, that the enhanced glucose absorbance capacity and reduction of amylase activity of dietary fiber of carrot help control postprandial serum glucose level. The recent research advocates that orange carrot with α- and β-carotene might help diabetics to succeed in their illness [97, 215]. Purple carrots, rich in anthocyanins and low in carotenoids, were also recently associated with reduction in impaired glucose tolerance [96].

Cucurbitaceae is a very important family for diabetics since it includes several vegetables with antidiabetic properties. Bitter gourd (Momordica charantia) has been intensively studied for its antidiabetic attributes. Different studies reported hypoglycemic and antihyperglycemic properties of bitter gourd [209, 216–218]. Clinical surveys on diabetic patients using pulp and juice extracts of bitter gourd were reported to bring down serum insulin levels, to lower fasting blood glucose levels, and to ameliorate glucose tolerance [219]. Vicine, charantin, and polypep- tide-p are the principal hypoglycemic bioactive compounds from bitter gourd [220]. But there are also carotenoids (β-carotene, lutein, and zeaxanthin), triterpenoids (momordicin), alkaloids, and saponins, responsible for their side effect on glycemic control [221]. Momordicin possess insulin-like activity [222].

Besides bitter gourd other non-sweet Cucurbitaceae that have antidiabetic properties are ivy gourd (Coccinia grandis), snake gourd (Trichosanthes cucumerina), and ridge gourd (Luffa acutangula). In ivy gourd, immature fruits have antihyperglycemic properties since they help regulate blood sugar levels [223]. In India, they are used to prevent or treat diabetes [223]. Bioactive compounds in the ivy gourd inhibit glucose-6-phosphatase [209], a liver enzyme involved in the regulation of sugar metabolism. Snake gourd is also considered to be useful in treating type 2 diabetes [209]. Ridge gourd contains insulin like peptides and alkaloids that help to lower fasting blood glucose levels [209, 217].

Legume consumption is also colligated with reduced risk of type 2 diabetes since they are the ideal carbohydrate source [3, 90, 224]. They are low in glycemic load due to their moderate protein and abundant dietary fiber and resistant starch (that is fermented by bacteria in the colon). This chemical composition of legumes decreases the number of calories that can be absorbed which contribute to the control of blood sugar levels.

Kwon et al. [193] presented eggplant phenolics as inhibitors of key enzymes relevant for type 2 diabetes and hypertension.

Conclusions

Consumption of a vegetable-rich diet has unquestionable positive effects on nutrition and health since vegetables are rich in bioactive compounds such as dietary fiber, vitamins, minerals, and phytochemicals that can protect the human body from several types of chronic and degenerative diseases. The mechanism by which vegetable bioactive compounds decrease the risk of some of these diseases is complex and sometimes unknown. In this chapter, some experimental research evidences that the bioactive compounds are responsible for mitigating some human diseases were presented. All the different bioactive compounds may contribute to the overall health benefit. Each vegetable family and each vegetable contain a unique combination of bioactive compounds. So, the health benefit of vegetables should not be linked to only one bioactive compound or one type of vegetable but rather with a balanced diet that includes more than one type of vegetable. Antioxidative, anticarcinogenic, antidiabetic, and cardiovascular disease-lowering effects of vegetables have been reported. Nutrition is both a quantity and quality issue. The availability of a large diversity of vegetables all year-round allied to increase in mean per capita incomes in recent years, and knowledge of vegetable nutritional quality and health benefits should enable consumers to include more and more a great variety of health-promoting vegetables in their diet.

Conflict of interest

There is no "conflict of interest."

Author details

João Silva Dias
Instituto Superior de Agronomia, University of Lisbon, Lisbon, Portugal

*Address all correspondence to: mirjsd@gmail.com

References

[1] Dias JS, Ryder E. World vegetable industry: Production, breeding, trends. Horticultural Reviews. 2011;**38**:299-356

[2] Dias JS. Major classes of phytonutriceuticals in vegetables and health benefits: A Review. Journal of Nutritional Therapeutics. 2012;**1**:31-62

[3] Dias JS. Vegetable breeding for nutritional quality and health benefits. In: Carbone K, editor. Cultivar: Chemical Properties, Antioxidant Activities and Health Benefits. Hauppauge, New York: Nova Science Publishers Inc.; 2012. pp. 1-81

[4] Prior RL, Cao G. Antioxidant phytochemicals in fruit and vegetables, diet and health implications. Hortscience. 2000;**35**:588-592

[5] Hyson D. The Health Benefits of Fruit and Vegetables. A Scientific Overview for Health Professionals. Wilmington, DE: Produce for Better Health Foundation; 2002

[6] Golberg G, editor. Plants: Diet and Health. The Report of a British Nutrition Foundation Task Force. Oxford: Blackwell Science; 2003

[7] IFAVA. Fruit, vegetables and health: A scientific overview. International Fruit and Vegetable Alliance (IFAVA). Fruit, vegetables and health: a scientific overview. International Fruit and Vegetable Alliance. Ottawa, Canada; 2006

[8] Malaterreb AS, Remizeb F, Pouchereta P. Fruits and vegetables, as a source of nutritional compounds and phytochemicals. Changes in bioactive compounds during lactic fermentation. Food Research International. 2018;**104**:86-99

[9] Saura-Calixto F, Goñi I. Antioxidant capacity of the Spanish Mediterranean diet. Food Chemistry. 2006;**94**(3):442-447

[10] Saura-Calixto F, Serrano J, Goñi I. Intake and bioaccessibility of total polyphenols in a whole diet. Food Chemistry. 2007;**101**:492-501

[11] Kays SJ, Dias JS. Common names of commercially cultivated vegetables of the world in 15 languages. Economic Botany. 1995;**49**:115-152. DOI: 10.1007/BF02862917

[12] Kays SJ. Cultivated Vegetables of the World: A Multi-lingual Onomasticon. The Netherlands: Wageningen Academic Publishers; 2011. DOI: 10.3920/978-90-8686-720-2

[13] Dias JS. Major classes of phytonutriceuticals in vegetables and health benefits: A review. In: Nath P, editor. The Basics of Human Civilization-Food, Agriculture and Humanity, Volume- II-Food. New Delhi, India: Prem Nath Agricultural Science Foundation (PNASF), Bangalore & New India Publishing Agency (NIPA); 2014. pp. 305-370

[14] Nielsen SE, Young JF, Daneshvar B, Lauriden ST, Knuthsen P, Sandrstromand B, et al. Effect of parsley (*Petroselinum crispum*) intake on urinary apigenin excretion, blood antioxidant enzymes and biomarkers for oxidative stress in human subjects. The British Journal of Nutrition. 1999;**81**:447-455

[15] Horbowicz M, Kosson R, Grzesiuk A, Bski HD. Anthocyanins of fruits and vegetables—Their occurrence analysis and role in human nutrition. Vegetable Crops Research Bulletin. 2008;**68**:5-22

[16] Lila MA. Anthocyanins and human health: An in vitro investigative approach. Journal of Biomedicine and Biotechnology. 2004;**5**:306-313

[17] Ching LS, Mohamed S. Alpha- tocopherol content of 62 edible tropical plants. Journal of Agricultural and Food Chemistry. 2001;**49**:3101-3105

[18] Crozier A, Burns J, Aziz AA, Stewart AJ, Rabiasz HS, Jenkins GI, et al. Antioxidant flavonols from fruits, vegetables and beverages: Measurements and bioavailability. Biological Research. 2000;**33**:79-88

[19] Prakash D, Nath P, Pal M. Composition, variation of nutritional contents in leaves, seed protein, fat and fatty acid profile of *Chenopodium* species. Journal of the Science of Food and Agriculture. 1993;**62**:203-205

[20] Sienera R. Oxalate contents of species of the *Polygonaceae*, *Amaranthaceae* and *Chenopodiaceae* families. Food Chemistry. 2006;**98**:220-224

[21] Dhillon NPS, Monforte AJ, Pitrat M. Melon landraces of India: Contributions and importance. Plant Breeding Reviews. 2012;**35**:85-150

[22] Burger Y, Yeselson Y, Saar U, Paris HS, Katzir N, Tadmor Y, et al. Screening of melon (*Cucumis melo*) germplasm for consistently high sucrose content and for high ascorbic acid content. In: Lebeda A, Paris HS, editors. Progress in Cucurbit Genetics and Breeding Research. Proc Cucurbitaceae 2004. Olomouc, Czech Republic: Palacky University; 2004. pp. 151-155

[23] Crosby KM, Lester GE, Leskovar DI. Genetic variation for beneficial phytochemical levels in melons (*Cucumis melo*). In: Holmes GJ, editor. Cucurbitaceae 2006. Raleigh, NC: Universal Press; 2006. pp. 70-76

[24] Misra SK. Anti-nutritive bioactive compounds present in unconventional pulses and legumes. Research Journal of Pharmaceutical, Biological and Chemical Sciences. 2012;**3**:586-597

[25] Mallillin AC, Trinidad TP, Raterta R, Dagbay K, Loyola AS. Dietary fiber and fermentability characteristics of root crops and legumes. The British Journal of Nutrition. 2008;**100**:485-488

[26] Trinidad TP, Mallillin AC, Loyola AS, Sagum RS, Encabo RR. The potential health benefits of legumes as a good source of dietary fiber. The British Journal of Nutrition. 2010;**103**:569-574

[27] Dias JS. World importance, marketing and trading of vegetables. Acta Horticulturae. 2011;(921):153-169

[28] Fahey JW, Zalcmann AT, Talalay P. The chemical diversity and distribution of glucosinolates and isothiocyanates among plants. Phytochemistry. 2001;**56**:5-51

[29] VanEtten CH, Dzenbichler ME, Williams P, Kwolek WF. Glucosinolates and derived products in cruciferous vegetables. Analysis in the edible part from twenty-two varieties of cabbage. Journal of Agricultural and Food Chemistry. 1976;**24**:452-455

[30] Carlson DG, Daxenbichler ME, Van Etten CH, Tookey HL, Williams PH. Glucosinolates in crucifer vegetables: Turnip and rutabagas. Journal of Agricultural and Food Chemistry. 1981;**29**:1235-1239

[31] Carlson DG, Daxenbichler ME, VanEtten CH, Hill CB, Williams PH. Glucosinolates in radish cultivars. Journal of the American Society for Horticultural Science. 1985;**110**:634-638

[32] Carlson DG, Daxenbichler ME, VanEtten CH, Kwolek WF, Williams PH. Glucosinolates in crucifer vegetables: Broccoli, Brussels sprouts, cauliflower, collards, kale, mustard green, and kohlrabi. Journal of the American Society for Horticultural Science. 1987a;**112**:173-178

[33] Carlson DG, Daxenbichler ME, VanEtten CH, Kwolek WF, Hill CB, Williams PH. Glucosinolates in turnip tops and roots: Cultivars grown for greens and/or roots. Journal of the American Society for Horticultural Science. 1987b;**112**:179-183

[34] Kushad MK, Brown AF, Kurillicn AC, Juvik JA, Klein BP, Wallig MA, et al. Variation in glucosinolates in vegetable crops of *Brassica oleracea*. Journal of Agricultural and Food Chemistry. 1999;**47**:1541-1548

[35] Ciska E, Martyniak-Przybyszewska B, Kozlowska H. Content of glucosinolates in cruciferous vegetables grown at the same site for two years under different climatic condition. Journal of Agricultural and Food Chemistry. 2000;**48**:2862-2867

[36] Vallejo F, Tomas-Barberan FA, Banavent-Garcia AG, Garcia-Viguera C. Total and individual glucosinolate contents in inflorescences of eight broccoli cultivars grown under various climatic and fertilization conditions. Journal of the Science of Food and Agriculture. 2003;**83**:307-313

[37] Nilsson J, Olsson K, Engqvist G, Ekvall J, Olsson M, Nyman M, et al. Variation in the content of glucosinolates, hydroxycinnamic acids, carotenoids, total antioxidant capacity and low-molecular-weight carbohydrates in *Brassica* vegetables. Journal of the Science of Food and Agriculture. 2006;**86**:528-538

[38] Borkowski J, Szajdek A, Borkowska EJ, Ciska E, Zielinski H. Content of selected bioactive components and anti oxidant properties of broccoli (*Brassica oleracea* L.). European Food Research and Technology. 2008;**226**:459-465

[39] Cartea ME, Velasco P, Obregón S, Padilla G, de Haro A. Seasonal variation in glucosinolate content in *Brassica oleracea* crops grown in northwestern Spain. Phytochemistry. 2008;**69**:403-410

[40] Hansen M, Bengtsson GB, Borge GI, Berge L, Wold AB. Red cabbage, a vegetable rich in health-related glucosinolates. Acta Horticulturae. 2010;**867**:61-65

[41] Fahey JW, Zhang YS, Talalay P. Broccoli sprouts: An exceptionally rich source of inducers of enzymes that protects against chemical carcinogens. Proceedings of the National Academy of Sciences of the United States of America. 1997;**94**:10367 10372

[42] Goodrich RM, Anderson JL, Stoewsand G. Glucosinolate changes in blanched broccoli and brussels sprouts. Journal of Food Processing and Preservation. 1989;**13**:275-280

[43] Vallejo F, Tomas-Barberan FA, Garcia-Viguera C. Potential bioactive compounds in health promotion from broccoli cultivars grown in Spain. Journal of the Science of Food and Agriculture. 2002;**82**:1293-1297

[44] Kusznierewics B, Bartoszek A, Wolska L, Drzewiwcki J, Gorinstein S, Namiesnik J. Partial characterization of white cabbages (*Brassica oleracea* var. *capitata* f. *alba*) from different regions by glucosinolates, bioactive compounds, total antioxidant activities and proteins. LWT- Food Science and Technology. 2008;**41**:1-9

[45] Cao G, Sofic E, Prior RL. Antioxidant capacity of tea and common vegetables. Journal of Agricultural and Food Chemistry. 1996;**44**:3426-3431

[46] Scott J, Releille F, Fletcher J. Folic acid and folates: The feasibility for nutritional enhancement in plant foods. Journal of Science and Food Agriculture. 2000;**80**:795-824

[47] Konings EJM, Roomans HH, Dorant E, Goldbohm RA, Saris WH, van den Brandt PA. Folate intake of the Dutch population according to newly established liquid chromatography data for foods. The American Journal of Clinical Nutrition. 2001;**73**:765-776

[48] Banuelos G, Meek D. Selenium accumulation in selected vegetables. Journal of Plant Nutrition. 1989;**12**:1255-1272

[49] Nencini C, Cavallo F, Capasso A, Franchi GG, Giorgio G, Micheli L. Evaluation of antioxidative properties of *Allium* species growing wild in Italy. Phytotherapy Research. 2007;**21**:874-878

[50] Kalra N, Arora A, Shukla Y. Involvement of multiple signaling pathways in diallyl sulfide mediated apoptosis in mouse skin tumors. Asian Pacific Journal of Cancer Prevention. 2006;7:556-562

[51] Rose P, Whiterman M, Moore PK, Zhu YZ. Bioactive S-alk(en)yl cysteine sulfoxide metabolites in the genus *Allium*: The chemistry of potential therapeutic agents. Natural Product Reports. 2005;**22**:351-368

[52] Rubec R, Svobodovaand M, Velisek J. Gas chromatographic determination of S-alk(en)yl-L-cysteine sulfoxides. Journal of Chromatography. 1999;**862**:85-94

[53] Thomas DJ, Parkin KL. Quantification of alk(en)yl-L- cysteine sulfoxide and related amino acids in alliums by high-performance liquid chromatography. Journal of Agricultural and Food Chemistry. 1994;**42**:1632-1638

[54] Yoo KS, Pike LM. Determination of flavor precursor compound S-alk(en) yl-L-cysteine sulfoxides by HPLC method and their distribution in *Allium* species. Scientia Horticulturae. 1998;**75**:1-10

[55] Kubec R, Svobodova M, Velisek J. Gas-chromatographic determination of S-alk(eny)lylcysteine sulfoxide. Journal of Chromatography. 1999;**862**:85-94

[56] Miean KH, Mohamed S. Flavonoid (myricetin, quercetin, kaempferol, luteolinand apigenin) content of edible tropical plants. Journal of Agricultural and Food Chemistry. 2001;**49**:106-112

[57] Hertog MG, Hollman PC, Katan MB. Content of potentially anticarcinogenic flavonoids of 28 vegetables and fruits commonly consumed in The Netherlands. Journal of Agricultural and Food Chemistry. 1992;**40**:2379-2383

[58] Bilyk A, Sapers GM. Distribution of quercetin and kaemperol in lettuce, kale, chive, garlic chive leek, horseradish, red radish and red cabbage tissue. Journal of Agricultural and Food Chemistry. 1985;**33**:226-228

[59] Ip C, Lisk DJ. Enrichment of selenium in allium vegetables for cancer prevention. Carcinogenesis. 1994;**15**:1881-1885

[60] Clinton S. Lycopene: Chemistry, biology and implication for human health and disease. Nutrition Reviews. 1998;**56**:35-51

[61] Scott KJ, Hart DJ. Development and evolution of an HPLC method for the analysis of carotenoids food and the measurement of the carotenoid content vegetables and fruits commonly consumed in the UK. Food Chemistry. 1995;**54**:101-111

[62] Tonucci LH, Holden JM, Beecher GR, Khachik F, Davis CS, Mulokozi G. Carotenoid content of thermally processed tomato-based food products. Journal of Agricultural and Food Chemistry. 1995;**43**:579-586

[63] Gerster H. The potential role of lycopene for human health. Journal of the American College of Nutrition. 1997;**16**:109-126

[64] Agarwal S, Rao AK. Tomato lycopene and its role in human health and chronic diseases. Canadian Medical Association Journal. 2000;**163**:739-744

[65] Rao AV, editor. Tomatoes, Lycopene and Human Health Preventing Chronic Diseases. Stranraer, Scotland: Caledonian Science Press; 2006

[66] Leonardi C, Ambrosino P, Esposito F, Fogliano V. Antioxidant activity and carotenoid and tomatine contents in different typologies of fresh consumption tomatoes. Journal of Agricultural and Food Chemistry. 2000;**48**:4723-4727

[67] Arab L, Steck S. Lycopene and cardiovascular disease. The American Journal of Clinical Nutrition. 2000;**71**:1691S-1695S

[68] Rao AV, Rao LG. Carotenoids and human health. Pharmacological Research. 2007;**55**:207-216

[69] Albushita AA, Daood HG, Biacs PA. Change in carotenoids and antioxidant vitamins in tomato as a function of varietal and technological factors. Journal of Agricultural and Food Chemistry. 2000;**48**:2075-2081

[70] Albushita AA, Hebshi EA, Daood HG, Biacs PA. Determination of antioxidant vitamins in tomato. Food Chemistry. 1997;**60**:207-212

[71] Crozier A, Lean ME, McDonaldand MS, Black C. Quantitative analysis of the flavonoid content of commercial tomatoes, onions, lettuce and celery. Journal of Agricultural and Food Chemistry. 1997;**45**:590-595

[72] Stewart AJ, Bozonnet S, Mullen W, Jenkins GI, Lean ME, Crozier A. Occurrence of flavonols in tomatoes and tomato-based products. Journal of Agricultural and Food Chemistry. 2000;**48**:2663-2669

[73] Craig W, Beck L. Phytochemicals: Health protective effects. Canadian Journal of Dietetic Practice and Research. 1999;**60**:78-84

[74] Dias JS. Nutritional quality and health benefits of vegetables: A review. Food and Nutrition Sciences. 2012;**3**:1354-1374. DOI: 10.4263/ fns.2012.310179

[75] Bosland PW. Capsicums: Innovative uses of an ancient crop. In: Janick J, editor. Progress in New Crops. Arlington, VA: ASHS Press; 1996. pp. 479-487

[76] Howard LR, Talcott ST, Brenes CH, Villalon B. Changes in phytochemical and antioxidant activity of selected pepper cultivars (*Capsicum* species) as influenced by maturity. Journal of Agricultural and Food Chemistry. 2000;**48**:1713-1720

[77] Howard LR, Smith RT, Wagner AB, Villalon B, Burns EE. Provitamin A and ascorbic acid content of fresh pepper cultivars (*Capsicum annum*) and processed jalapenos. Journal of Food Science. 1994;**59**:362-365

[78] Lee Y, Howard R, Villalon B. Flavonoids and antioxidant activity of fresh pepper (*Capsicum annum*) cultivars. Journal of Food Science. 1995;**60**:473-476

[79] Suzuki T, Iwai K. The alkaloids. In: Brossi A, editor. The Alkaloids Chemistry and Pharmacology. Vol. XXIII. San Diego, CA: Academic Press; 1984. pp. 227-229

[80] Thomas BV, Schreilber AA, Weisskopf CP. Simple method for quantitation of capsaicinoids in pepper using capillary gas chromatography. Journal of Agricultural and Food Chemistry. 1998;**46**:2655-2663

[81] Frei B, Lawson S. Vitamin C and cancer revisited. Proceedings of the National Academy of Sciences of the United States of America. 2008;**105**:11037-11038

[82] Noda Y, Kaneyuki T, Igarashi K, Moriand A, Pacer L. Antioxidant activity of nasunin, an anthocyanin in eggplant. Research Communications in Molecular Pathology and Pharmacology. 1998;**102**:175-187

[83] Kayamori F, Igarashi K. Effect of dietary nasunin on the serum cholesterol level in rats. Bioscience, Biotechnology, and Biochemistry. 1994;**58**:570-571

[84] Noda Y, Kneyuki T, Igarashi K. Antioxidant activity of nasunin, an anthocyanin in eggplant peels. Toxicology. 2000;**148**:119-123

[85] Matsuzoe N, Yamaguchi M, Kawanobu S, Watanabe Y, Higashi H, Sakata Y. Effect of dark treatment of the eggplant on fruit skin color and its anthocyanin components. The Japanese Society for Horticultural Science. 1999;**68**:138-145

[86] Whitaker BD, Stommel JR. Distribution of hydroxycinnamic acid conjugates in fruit of commercial eggplant (*Solanum melongena* L.) cultivars. Journal of Agricultural and Food Chemistry. 2003;**51**:3448-3454

[87] Ben-Amos A, Fishler R. Analysis of carotenoids with emphasis on 9-cis β-carotene in vegetables and fruits commonly consumed in Israel. Food Chemistry. 1998;**62**:515-520

[88] Assimos DG, Holmes RP. Role of diet in the therapy of urolithiasis. The Urologic Clinics of North America. 2000;**27**:255-268

[89] Britton G, Khachik F. Carotenoids in food. In: Britton G, Pfander H, Liaaen- Jensens S, editors. Carotenoids. Baseline: Birkhäuser; 2009. pp. 45-66

[90] Fuhrman J. The End of Diabetes: The Eat to Live Plan to Prevent and Reverse Diabetes. New York: Harper Collins Publishers; 2013

[91] Pyo YH, Lee TC, Logendrac L, Rosen RT. Antioxidant activity and phenolic compounds of Swiss chard (*Beta vulgaris* subspecies *cycla*) extracts. Food Chemistry. 2004;**85**:19-26. DOI: 10.1016/S0308-8146(03)00294 -2

[92] Bolkent S, Yanarda R, Tabakolu- Oguz A, Ozsoy-Sacan O. Effects of chard (*Beta vulgaris* L. var. *cicla*) extract on pancreatic β cells in streptozotocin-diabetic rats: A morphological and biochemical study. Journal of Ethnopharmacology. 2000;**73**:251-259. DOI: 10.1016/S0378-8741(00)00328 -7

[93] Mateljan G. The World's Healthiest Foods. Glendale, California: George Mateljan Foundation; 2016

[94] Kugler F, Stintzing FC, Carle R. Identification of betalains from petioles of differently colored Swiss chard (*Beta vulgaris* L. ssp. *cicla* [L.] Alef. cv. Bright Lights) by high-

performance liquid chromatography- electrospray ion. Journal of Agricultural and Food Chemistry. 2004;**52**: 2975-2981. DOI: 10.1021/jf035491w

[95] Dias JS, Imai S. Vegetables consumption and its benefits on diabetes. Journal of Nutritional Therapeutics. 2017;**6**:1-10

[96] Poudyal H, Panchal S, Brown L. Comparison of purple carrot juice and β-carotene in a high-carbohydrate, high-fat diet-fed rat model of the metabolic syndrome. The British Journal of Nutrition. 2010;**104**:1322-1332. DOI: 10.1017/S0007114510002308

[97] Dias JS. Nutritional and health benefits of carrots and their seed extracts. Food and Nutrition Sciences. 2014;**5**:2147-2156. DOI: 10.4236/ fns.2014.522227

[98] Ferracane R, Pellegrini N, Visconti A, Graziani G, Chıavaro E, Miglio C, et al. Effects of different cooking methods on antioxidant profile, antioxidant capacity, and physical characteristics of artichoke. Journal of Agricultural and Food Chemistry. 2008;**56**:8601-8608

[99] World Health Organization (WHO). Increasing Fruit and Vegetable Consumption to Reduce the Risk of Non- Communicable Diseases. World Health Organization. e-Library of Evidence for Nutrition Actions (eLENA). World Health Organization. Geneva, Switzerland; 2018

[100] Fergunson LR. Prospect of cancer prevention. Mutation Research. 1999;**428**:329-338

[101] American Institute of Cancer Research (AICR). Food, Nutrition, Physical Activity, and the Prevention of Cancer: A Global Perspective. Washington, DC: AIRC/World Cancer Research Fund; 2007

[102] Potter JD, Slattery ML, Bostick RM. Colon cancer: A review of the epidemiology. Epidemiologic Reviews. 1993;**15**:499-545

[103] van Duijnhoven FJ, Bueno-de- Mesquita HB, Ferrari P, Jenab M, Boshuizen HC, Ros MM, et al. Fruit, vegetables and colorectal cancer risk: The European prospective investigation into cancer and nutrition. The American Journal of Clinical Nutrition. 2009;**89**:1441-1452

[104] Trock B, Lanza E, Greenwald P. Dietary fiber, vegetables, and colon cancer: Critical review and meta-analysis of the epidemiologic evidence. Journal of the National Cancer Institute. 1990;**82**:650-661

[105] Neugut AI, Jacobson JS, DeVivo L. Epidemiology of colorectal adenomas: Macronutrients, cholesterol and fiber. Journal of the National Cancer Institute. 1993;**85**:884-891

[106] Steinmetz KA, Kushi LH, Bostick R, Folisom AR, Potter JD. Vegetable, fruit and colon cancer in the Iowa women's health study. American Journal of Epidemiology. 1994;**139**:1-15

[107] Witte JS, Longnecker MP, Bird SL, Lee ER, Frakl HD, Haile RW. Relation of vegetable, fruit and grain consumption to colorectal adenomatous polyps. American Journal of Epidemiology. 1996;**144**:1015-1025

[108] Iscovich JM, L'Abbe KA, Castelleto R, Calzona A, Bernaedo A, Chopita NA, et al. Colon cancer in Argentina. Risk from intake of dietary items. International Journal of Cancer. 1992;**51**:851-857

[109] Zaridize D, Filipchenco V, Kustov V. Diet and colorectal cancer: Results of two case-control studies in Russia. European Journal of Cancer. 1993;**29A**:113-115

[110] Tanaka S, Haruma K, Yoshihara M, Kajiyama G, Kira K, Amagase H, et al. Aged garlic extract has potential suppressive effect on colorectal adenomas in humans. The Journal of Nutrition. 2006;**136**:821S-826S

[111] Radhika G, Sudha V, Sathya RM, Ganesan A, Mohan V. Association of fruit and vegetable intake with cardiovascular risk factors in urban south Indians. The British Journal of Nutrition. 2008;**99**:398-405. DOI: 10.1017/S0007114507803965

[112] Soh Y, Shin M, Lee J, Jang J, Kim OH, Kang H, et al. Oxidative DNA damage and glioma cell death induced by tetrahydropapaveroline. Mutation Research. 2003;**544**:129-142. DOI: 10.1016/j.mrrev.2003.06.023

[113] Tao J, Li Y, Li S, Li HB. Plant foods for the prevention and management of colon cancer. Journal of Functional Foods. 2018;**42**:95-110. DOI: 10.1016/j.jff.2017.12.064

[114] Tewani R, Sharma JK, Rao SV. Spinach (Palak) natural laxative. International Journal of Applied Research and Technology. 2016;**1**:140-148. DOI: 10.4172/2157-7471.1000110

[115] Verhoeven DTH, Goldbohm RA, van Poppel G, Verhagen H, van den Brandt PA. Epidemiological studies on *Brassica* vegetables and cancer risk. Cancer Epidemiology, Biomarkers and Prevention. 1996;**5**:733-751

[116] Ambrosone CB, McCann SE, Freudenheim JL, Marshall JR, Zhang Y, Shields PG. Breast cancer risk in premenopausal women is inversely associated with consumption of broccoli, a source of isothiocyanates, but is not modified by GST genotype. The Journal of Nutrition. 2004;**134**:1134-1138

[117] Brennan P, Hsu CC, Moullan N, Szeszenia-Dabrowska N, Lissowska J, Zaridze D, et al. Effect of cruciferous vegetables on lung cancer in patients stratified by genetic status: A mendelian randomisation approach. Lancet. 2005;**366**:1558-1560

[118] Kirsh VA, Peters U, Mayne ST, Subar AF, Chatterjee N, Johnson CC, et al. Prospective study of fruit and vegetable intake and risk of prostate cancer. Journal of the National Cancer Institute. 2007;**99**:1200-1209

[119] Traka M. Broccoli consumption interferes with prostate cancer progression: Mechanisms of action. Acta Horticulturae. 2010;**867**:19-25

[120] Seow A, Yuan JM, Sun CL, Van Den Berg D, Lee HP, Yu MC. Dietary isothiocyanates, glutathione S-transferase polymorphisms and colorectal cancer risk in the Singapore Chinese health study. Carcinogenesis. 2002;**23**:2055-2061

[121] London SJ, Yuan JM, Chung FL, Gao YT, Coetzee GA, Ross RK, et al. Isothiocyanates, glutathione S-transferase M1 and T1 polymorphisms, and lung-cancer risk: A propective study of men in Shanghai, China. Lancet. 2000;**356**:724-729

[122] Fowke JH, Chung FL, Jin F, Qi D, Cai Q , Conaway C, et al. Urinary isothiocyanate levels, brassica, and human breast cancer. Cancer Research. 2003;**63**:3980-3986

[123] Joseph MA, Moysich KB, Freudenheim JL, Shields PG, Bowman ED, Zhamg Y, et al. Cruciferous vegetables, generic polymorphism in glutathione S-transferases M1 and T1, and prostate cancer risk. Nutrition and Cancer. 2004;**50**:206-213

[124] Juge N, Mithen RF, Traka M. Molecular basis for chemoprevention by sulforaphane: A comprehensive review. Cellular and Molecular Life Sciences. 2007;**64**:1105-1127

[125] Zhang Y, Talalay P. Anticarcinogenic activities of organic isothiocyanate : Chemistry and mechanisms. Cancer Research. 1994;**54**:1976s-1981s

[126] Mithen R, Faulkner K, Magrath R, Rose P, Williamson G, Marquez J. Development of isothiocyanate enriched broccoli and its enhanced ability to induce phase 2 detoxification enzymes in mammalian cells. Theoretical and Applied Genetics. 2003;**106**:727-734

[127] Rosa EAS, Heaney RK, Fenewick GR, Portas CAM. Glucosinolates in crop plants. Horticultural Reviews. 1997;**19**:99-215

[128] Abbaoui B, Lucas CR, Riedl KM. Cruciferous vegetables, isothiocyanates, and bladder cancer prevention. Molecular Nutrition and Food Research. 2018;**62**:1-50

[129] Dorant E, van Den Brandt PA, Goldbohm RA, Sturnmans F. Consumption of onions and a reduced risk of stomach carcinoma. Gastroenterology. 1996;**110**:12-20

[130] You WC, Li JY, Zhang L, Jin ML, Chang YS, Ma JL, et al. Etiology and prevention of gastric cancer: A population study in high risk area of China. Chinese Journal of Digestive Diseases. 2005;**6**:149-154

[131] Galeone C, Pelucchi C, Levi F, Negri E, Franceschi S, Talamini R, et al. Onion and garlic use and human cancer. The American Journal of Clinical Nutrition. 2006;**84**:1027-1032

[132] Grant WB. A multicountry ecologic study of risk and risk reduction factors for prostate cancer mortality. European Urology. 2004;**45**:271-279

[133] Shon MY, Choi SD, Kahng GG, Nam SH, Sung NJ. Antimutagenic, antioxidant and free radical scavenging activity of ethyl acetate extracts from white, yellow and red onions. Food and Chemical Toxicology. 2004;**42**:659-666

[134] Yang J, Meyers KJ, vander Heide J, Liu RH. Varietal differences in phenolic content and antioxidant and antiproliferative activities of onions. Journal of Agricultural and Food Chemistry. 2004;**52**:6787-6793

[135] Kim JY, Kwon O. Garlic intake and cancer risk: An analysis using the Food and Drug Administration's evidence- based review system for the scientific evaluation of health claims. The American Journal of Clinical Nutrition. 2009;**89**:257-264

[136] Salem S, Salahi M, Mohseni M, Ahmadi H, Mehrsai A, Jahani Y, et al. Major dietary factors and prostate cancer risk: A prospective multicenter case-control study. Nutrition and Cancer. 2011;**63**:21-27

[137] Iciek M, Kwiecien I, Wlodek L. Biological properties of garlic and garlic-derived organosulfur compounds. Environmental and Molecular Mutagenesis. 2009;**50**:247-265

[138] Melino S, Sabelli R, Paci M. Allyl sulfur compounds and cellular detoxification system: Effects and perspectives in cancer therapy. Amino Acids. 2011;**41**:103-112

[139] You WC, Zhang L, Gail MH, Ma JL, Chang YS, Blot WJ, et al. *Helicobacter pylori* infection, garlic intake and precancerous lesions in a Chinese population at low risk of gastric cancer. International Journal of Epidemiology. 1998;**27**:941-944

[140] Tanaka S, Haruma K, Kunihiro M, Nagata S, Kitadai Y, Manabe N, et al. Effects of aged garlic extract (AGE) on colorectal adenomas: A double-blinded study. Hiroshima Journal of Medical Sciences. 2004;**53**:39-45

[141] Fleischauer AT, Poole C, Arab L. Garlic consumption and cancer prevention: Meta-analyses of colorectal and stomach cancers. The American Journal of Clinical Nutrition. 2000;**72**:1047-1052

[142] Hsing AW, Chokkalingam AP, Gao YT, Madigan MP, Deng J, Gridley G, et al. Allium vegetables and risk of prostate cancer: A population-based study. The Journal of the National Cancer Institute. 2002;**94**:1648-1651

[143] Challier B, Perarnau JM, Viel JF. Garlic, onion and cereal fibre as protective factors for breast cancer: A French case-control study. European Journal of Epidemiology. 1998;**14**:737-747

[144] Galeone C, Pelucchi C, Dal Maso L, Negri E, Montella M, Zucchetto A, et al. Allium vegetables intake and endometrial cancer risk. Public Health Nutrition. 2009;**12**:1576-1579

[145] Satia JA, Littman A, Slatore CG, Galanko JA, White E. Associations of herbal and specialty supplements with lung and colorectal cancer risk in the vitamins and lifestyle study. Cancer Epidemiology, Biomarkers and Prevention. 2009;**18**:1419-1428

[146] Wang Y, Tian W, Ma X. Inhibitory effects of onion (*Allium cepa* L.) extract on proliferation of cancer cells and adipocytes via inhibiting fatty acid synthase. Asian Pacific Journal of Cancer Prevention. 2012;**13**:5573-5579. DOI: 10.7314/APJCP.2012.13.11.5573

[147] Burney PG, Comstock GW, Morris JS. Serologic precursors of cancer: Serum micronutrients and the subsequent risk of pancreatic cancer. The American Journal of Clinical Nutrition. 1989;**49**:895-900

[148] Van Eenwyk J, Davis FG, Bowen PE. Dietary and serum carotenoids and cervical intraepithelial neoplasia. International Journal of Cancer. 1991;**48**:34-38

[149] Franceschi S, Bidoli E, La Vecchia C, Talamini R, D'Avanzo B, Negri E. Tomatoes and risk of digestive-tract cancers. International Journal of Cancer. 1994;**59**:181-184

[150] Helzlsouer KJ, Comstock GW, Morris JS. Selenium, lycopene, alpha- tocopherol, beta-carotene, retinol, and subsequent bladder cancer. Cancer Research. 1989;**49**:6144-6148

[151] Gann PH, Ma J, Giovannucci E. Lower prostate cancer risk in men with elevated plasma lycopene levels: Results of a prospective analysis. Cancer Research. 1999;**59**:1225-1230

[152] Yuan JM, Ross RK, Gao YT, Qu YH, Chu XD, Yu MC. Prediagnostic levels of serum micronutrients in relation to risk of gastric cancer in Shanghai, China. Cancer Epidemiology, Biomarkers and Prevention. 2004;**13**:1772-1780

[153] Wakai K, Ando M, Ozasa K. Updated information on risk factors for lung cancer: Findings from the JACC Study. Journal of Epidemiology. 2005;**15**:S134-S139

[154] Giovannucci E. Tomatoes, tomato based products, lycopene and cancer: Review of the epidemiological literature. The Journal of the National Cancer Institute. 1999;**91**:317-331

[155] Jang J, Surh Y. Potentiation of cellular antioxidant capacity by Bcl-2: Implications for its antiapoptotic function. Biochemical Pharmacology. 2003;**66**:1371-1379. DOI: 10.1016/ S0006-2952(03)00487-8

[156] Hadley CW, Miller EC, Schwartz SJ, Clinton SK. Tomatoes, lycopene, and prostate cancer: Progress and promise. Experimental Biology and Medicine. 2002;**227**:869-880. DOI: 10.1177/153537020222701006

[157] Giovannucci E, Ashcerio A, Rimm EB. Intake of carotenoids and retinol in relation to risk of prostate cancer. Journal of the National Cancer Institute. 1995;**87**:1767-1776

[158] Clark R, Lee SH. Anticancer properties of capsaicin against human cancer. Anticancer Research. 2016;**36**:837-844

[159] Nagase H, Sasaki K, Kito H, Haga A, Sato T. Inhibitory effect of delphinidin from *Solanum melongena* on human fibrosarcoma HT-1080 invasiveness in vitro. Planta Medica. 1998;**64**:216-219

[160] Goldwyn S, Lazinskyand A, Wei H. Promotion of health by soy isoflavones: Efficacy, benefit and safety concerns. Drug Metabolism and Drug Interactions. 2000;**17**:261-289

[161] Sarkar FH, Li Y. Isoflavones, soybean phytoestrogens, and cancer. In: Awad AB, Bradford PG, editors. Nutrition and Cancer Prevention. Boca Raton, FL: CRC Press; 2006. pp. 295-312

[162] Ziegler RG, Hooverand RN, Hildeshein RN. Migration patterns and breast cancer risk in Asian-America women. The Journal of the National Cancer Institute. 1993;**85**:1819-1827

[163] Lamartiniere C. Protection against breast cancer with genistein: A component of soy. The American Journal of Clinical Nutrition. 2000;**71**:1705S-1707S

[164] Steiner C, Arnould S, Scalbert A, Manach C. Isoflavones and the prevention of breast and prostate cancer: New perspectives opened by nutrigenomics. The British Journal of Nutrition. 2008;**99**:78-108

[165] Messina MJ, Wood CE. Soy isoflavones, estrogen therapy, and breast cancer risk: Analysis and commentary. Nutrition Journal. 2008;**7**:17. DOI: 10.1186/1475-2891 7 17

[166] Dong JY, Qin LQ. Soy isoflavones consumption and risk of breast cancer incidence or recurrence: A meta- analysis of prospective studies. Breast Cancer Research and Treatment. 2011;**125**:315-323

[167] Jiang HY, Lv FJ, Tai JQ. Bioactive components of soybean and their function. Soybean Science. 2000;**19**:160-164

[168] Sarkar FH, Li Y. Soy isoflavones and cancer prevention. Cancer Investigation. 2003;**21**:744-757

[169] Zaini R, Clench MR, Maitre CL. Bioactive chemicals from carrot (*Daucus carota*) juice extracts for the treatment of leukemia. Journal of Medicinal Food. 2011;**14**:1303-1312. DOI: 10.1089/jmf.2010.0284

[170] Larsen MK, Christensen LP, Vach W, Hoitinga RJ, Brant K. Inhibitory effects of feeding with carrots or falcarinol on development of azoxymethane-induced preneoplastic lesions in the rat colon. Journal of Agricultural and Food Chemistry. 2005;**53**:1823-1827. DOI: 10.1021/jf048519s

[171] Purup S, Larsen E, Christesen LP. Differential effects of falcarinol and related aliphatic C17-polyacetylenes on intestinal cell proliferation. Journal of Agricultural and Food Chemistry. 2009;**57**:8290-8296. DOI: 10.1021/ jf901503a

[172] Pisani P, Berrino F, Macaluso M, Pastorino U, Crosignani P, Baldasseroni A. Carrots, green vegetables and lung cancer: A case-control study. International Journal of Epidemiology. 1986;**15**:463-468. DOI: 10.1093/ ije/15.4.463

[173] Mullie P, Clarys P. Association between cardiovascular disease risk factor knowledge and lifestyle. Food and Nutrition Sciences. 2011;**2**:1048-1053

[174] Roth GA, Forouzanfar MH, Moran AE, Barber R, Nguyen G, Feigin VL, et al. Demographic and epidemiologic drivers of global cardiovascular mortality. The New England Journal of Medicine. 2015;**372**:1333-1341. DOI: 10.1056/NEJMoa1406656

[175] Liu S, Lee IM, Ajani U, Cole SR, Buring JE, Manson JE. Intake of vegetables rich in carotenoids and risk of coronary heart disease in men: The physicians' health study. International Journal of Epidemiology. 2001;**30**:130-135

[176] American Heart Association (AHA). Heart and stroke statistical update. Dallas, Texas: American Heart Association; 2017

[177] Yeh YY, Liu L. Cholesterol- lowering effect of garlic extracts and organosulfur compounds: Human and animal studies. The Journal of Nutrition. 2001;**131**:989-993. DOI: 10.1093/jn/131.3.989S

[178] Moriguchi T, Takasugi N, Itakura Y. The effects of aged garlic extract on lipid peroxidation and the deformability of erythrocytes. The Journal of Nutrition. 2001;**131**:1016-1019. DOI: 10.1093/jn/131.3.1016S

[179] Chang HS, Yamato O, Yamasaki M, Maede Y. Modulatory influence of sodium 2-propenylthiosulfate from garlic on cyclooxygenase activity in canine platelets: Possible mechanism for the anti-aggregatory effect. Prostaglandins, Leukotrienes, and Essential Fatty Acids. 2005;**72**:351-355. DOI: 10.1016/j.plefa.2005.01.003

[180] Osmont KS, Arnt CR, Goldman IL. Temporal aspects of onion-induced antiplatelet activity. Plant Food for Human Nutrition. 2003;**58**:27-40

[181] Hubbard GP, Wolffram S, Lovegrove JA, Gibbins JM. Ingestion of quercetin inhibits platelet aggregation and essential components of the collagen-stimulated platelet activation pathway in man: A pilot study. Journal of Thrombosis and Haemostasis. 2006;**2**:2138-2145

[182] Briggs WH, Folts JD, Osman HE, Goldman IL. Administration of raw onion inhibits platelet-mediated thrombosis in dogs. The Journal of Nutrition. 2001;**131**:2619-2622. DOI: 10.1093/jn/131.10.2619

[183] Ried K, Frank OR, Stocks NP. Aged garlic extract reduces blood pressure in hypertensives: A dose–response trial. European Journal of Clinical Nutrition. 2013;**67**:64-70. DOI: 10.1038/ ejcn.2012.178

[184] Freudenheim JL, Graham S, Marshall JR, Haughey BP, Wilkinson G. A case-control study of diet and rectal cancer in western New York. American Journal of Epidemiology. 1990;**131**:612-624

[185] Knekt P, Jarvinen R, Reunanen A, Maatela J. Flavonoid intake and coronary mortality in Finland: A cohort study. British Medical Journal. 1996;**312**:478-481. DOI: 10.1136/ bmj.312.7029.478

[186] Rastogi T, Reddy KS, Vaz M, Spiegelman D, Prabhakaran D, Willett WC, et al. Diet and risk of ischemic heart disease in India. The American Journal of Clinical Nutrition. 2004;**79**:582-592. DOI: 10.1093/ ajcn/79.4.582

[187] Saluk J, Bijak M, Kołodziejczyk- Czepas J, Posmyk M, Janas K, Wachowicz B. Anthocyanins from red cabbage extract—Evidence of protective effects on blood platelets. Open Life Sciences. 2012;7:655-663. DOI: 10.2478/ s11535-012-0057-9

[188] Manchali S, Murthy KNC, Patil BS. Crucial facts about health benefits of popular cruciferous vegetables. Journal of Functional Foods. 2012;**4**: 94-106. DOI: 10.1016/j.jff.2011.08.004

[189] Jeffery EH, Araya M. Physiological effects of broccoli consumption. Phytochemistry Reviews. 2009;**8**:283-298. DOI: 10.1007/s11101-008-9106-4

[190] Murashima M, Watanabe S, Zhuo XG, Uehara M, Kurashige A. Phase 1 study of multiple biomarkers for metabolism and oxidative stress after one-week intake of broccoli sprouts. BioFactors. 2004;**22**:271-275. DOI: 10.1002/biof.5520220154

[191] Jorge PA, Neyra LC, Osaki RM. Effect of eggplant on plasma lipid levels, lipidic peroxidation and reversion of endothelial dysfunction in experimental hypercholesterolemia. Arquivos Brasileiros de Cardiologia. 1998;**70**:87-91

[192] Guimarães PR, Galvão AM, Batista CM, Azevedo GS, Oliveira RD, Lamounier R, et al. Eggplant (*Solanum melongena*) infusion has a modest and transitory effect on hypercholesterolemic subjects. Brazilian Journal of Medical and Biological Research. 2000;**33**:1027-1036

[193] Kwon YI, Apostolidis E, Shetty K. In vitro studies of eggplant (*Solanum melongena*) phenolics as inhibitors of key enzymes relevant for type 2 diabetes and hypertension. Bioresource Technology. 2008;**99**:2981-2988

[194] Anderson JW, Deakins DA, Floore TL, Smith BM, Whitis SE. Dietary fiber and coronary heart disease. Critical Reviews in Food Science and Nutrition. 1990;**29**:95-147

[195] Menotti A, Kromhout D, Blackburn H, Fidanza F, Buzina R, Nissinen A. Food intake patterns and 25-year mortality from coronary heart disease: Cross-cultural correlations in the seven countries study. European Journal of Epidemiology. 1999;**15**:507-515

[196] Nöthlings U, Schulze MB, Weikert C, Boeing H, Van der Schouw YT, Bamia C, et al. Intake of vegetables, legumes, and fruit, and risk for all-cause, cardiovascular, and cancer mortality in a European diabetic population. The Journal of Nutrition. 2008;**138**:775-781. DOI: 10.1093/jn/138.4.775

[197] Lattimer JM, Haub MD. Effects of dietary fiber and its components on metabolic health. Nutrients. 2010;**2**:1266-1289. DOI: 10.3390/ nu2121266

[198] Nicolle C, Cardinault N, Aprikian O, Busserolles J, Grolier P, Rock E, et al. Effect of carrot intake on cholesterol metabolism and on antioxidant status in cholesterol-fed rat. European Journal of Nutrition. 2003;**42**:254-261. DOI: 10.1007/s00394-003-0419-1

[199] Gramenzi A, Gentile A, Fasoli M, Negri E, Parazzini F, La Vecchia C. Association between certain foods and risk of acute myocardial infarction in women. British Medical Journal. 1990;**300**:771-773. DOI: 10.1136/ bmj.300.6727.771

[200] Gilani AH, Shaheeri F, Saeed SA, Bibi S, Irfamillah-Sadiq M, Faiz S. Hypotensive action of coumarin glycoside from daucus carot. Phytomedicine. 2000;**7**:423-426. DOI: 10.1016/S0944-7113(00)80064-1

[201] Carter P, Gray LJ, Troughton J, Khunti K, Davies MJ. Fruit and vegetable intake and incidence of type 2 diabetes mellitus: Systematic review and meta-analysis. British Medical Journal. 2010;**341**:c4229. DOI: 10.1136/bmj.c4229

[202] Bazzano LA, Li TY, Joshipura KJ, Hu FB. Intake of fruit, vegetables and fruit juices and risk of diabetes in women. Diabetes Care. 2008;**31**: 1311-1317. DOI: 10.2337/dc08-0080

[203] Khan BA, Abraham A, Leelamma S. Hypoglycemic action of *Murraya koenigii* (curry leaf) and *Brassica juncea* (mustard): Mechanism of action. Indian Journal of Biochemistry and Biophysics. 1995;**32**:106-108

[204] Tundis R, Loizzo MR, Menichini F. Natural products as alpha-amylase and alpha-glucosidase inhibitors and their hypoglycaemic potential in the treatment of diabetes: An update. Mini Reviews in Medicinal Chemistry. 2010;**10**:315-331

[205] Yoshikawa M, Murakami T, Kadoya M, Yamahara J, Matsuda H. Medicinal foodstuff. III. Sugar beet. Hypoglicemic oleanolic acid oligoglycosides, betavulgarosides I, II, III, and IV, from the root of *Beta vulgaris* L. (*Chenopodiaceae*). Chemical and Pharmaceutical Bulletin. 1996;**44**:1212-1217

[206] American Diabetes Association (ADA). Standards of Care. Diabetes Care, 2016;**39**:S1-S119

[207] Gu JF, Zheng ZY, Yuan JR, Zhao BJ, Wang CF, Zhang L, et al. Comparison on hypoglycemic and antioxidant activities of the fresh and dried *Portulaca oleracea* L. in insulin-resistant HepG2 cells and streptozotocin-induced C57BL/6J diabetic mice. Journal of Ethnopharmacology. 2015;**161**:214-223. DOI: 10.1016/j.jep.2014.12.002

[208] Wainstein J, Landau Z, Dayan YB, Jakubowicz D, Grothe T, Perrinjaquet- Moccetti T, et al. Purslane extract and glucose homeostasis in adults with type 2 diabetes: A double-blind, placebo-controlled clinical trial of efficacy and safety. Journal of Medicinal Food. 2016;**19**:133-140. DOI: 10.1089/ jmf.2015.0090

[209] Swamy KRM, Nath P, Ahuja KG. Vegetables for human nutrition and health. In: Nath P, editor. The Basics of Human Civilization-Food, Agriculture and Humanity, Volume-II-Food. New Delhi, India: Prem Nath Agricultural Science Foundation (PNASF), Bangalore & New India Publishing Agency (NIPA); 2013. pp. 145-198

[210] El-Demerdash FM, Yousef MI, El-Naga NA. Biochemical study on the hypoglycemic effects of onion and garlic in alloxan-induced diabetic rats. Food and Chemical Toxicology. 2005;**43**: 57-63. DOI: 10.1016/j.fct.2004.08.012

[211] Ogunmodede OS, Saalu LC, Ogunlade B, Akunna GG, Oyewopo AO. An evaluation of the hypoglycemic, antioxidant and hepatoprotective potentials of onion (*Allium cepa* L.) on alloxan-induced diabetic rabbits. International Journal of Pharmacology. 2012;**8**:21-29. DOI: 10.3923/ ijp.2012.21.29

[212] Yoshinari O, Shiojima Y, Igarashi K. Anti-obesity effects of onion extract in Zucker diabetic fatty rats. Nutrients. 2012;**4**:1518-1526. DOI: 10.3390/ nu4101518

[213] Wang H, Kruszewki A, Brautigan DL. Cellular chromium activation of insulin receptor kinase. Biochemistry. 2005;**44**:8167-8175. DOI: 10.1021/ bi0473152

[214] Chau CF, Chen CH, Lee MH. Comparison of the characteristics, functional properties, and in vitro hypoglycemic effects of various carrot insoluble fiber-rich fractions. Lebensmittel-Wissenshaff und Technologie. 2004;**37**:155-160. DOI: 10.1016/j.lwt.2003.08.001

[215] Coyne T, Ibiebele TI, Baade PD. Diabetes mellitus and serum carotenoids: Findings of a population-based study in Queensland, Australia. The American Journal of Clinical Nutrition. 2005;**82**:685-693

[216] Chen Q , Chan LLY, Li ETS. Bitter melon (*Momordica charantia*) reduces adiposity, lowers serum insulin and normalizes glucose tolerance in rats fed a high fat diet. The Journal of Nutrition. 2003;**133**:1088-1093

[217] Patil B, Jayaprakasha GK, Vikram A. Indigenous crops of Asia and Southeast Asia: Exploring health-promoting properties. Hortscience. 2012;**47**:821-827

[218] Chao PM. One more support for recruiting bitter melon in therapeutic diet for diabetes and its comorbidity management—Bitter melon ameliorates hepatic steatosis related with hyperglycemia. BIT's 4th Annual World Congress of Diabetes–2015, Kaohsiung, Taiwania 2015; p. 236

[219] Ahmad N, Hassan M, Halder H, Bennoor K. Effect of *Momordica charantia* (Karolla) extracts on fasting and postprandial serum glucose levels in NIDDM patients. Bangladesh Medical Research Council Bulletin. 1999;**25**:11

[220] Yeh G, Eisenberg D, Kaptchuk T, Phillips R. Systematic review of herbs and dietary supplements for glycemic control in diabetes. Diabetes Care. 2003;**26**:1277. DOI: 10.2337/ diacare.26.4.1277

[221] Chen J, Tian R, Qiu M, Lu L, Zheng Y, Zhang Z. Trinorcucurbitane and cucurbitane triterpenoids from the roots of *Momordica charantia*. Phytochemistry. 2008;**69**:1043-1048. DOI: 10.1016/j.phytochem.2007.10.020

[222] Saxena A, Vikram N. Role of selected Indian plants in management of type 2 diabetes: A review. The Journal of Alternative and Complementary Medicine. 2004;**10**:369-378. DOI: 10.1089/107555304323062365

[223] Singh LW. Traditional medicinal plants of Manipur as anti-diabetics. Journal of Medicinal Plant Research. 2011;**5**:677-687

[224] Villegas R, Gao YT, Yang G, Li HL, Elasy TA, Zheng W, et al. Legume and soy food intake and the incidence of type 2 diabetes in the Shanghai women's health study. The American Journal of Clinical Nutrition, 2008;**87**:162-167. DOI: 10.1093/ajcn/87.1.162

10

Sports Nutrition and Performance

Raúl Arcusa Saura, María Pilar Zafrilla Rentero and Javier Marhuenda Hernández

Abstract

Nutrition plays an essential role on sports performance. Following an adequate nutrition pattern determines winning the gold medal or failing in the attempt. That is why it is commonly referred to as "invisible training." However, regarding food and performance, it is not only referred to professional athletes. Nowadays, a large number of amateur athletes perform daily physical activity both recreationally and semiprofessionally. That population also seeks to achieve an improvement in their personal brands, which can be reached following proper nutritional guidelines. In athlete population, nutrient requirements are incremented compared with non-athlete population. Therefore, it is essential to carry out a nutritional approach adapted to the athlete and training sessions. In addition, other advantages of adequate food intake in sports are related to changes in body composition, reduction of injuries, and prolongation of professional career length. The objective of this chapter is to determine the nutritional requirements of athlete population that allow to achieve their sporting goals. Nutritional strategies will be addressed in terms of macronutrients consumption, hydration, and timing depending on type and intensity of exercise.

Keywords: nutrition, sports performance, intake, nutrients, hydration

Introduction

Nutrition is strongly linked to health, especially when sports are concerned, due to the increase in energy and nutrient demands. It is necessary to know the physiology of the exercise in order to know the different metabolic pathways that coexist during sports practice. In this way, you can predict the changes that occur in the organism during physical effort, in order to achieve some dietary recommendations.

The nutritional practices of athletes are multifactorial and depend on the habits, culture, or nutritional knowledge of the athlete. So the work of a sports nutritionist is to advise the athlete and his environment to make the necessary changes in his intake and thereby improve sports performance (SP).

Nutrition is determinant in achieving an adequate SP, which is defined by three variables: training, rest, and feeding. However, the main objective of sports nutrition must be preserving the health of the athlete, which can be achieved with an adequate intake adapted to the type of training performed. Optimal nutrition provides the energy necessary to perform physical exercise while reducing injury rate, a factor that together makes the SP increase by itself.

Two of the aspects that can limit the SP are the state of hydration and the energy contribution. Hypohydration states produce alterations in homeostasis, decreased blood volume, increased heart rate, lower rate of sweating, increased organism temperature, and greater perception of effort which translates into SP deterioration. Likewise, a low energy consumption accentuates fatigue, immunosuppression, and predisposition for injuries, which can interfere in the development of SP.

Nowadays, an exponential increase in the population that performs physical activity has been reported. In the USA, the total number of runners endorsed in marathon events is 541,000 in 2013, which represents 27% more participants than observed in 2008 in the same trend observed in many countries. For example, in Spain the number of participants increased from 28,000 (2008) to 57,931 (2013), which represented an increase of 101%. These increases far from ceasing have continued growing in the last 5 years. Specifically, marathons of Sevilla and Valencia have reached 14,500 and 20,000 runners in 2018, which contrast with the previous participation observed in 2013 (5963 and 9653 participants, respectively).

Unfortunately, sports nutrition is often referenced to sports supplements or "magical" strange diets. In fact 40–70% of athletes use sports supplements without even analyzing if their use is really necessary.

Body composition

The body composition (BC) of the athletes is related to the SP, as it can be modified throughout the season. There is no single BC for each group of athletes; however, it can serve as a guide for athletes and coaches [1].

The season of the athlete will be divided into different phases throughout the competitive period. Competitive season can be divided in preseason, competitive period, transition period, and in the worst case injury period. Due to different intensities, timing, and types of training, the BC is normally different in the competitive season. Therefore, it is vital to know the BC of the athletes in order to determine the adequacy of the current season stage [2].

Apart from a higher body mass index (BMI), there are several methods for the evaluation of BC [2]. Dual-energy X-ray absorptiometry (DEXA) is considered the gold standard for the assessment of body fat, mainly due to its high reproducibility and accuracy. However, DEXA has high economic cost, is not portable, and also emits a small radiation, so its use is not very common [3].

Among the most used methods are bioelectrical impedance analysis (BIA) and anthropometry. Impedance is defined as the opposition shown by biological materials to the passage of an electric flow. Tissues with high impedance offer greater resistance (adipose tissue, bone, air in the lungs) and contain less amount of water [4]. The greater the amount of water, the better this electrical flow, will pass through. Therefore, the hydration sate of the individual is the determinant for the BC measurement by BIA. In addition, in order to standardize previous conditions and dismiss errors, certain protocols must be followed prior to the measurement of BC by BIA. That fact makes BIA a rather imprecise method [5].

Anthropometry allows the evaluation of different body dimensions and the overall composition of the body. It consists of the measurement of skinfolds, perimeters of the muscles, and bone diameters. This technique must be carried out by experts qualified by the International Society for the Advancement of Kinanthropometry (ISAK) [4]. It is the most widely used method in the sports field, from which the percentages of fat, muscle mass, and bone mass can be obtained by means of mathematic formulas [5]. The most effective way to monitor an athlete using this technique is performing a sum of six bodyfolds (triceps, subscapular, supraspinal, abdominal, thigh, and medial leg) that gives an absolute value [6].

In summary mode, the values for said summation of folds are estimated in physically active people (75 mm men and 100 mm in women), footballers (<50 mm men and <65 mm women), and endurance athletes (<35 mm men and 50 mm women). The minimum values seen in the healthy sports population were 25 mm for men and 42 mm for women (**Table 1**).

Table 1. *Summary of summation folds of the athletes.*

Population	Men (Σsix skinfolds)	Women (Σsix skinfolds)
Physically active people	75	10
Footballers	<50	<65
Runners	<35	50
Minimum value	25	42

However, it must be taken into account that BC is not the only thing that will measure sports performance, but it is one more parameter of the measurements that must be made in the athlete.

Metabolic pathways and exercise

Prior to establishing requirements regarding quantity and timing of macronutrients, a brief approach about different metabolic pathways that provides energy during exercise is necessary. The energy systems are integrated by a set of metabolic pathways that come into operation during exercise, depending on the intensity and duration. In summary, they can be divided into non-oxidative pathways (phosphogenic and glycolytic pathways) and aerobic pathways (nutrient oxidation) [1].

Both pathways aim to generate ATP that will be consumed during the exercise. The non-oxidative pathways occur in the cellular cytosol, do not require oxygen, and are activated during short-time periods (seconds). Phosphagen route uses ATP and phosphocreatine, lasting between 1 and 10 s, and is a route that does not need oxygen and does not generate lactate. Glycolytic pathways metabolize glucose, muscle, and liver glycogen through glycolysis and occur in high-intensity exercises up to 3 min. These glycolytic pathways generate lactate and hydrogen bonds, generating an acidity in the muscle cell—this acidity being one of its limitations [7].

The aerobic pathway occurs inside the mitochondria, so it requires the presence of oxygen to metabolize fuels. It is typical of resistance exercises with medium-low intensity and long duration. It includes the oxidation of CHOs, fats, and to a lesser extent proteins. This route generates much more ATP than the anaerobic path but more slowly, speed being the limitation of this path [7].

Energy needs

The key to success for any athlete will be to adapt energy intake to energy expenditure, which allows the correct functioning of the organism while improving BC [1]. However, it can be complicated due to multiple changes in periodization of training and competitions.

The energy demands of athletes differ widely depending on the type of sport, duration, intensity, competitive level, and individual variability of each athlete. The more demanding the competitive levels of the athlete are, the greatest increase in the intensity of both training and competition occurs, which will result in a significant reduction energy reserves that must be replaced by an adequate diet [8].

The objectives of the athletes' diet are the following: provide the necessary energy for exercise, regulate body metabolism, and provide nutrients to maintain and repair tissues [9]. Due to variation among athletes, different available food options, and individual food patterns, there is no single feeding pattern for athletes, so there are a large number of strategies and options to assess [2].

Caloric intakes below the basal metabolic rate (BMR) are not recommended because it can compromise organism functions. Depending on the type of training energy requirement, the following recommendations for athletes can be approached: moderate training 1.7 × BMR, intense training 2.1 × BMR, extreme training 3 × BMR, and with the maximum recommended limit being 4 × BMR.

Athletes should bear in mind that it is not enough to pay attention to food only on the day of competition, but daily. Appropriate nutritional guidelines will optimize SP, improve recovery, and reduce the risk of injury and illness [2]. For example, in women daily intake below 30 kcal/kg body mass/day can induce damage to metabolic and hormonal functions that affect SP, growth, and health [10].

A varied diet is recommended, covering energetic requirements, and is based on foods as fruits, vegetables, legumes, cereals, dairy products, eggs, fish, and lean meat, in order to provide vitamins and minerals. A poor choice of foods cannot be compensated by the use of supplements [2].

Macronutrients

In order to establish recommendations for macronutrients, it is preferable taking into account the body weight (BW) of the athlete, instead of giving the typical percentages based on the total caloric intake of the diet [2]. For this purpose the recommendations will be provided by grams of nutrient/kg of BW.

Main energy substrates used for physical exercise are carbohydrates (CHO) and lipids, while proteins as energy substrate are reserved for extreme conditions. The use of energy substrate varies depending on the intensity and duration of the exercise, level of training of the athlete, and the state of pre-workout CHO stores. The use of CHO as energy substrate is produced mainly during high- intensity and short-duration exercises. Meanwhile, less intense and long-term exercises use fats' main energy substrate [11]. However the use of CHO will also have a great impact on exercises of less intensity and longer duration such as resistance test, showing that depletion of CHO together with dehydration is a major limitation of the SP [12].

One of the big differences between CHO and lipids is their storage in the body. While CHOs have a limited reserve which leads to around 1600–2000 kcal, fats suppose a practically unlimited energy reserve close to 70,000 kcal (depending on fat mass) [7, 11].

Carbohydrate

Currently, there are a large number of myths related to nutrition, which causes great confusion in general population. One of the most widespread errors is the demonization suffered by the CHO, which has generated some carbophobia in society, including the athlete population [13]. This is a mistake, due to the importance of CHO as energy substrate for the brain and central nervous system. Moreover, they can also be used at different intensities both by anaerobic and aerobic pathways [1].

CHO are an energy fuel that provides 4 kcal/g of dry weight. They are stores in liver and muscle in the form of glycogen. Although, these deposits are limited to around 400-500 g, providing 1600- 2000 kcal, they can be depleted if the diet does not contain enough CHO. Glycogen stores in the organism are divided into 350–400 g in the muscle, 75–100 g in the liver, and around 5 g in the plasma [14]. In addition to size differences, the liver is really a store of glycogen, responsible for maintaining blood glucose. Meanwhile, the muscle can be considered a "false" store since it only uses glucose for its own needs. In other words, the liver can contribute to the replacement of muscle glycogen in the event of depletion, something that does not happen in reverse, which can lead to hypoglycemia and considerably affect SP due to fatigue [15].

It is vitally important to maintain high levels of glycogen so as not to compromise the physical demands of physical activity, since low availability can be associated with loss of abilities and impaired decision-making and increases risk of injury and decreases SP. Therefore, it is essential to provide CHO before exercise, as well as during, in order to improve the SP and delay the onset of fatigue [14, 16].

A good strategy in order to optimize increased glycogen reserves for a competition is the "CHO overload" in the hours or even days before. In athletes with good training status, it is not necessary to deplete these deposits previously, as was believed decades ago. In fact an intake or around 10 g CHO/kg/day during the previous 36–48 h would be enough [17]. Athletes are advised to test how many CHOs are able to inatek without gastric problems. On the other hand, it is also advisable not to try new things on competition days [14].

In general, the CHO recommendations based on the intensity and duration of physical activity can be summarized as follows [1, 18]:

- 3–5 g/kg/d of low-intensity training such as recovery days or tactical skills
- 5–7 g/kg/d for moderate intensity training of 1 h duration
- 6–10 g/kg/d for moderate–high intensity exercises between 1 and 3 h
- 8–12 g/kg/d for workouts of more than 4–5 h of moderate-high intensity

During competition as well as during high-intensity training, a high intake of CHO between 3 and 4 h before the beginning of the exercise is convenient, in order to complete glycogen levels [14]. In case of CHO overload, the recommendation ranges from 200 g CHO to 300 g CHO of moderate glycemic index. The intake should be light, easily digestible, and low in fat, protein, and fiber, in order not to decrease glycemia. Also, an intake of 1–4 g/kg of CHO between the previous 1 and 4 h would be recommended. However, some athletes should be careful with the intake of simple CHOs in the hour before the competition, which can cause a reactive hypoglycemia that affects the SP [18].

The type of exercise, length, and provisioning are determinant factors for the physical exercise. Depending on all the variables, the nutritional strategies will be adapted to the athlete as personalized as possible. To summarize, the recommendations of CHO during the exercise are [19, 20]:

- In an exercise of less than 30 min, CHO intake is not necessary.
- In exercise lasting 45–75 min, it seems that the intake of CHOs is not necessary and it would be enough to perform mouth rinses. However, ingesting this liquid can promote hydration.
- In exercises lasting 1–2 h, the intake of 30 g/h seems to be sufficient, increasing CHO intake up to 60 g/h in case of more delayed sports.
- In exercises lasting more than 2.5 h, the intake of CHO should be 90 g/h. High CHO amounts can cause digestive problems; therefore, a previous intestine training is determinant to tolerate such CHO intake.

The rate of glucose oxidation is estimated at 60 g/h. Therefore, the CHO composition must be formed by a combination of CHOs that use different transporters and increase the oxidation rate, such as maltodextrin or sucrose, among others [20]. Consuming 90 g CHOs/h can cause gastrointestinal problems in sports such as continuous running. These gastrointestinal problems may be due to the redistribution of blood flow to the muscles during exercise. Therefore, strategies for bowel training have been proposed to increase the rate of gastric emptying as well as reduce possible discomfort [21]. When it is proposed to reach recommendations, it seems beneficial to alternate different types of drinks, gels, or bars, so that the taste is not monotonous.

The reposition of CHO is determinant in approaching the following training or competitive sessions. After the completion of physical activity, it is vitally important to replenish CHO stores after the training and competition sessions. These replacements of CHO levels can be approached by different methods, depending on the closeness and intensity of the next sporting event. It will be necessary to rehydrate and to ensure glycogen recovery as well as muscle tissue. The optimum approach is a recovery of 150% of BW lost and a CHO intake between 1 and 2 g/kg/h during the following 6 h after exercise. Moreover, it is advisable to take advantage of the first 2 h afterward where the glycogen resynthesis rate is maximum [14, 22].

The contribution of 1 g/kg BW of CHO after the first hour post-exercise has anticatabolic effect, increases insulin secretion, and increases muscle protein synthesis. Moreover, the addition of protein may also increase the glycogen resynthesis, so a less aggressive pattern can be reached by combining a consumption of 0.8 g kg BW/h of CHO together with protein intake of 0.2–0.4 g/kg BW/h [19].

The appropriate intake of CHO before, during and, after exercise ensures a satisfactory energy intake to face both training and competitions. Most CHOs are found in cereals, fruits, legumes, and vegetables and can be found in smaller quantities in dairy products, unless they could have added sugars. Given the importance of CHO, it is considered essential that athletes ingest enough CHO complexes during the course of the day, leaving simple CHOs during and after exercise [2].

However, in some circumstances in which physiological adaptations to training are the target, different strategies can be handled to those previously mentioned. For example, training with low availability of glycogen induces mitochondrial biogenesis (increase in the number of mitochondria) and thereby enhances lipid oxidation [23]. This strategy can make the athlete more profitable metabolically, allowing a saving of glycogen reserves during exercise and thereby delaying the onset of fatigue. Another purpose of this strategy can be to accustom the athlete to know the feeling of emptiness that can have at the end of a competition and know in advance how to deal with it [24].

Because a reduction in the availability of CHO will affect the quality of the training, these strategies should be carried out with extreme caution and under the supervision of nutritionist and coach. The performance of training under low availability of CHO will be done during low-intensity sessions due to the perception of effort is greater, the immune system can be affected, and the athlete is at greater risk of injury [24].

Proteins

The proteins are composed of amino acid (AA) chains. There are 20 types of AA, divide into nonessential AAs (can be synthetized by the organism) and essential AAs (must be contributed by the diet) [2]. Within the essential AAs, there are three types of AAs called branched (leucine, valine, and isoleucine). Among them, leucine stands out as a stimulator of the mammalian target of rapamycin (mTOR) pathway, which is related to protein synthesis and hypertrophy [25].

Although proteins can contribute between 5 and 10% to the total energy used during physical activity, they are not considered as energy source. Proteins constitute the base of muscle tissue and of the immune system and are the major component of muscle enzymes and play a large role in SP [14].

Regarding sedentary population, the estimated consumption rate is 0.8 g/ kg BW/day. In the athlete population, these requirements are increased to repair muscle damage caused by exercise, enhance metabolic adaptations to training, and avoid possible muscle catabolism [2]. The focus of protein consumption is on estimating an adequate protein intake for each given moment [1].

The current recommendations for athlete population range between 1.2 and 2.0 g/kg BW/day depending on the type of sports performed [1]. Moreover, higher amounts may be reached at exceptional times such as injurious period, high- intensity training, or weight loss plans with caloric restriction. The purpose of this increase is to maintain maximum muscle mass integrity [26].

Although the most important factor in terms of protein consumption is the overall consumption throughout the day, it may be advisable to divide the protein intake into several intakes. For example, four doses of 0.4 g/kg BW ensuring a total of 1.6 g/kg BW a day [25]. Likewise, it is recommended to ensure a contribution of 3 g of leucine every meal [27]. The optimal timing seems to adjust the intake depending on the moment, type of training, as well as availability of the rest of nutrients and energy. It is important to have an adequate energy and CHO consumption, so that dietary amino acid are used for protein synthesis and not oxidized to obtain energy [28].

Protein-rich diets are associated with increased risk of dehydration due to elimination of nitrogenous waste products, an increased cardiovascular disease risk due to the association of fat with protein products, or a shift of CHO [2]. However, even at high doses, no negative effects on renal function have been reported in healthy subjects.

Regarding timing of protein intake along with exercise, it seems that the most optimal time is the period after exercise. Better doses ranged between 0.25 and 0.3 g/protein/kg BW (approximately 15–25 g protein) [1]. However, high protein intake is discouraged close to physical exercise, due to possible digestive problems as a result of its long time of gastric emptying. However, in very long duration exercise, there is not such limitation.

In order to stimulate muscle protein synthesis, the intake of 30–40 g of casein is beneficial prior to going to bed, promoting nocturnal recovery due to its slow digestion [29].

To choose protein sources, it is important that animal proteins may be of greater interest. In fact, animal proteins are considered as a complete protein due to the presence of all essential AAs [30].

The main protein sources are lean meat products, fish, eggs, dairy products, and legumes that provide vegetable protein and reduce animal consumption.

The use of protein supplements does not seem to be necessary because protein requirements are usually reached with diet in Western population. However, population that may find it difficult to reach such recommendations should be monitored. These groups includes: vegetarian athletes, young athletes in the growth phase, and athletes who restrict their diet due to religious or cultural reason. can be included [2]. If protein supplementation is chosen, the best option is whey protein for its high content on AAs and leucine content.

Lipids

Along with the CHO, lipids are major energy substrates during exercise [27]. The difference is that fats are not as profitable per unit of time as CHO and high fat consumption is not associated with improvements in SP [31].

Lipid consumption is important for both energy intake and essential nutrients such as fat-soluble vitamins A, D, E, and K. Both quantity and quality of fats are determinant in the diet. The quality is often referred by its content on inflammatory fatty acids [2].

The recommendation regarding fat consumption in athletes is similar to that of the general population. It is advisable not to make restrictive consumption of fat, as it can lead to deficit of nutrients such as fat-soluble vitamins and omega-3 fatty acids [1].

Fatty acid requirements, according to the American College of Sports Medicine (ACSM), are 20–35% of the total kcal of the diet, where 7–10% should correspond to saturated fatty acids, 10% to polyunsaturated fatty acids, and 10–15% to mono- unsaturated fatty acids [32].

Adequate intake of omega-3 fatty acids should be ensured due to its anti- inflammatory effects, improvements in the organism's coagulation, or increase in omega-3/omega-6 ratio [33].

In particular, food as avocado or olive oil is recommended, due to their high content on monounsaturated fatty acids, which have less susceptible to oxidation.

It is recommended to reduce the consumption of fatty meats, substituting them for lean meats, fish, and legumes. It is also advisable to eliminate the consumption of processed products such as sausages [2].

An excess of polyunsaturated fatty acids carries a risk of lipid peroxidation, so a joint intake with vitamin E is recommend. Moreover, the ratio omega-3/omega-6 series should be greater as possible, because of the greater pro-inflammatory character of omega-6. The recommendations regarding the omega-6/omega-3 range oscillate between 2 and 4/1 in favor of the omega-6, something that is far from the inflammatory level that this entails [33]. In order to reduce the omega-6/omega-3 ratio, it is advisable to reduce consumption of meats and increase consumption of blue fish such as sardines, salmon, tuna, anchovy, and mackerel.

Hydration

During exercise, increments of energy requirements are associated to larger production of metabolic heat [34]. Human organism dissipates that extra heat mainly by the mechanism of evaporation, which ultimately induces dehydration [35, 36].

One of the greatest limitations of SP is dehydration. It is estimated that each kg of BW lost during exercise corresponds to 1 L of sweat [35]. The sensitivity to dehydration is personal, but generally no losses greater than 2% of the BW are recom- mended in order not to compromise the SP [37]. In fact, 1% of BW lost leads to SP decrease by 10%. Some authors have raised the possibility of training dehydration, but there is some controversy about it [38, 39].

The consumption of water is the only method to prevent dehydration and will be essential before, during, and after exercise. However, a large number of athletes usually begin the exercise in a state of hypohydration [40]. Therefore, it is necessary to instruct the athlete to acquire correct hydration habits according to the type of sports, so that the SP is affected as little as possible [12].

Losses of electrolytes, especially sodium, occur along with water losses. It has been seen that well-trained athletes "sweat more but swear better," that is, they sweat more water, but the loss of electrolytes is lower [41]. Recent studies have compared both the rate of sweating and the concentration of sodium in tattooed people versus non-tattooed people, concluding that the most tattooed skin presented lower sweating rate and higher sodium concentration [42].

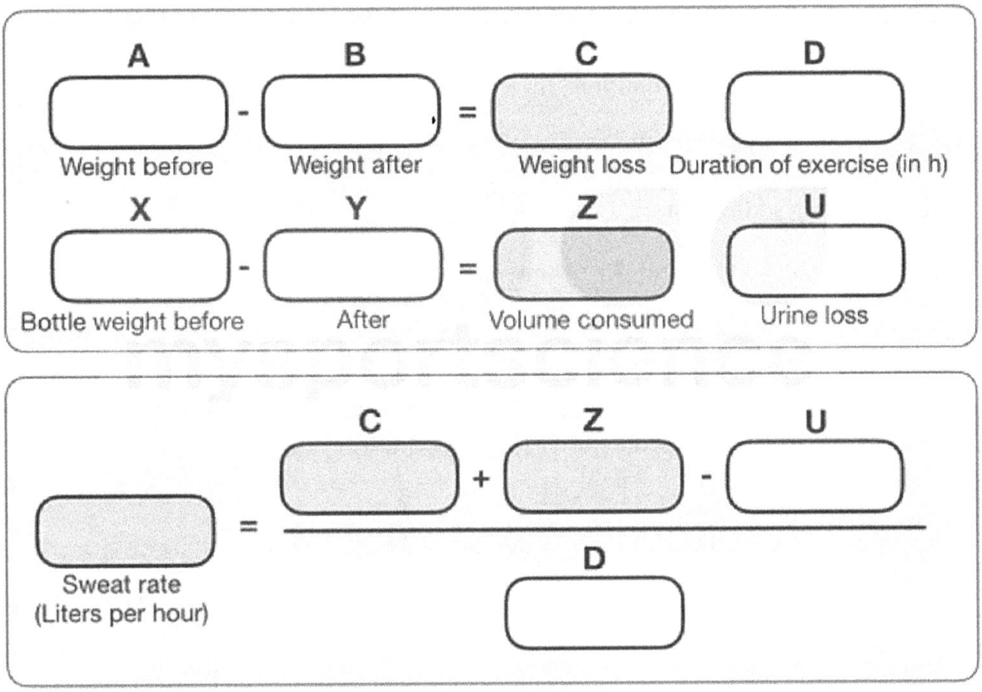

Figure 1. *How to calculate sweat rate? [43].*

It seems interesting to perform a sweat test to athletes, in order to know their rate of sweating (liters/hour). To accomplish it, weighing the athlete before and after the exercise session is enough. This data reveals the amount of sweat that is lost at the time, so it can serve to adjust the athlete's water intake (**Figure 1**). [43]. In general, the rate of sweating is usually greater than that of gastric emptying. However athletes can be trained to increase gastric emptying during workouts and thereby reduce dehydration as possible [21]. In conditions of higher temperature and humidity, this rate of sweating will rise higher. Another simpler way to determine the state of hydration in athletes is controlling the color of urine (darker colors are associated with enhanced dehydration states) [2].

Wherein some cases, athletes must acclimatize to different temperatures they accustomed. It has been reported that among all factors, the most important factor is the previous state of hydration.

In healthy non-athlete population, the sensation of thirst is an ancestral mechanism that informs of the need to ingest liquid. However, in children, elderly people, and athletes, this mechanism is altered and liquid should be ingested before presenting thirst sensation. In the case of athletes, thirst appears when there is a deficit of 2% dehydration [27]. However, special care should be taken to amateur athletes, who increase their water intake above their needs, which can suffer dilutional hyponatremia "leading to serious problems and even lead to death" [44].

Regarding the drink to be used for sports, it is advisable to use replacement drinks instead of water, due to the CHO and sodium content. Both salts and CHO improve intestinal transport, which facilitates the arrival of fluid in the blood. Prepositional beverages should present an isotonic composition, with the following characteristics [12]:

- 80–35 kcal
- At least 75% of the kcal should be high glycemic index CHO
- No more than 90 g CHO/liter
- 460–1150 mg sodium/liter
- Osmolality 200–330 mOsm/kg of water

As commented before, it is advisable to use drink with different CHOs as glucose, sucrose, and maltodextrinas, in order to facilitate the absorption of liquid due to the use of different intestinal transporters. Moreover, the fructose content should not be very high, due to quantities between 20 and 30% can cause intestinal problems [22]. The hydration guidelines indicated for performing physical exercise are [12, 14]:

- Ingest between 400 and 600 ml of water along the 4 h before the start of the exercise.
- Just at the beginning of the activity, ingest 200–400 ml of water with CHO (5–8%).
- During the exercise, ingest 100–200 ml of water every 15–20 min.
- After physical activity consume 150% of the BW lost in the 6 h after.
- In low-intensity training and short-duration, the intake of water alone is sufficient
- The ideal temperature of drinks oscillates between 15 and 21°C
- The taste should be pleasant to the palate of the athlete.

In a situation where the environment is very hot and has high humidity, the recommendations of intake of liquid and sodium will be higher [22]. A good strategy can be to make salted snacks in the hours before the exercise or add more salt content to the meals before and after the exercise. Such increase of sodium has a double purpose, on the one hand to increase the intake of liquid through thirst and on the other to favor the retention of that liquid in the organism. Finally, alcohol consumption is discouraged in both athletes and non-athletes. However, there seems to be a high consumption of this substance in team sports and greater consumption in men than women [45]. Among the harmful effects of alcohol consumption, the following can be highlighted: reduction of SP due to decrease in strength, power, speed, and resistance; diuretic effect that affects hydration [46]; diminution of sleep quality, mood, and immune system [47]; elevation of cortisol concentration; and reduction of muscle synthesis up to 24% even when consumed right at the end of the exercise [48].

Diabetes in sports

First, the effect of exercise between insulin-dependent (type 1) and insulin- dependent (type 2) diabetes should be differentiated. In type 2, you do the exercise to improve insulin resistance, while in type 1, you should adjust and modify the amount of insulin administered, along with the CHO intake.

Physical exercise is one of the most difficult activities to adapt to diabetes, due to the increase in the frequency of hypoglycemia. People with diabetes who perform physical activity on a regular basis have less need for insulin, but this does not ensure adequate glycemic control. The blood glucose value is of multifactorial origin, and one should take into account the CHO intake and type of sports performed as well as adjust the dose of insulin used [49].

In order to avoid hypoglycemia, during the exercise the dose of insulin will be reduced but in no case will be completely eliminated, because the lack of insulin prevents the entry of a sufficient amount of glucose into the cells for obtaining energy. A greater use of fats as fuel can generate an accumulation of ketone bodies and cause ketoacidosis. In the presence of glucose values (>250 mg/dL), ketone levels should be checked, and if elevated (>0.5 mmol/l), postpone the activity [49].

The type of exercise performed by the athlete should be taken into account, since aerobic exercise increases the risk of hypoglycemia during and after exercise, while anaerobes cause hyperglycemia due to counterregulatory hormones (glucagon, cortisol, and catecholamines) [49].

Physical exercise has some ability to introduce glucose into the muscle cell without the need for insulin action. This effect can occur during the 48 h after exercise, so there is a certain risk of suffering hypoglycemia in that period depending on the sports performed. This is due to the fact that during the physical exercise, the reserves of the muscle and liver glycogen have been emptied. Once the exercise is finished and after the intake of CHO, the glucose will be destined to replace the glycogen reserves instead of the blood, which can cause hypoglycemia, so that the high blood glucose value after a type of anaerobic exercise can be deceptive. Therefore, higher consumption of CHO or decreased insulin dose can prevent such hypoglycemia [49].

Supplements

An ergonomic aid is a product that contains a nutrient or a group of nutrients that improve the SP without taking into account the harmful effects in athletes, while a supplement is a nutritional aid to complete the diet associated with the practice of physical exercise [50].

When an athlete seeks to improve in the SP, his ability to tolerate intense workouts and hard competitions is crucial to avoid falling into injury or chronic fatigue. To achieve this purpose, an adequate supply of nutrients is essential. However, many times this does not happen, and the use of dietary supplements is resorted to [50].

These supplements must be prescribed individually according to the needs of each person (sex, age, fitness, intensity and duration of the exercise, season, etc.), in order to maintain both the state of health and the improvement of the SP. Dietary supplements must offer maximum possible safety and have a degree of scientific evidence to support their effect [50].

Currently between 40 and 70% of athletes make use of supplements without previously analyzing if necessary. In addition, a large number of sports supplements have not shown empirical evidence to improve SP. Likewise, there is a certain legal vacuum with the labeling of these substances, where 80% of these products do not contain the quantities declared on the label. In addition, 10–15% of these contain prohibited substances, and this can generate a high risk of committing an offense involuntarily by the athlete [51].

According to the Australian Institute of Sport, supplements are classified into four groups, based on effectiveness and safety [52]:

- Group A: based on the evidence. Recommended for athletes.
    - Useful and timely source of energy or nutrients in the diet of athlete
    - Scientifically proven their evidence for the improvement of the SP, when they are used with a protocol and specific situation

In this group we can find:

- Food for athletes (gels, bars, electrolytes, isotonic drinks, maltodextrins, whey protein)
- Medical supplements (vitamin D, probiotics, iron/calcium supplements)
- Substances to improve SP (creatine monohydrate, caffeine, beta-alanine, bicarbonate, beet juice)
- Group B: more research deserved and advised under research or monitoring protocol.
    - Some benefit in non-athlete population or have data that suggest possible benefit of SP.
    - Of particular interest to athletes and coaches.

In this group we can find (quercetin, HMB, glutamine, BCCA, CLA, carnitine).

- Group C: few tests of beneficial effect are not provided to athletes.
    - Not proven improvement RD despite its widespread use.
    - Very little or no benefit, and sometimes they even affect the RD in a negative way.

In this group supplements of group A and B may be included when used without an individualized protocol and without a basis in scientific evidence.

- Group D: should not be used by athletes.
    - Are prohibited or have risk of contamination with doping or positive substance by drug

In this group we can find glycerol, ephedrine, sibutramine, and tribulus terrestris.

Despite all this information, many athletes believe that supplements are the basis of the athlete's diet and believe that without that supplement, they will not reach their maximum level. This belief is one of the biggest mistakes in the world of sports nutrition, where the basic diet that is the true pillar on which sports nutrition is based is neglected.

Conclusions

The basis of sports nutrition is a varied diet and individually tailored to the requirements and appetency of each athlete. The athlete should be instructed about the importance of diet, called "invisible training," which is not only important on competition day. Prior to establishing nutritional guidelines, it is necessary to know and adapt the BC of the athlete in the different periods of the season and make revisions through the sum of six skinfolds.

It is necessary to know some physiology to know the different metabolic pathways that interact during the exercise. In this way depending on the type of sports performed, duration and intensity adapt dietary intake at expense. Macronutrient requirements will be established based on g/kg/BW. With respect to CHOs, recommendations vary between 3 and 12 g/kg/BW to avoid compromising the SP, and protein consumption can vary between 1.2 and 2.0 g/kg/BW, with the total daily intake being more important than the number of intakes. Regarding to fatty acids, quality will prevail, improving the inflammatory profile with an increase in the consumption of omega-3 compared to omega-6.

It is essential to maintain a state of hydration before, during, and after exercise to avoid compromising SP, so it is necessary to instruct the athlete with proper hydration guidelines. It is advisable to train the digestive system during workouts, both for hydration and testing different CHOs doses. It is important not to try new patterns on the day of competition.

Acronyms and abbreviations

SP sports performance

BC body composition

BMI body mass index

DEXA dual-energy X-ray absorptiometry

BIA bioelectrical impedance analysis

ISAK International Society for the Advancement of Kinanthropometry

CHOs carbohydrates

BMR basal metabolic rate

BW body weight

AA amino acid

mTOR mammalian target of rapamycin

ACSM American College of Sports Medicine

Author details

Raúl Arcusa Saura, María Pilar Zafrilla Rentero and Javier Marhuenda Hernández*

Faculty of Health Sciences, Universidad Católica San Antonio de Murcia (UCAM), Spain

*Address all correspondence to: jmarhuenda@ucam.edu

References

[1] Thomas DT, Erdman KA, Burke LM. American College of Sports Medicine Joint Position Statement. Nutrition and athletic performance. Medicine and Science in Sports and Exercise. 2016;**48**(3):543-568

[2] Benardot D. Nutrición deportiva avanzada: Cómo ajustar la ingesta de alimentos y fluidos a fin de conseguir un entrenamiento y rendimiento óptimos. 2ªed ed. Madrid: Tutor; 2008

[3] Ackland TR, Lohman TG, Sundgot- borgen J, Maughan RJ, Meyer NL, Stewart AD, et al. Current status of body composition assessment in sport. Sports Medicine. 2012;**42**(3):227-249

[4] Alvero JR, Cabañas MD, Herrero A, Martínez L, Moreno C, Porta J, et al. Protocolo de valoración de la composición corporal para el reconocimiento médico-deportivo.

Documento de consenso del grupo español de cineantropometría (GREC) de la federación española de medicna del deporte (FEMEDE). Versión 2010., Archivos de Medicina del Deporte. 2010;**27**(139):330-334

[5] Alonso-aubin DA, Moreira OC, Alonso-aubin DA, De OCEP, Candia- luján R. Métodos de evaluación de la composición corporal : Una revisión actualizada de descripción, aplicación, ventajas y desventajas. Archivos de Medicina del Deporte. 2015;**32**(6):387-394

[6] Holway F. Composición corporal en nutrición deportiva. [Internet]. 2014. Disponible en: https://www.researchgate.net/ publication/257141125_Composicion_ corporal_ en_nutricion_deportiva

[7] Teijón JM, Garrido A, Blanco D, Villaverde C, Mendoza C, Ramírez J. Fundamentos de Bioquímca Metabólica. 3ª ed. Madrid: Tébar; 2009

[8] Martínez JM, Urdampilleta A, Mielgo J. Necesidades energéticas, hídricas y nutricionales en el deporte. Motricidad. European Journal of Human Movement. 2013;**30**:37-52

[9] Burke L. Nutrición en el Deporte. Un enfoque práctico. Madrid: Editorial Médica Panamericana; 2007. pp. 1-28

[10] Daily JP, Stumbo JR. Female Athlete Triad. Prim Care Clin Off Pract [Internet]. 2018. Disponible en: https:// doi.org/10.1016/j.pop.2018.07.004

[11] Jeukendrup AE. Modulation of carbohydrate and fat utilization by diet, exercise and environment. Biochemical Society Transactions. 2003;**31** (Pt 6):1270-1273

[12] Gil-Antuñano NP, Bonafonte LF, Marqueta PM, González BM, García JAV. Consenso sobre bebidas para el deportista. Composición y pautas de reposición de líquidos—Documento de consenso de la federación Española de medicina del deporte. 2008;**25**(126):245-258

[13] Rodríguez-martín B, Alberto C. Hidratos de carbono y práctica deportiva: Una etnografría virtual en Twitter. Nutrición Hospitalaria. 2017;**34**(1):144-153

[14] Olivos C, Cuevas A, Alvarez V, Jorquera C. Nutrición para el entrenamiento y la competición. Revista Médica Clínica Las Condes. 2012;**23**(3):253-261

[15] Arasa M. Manual de Nutrición Deportiva. 1ª ed. Paidotribo: Badalona; 2005

[16] Murray B, Rosenbloom C. Fundamentals of glycogen metabolism for coaches and athletes. Nutrition Reviews. 2018;**76**(4):243-259

[17] Nikolaidis PT, Veniamakis E, Rosemann T, Knechtle B. Nutrition in ultra-endurance: State of the art. Nutrients. 2018;**10**(12). pii: E1995.DOI: 10.3390/nu10121995

[18] Burke LM, Hawley JA, Wong SHS, Jeukendrup AE. Carbohydrates for training and competition. Journal of Sports Sciences. 2011;**29**(Suppl 1): S17-S27

[19] Jeukendrup AE. Nutrition for endurance sports: Marathon, triathlon, and road cycling. Journal of Sports Sciences. 2011;**28**(Suppl 1):S91-S99

[20] Jeukendrup AE. A step towards personalized sports nutrition: Carbohydrate intake during exercise. Sports Medicine. 2014;**44**(Suppl 1): 25-33

[21] Jeukendrup AE. Training the gut for athletes. Sports Medicine. 2017;**28**(178):1-5

[22] Urdampilleta A, Martínez JM, Sanchez J, Álvarez J. Protocolo de hidratación antes, durante y después de la actividad físico-deportiva. Motricidad. European Journal of Human Movement. 2013;**31**:57-76

[23] Yeo WK, Paton CD, Garnham AP, Burke LM, Carey AL, Hawley JA, et al. Skeletal muscle adaptation and performance responses to once a day versus twice every second day endurance training regimens. Journal of Applied Physiology. 2008;**105**(5):1462-1470

[24] Hawley JA, Burke LM. Carbohydrate availability and training adaptation: Effects on cell metabolism. Exercise and Sport Sciences Reviews. 2010;**38**(4):152-160

[25] Schoenfeld BJ, Aragon AA. How much protein can the body use in a single meal for muscle-building? Implications for daily protein distribution. Journal of the International Society of Sports Nutrition. 2018;**15**:10. DOI: 10.1186/s12970-018-0215-1. eCollection 2018

[26] Mettler S, Mitchell N, Tipton KD. Increased protein intake reduces lean body mass loss during weight loss in athletes. Medicine and Science in Sports and Exercise. 2010;**42**(2):326-337

[27] Kerksick CM, Wilborn CD, Roberts MD, Smith-ryan A, Kleiner SM, Jäger R, et al. ISSN exercise & sports nutrition review update: Research & recommendations. Journal of the International Society of Sports Nutrition. 2018;**15**(1):1-57

[28] Bolster DR, Pikosky MA, Gaine PC, Martin W, Wolfe RR, Tipton KD, et al. Dietary protein intake impacts human skeletal muscle protein fractional synthetic rates after endurance exercise. American Journal of Physiology. Endocrinology and Metabolism. 2005;**289**(4):E678-E683

[29] Res PT, Groen B, Pennings B, Beelen M, Wallis GA, Gijsen AP, et al. Protein ingestion before sleep improves postexercise overnight recovery. Medicine and Science in Sports and Exercise. 2012;**44**(8):1560-1569

[30] Tipton KD, Wolfe RR. Protein and amino acids for athletes. Journal of Sports Sciences. 2004;**22**(1):65-79

[31] Onzari M. In: Fundamentos de nutrición en el deporte. Buenos Aires: El Ateneo; 2008. pp. 129-164

[32] Rodriguez NNR, Di Marco N, Langley S, DiMarco NM. American College of Sports Medicine, American Dietetic Association, and Dietitians of Canada joint position statement: Nutrition and athletic performance. Medicine and Science in Sports and Exercise. 2009;**41**(3):709-731

[33] Daley CA, Abbott A, Doyle PS, Nader GA, Larson S. A review of fatty acid profiles and antioxidant content in grass-fed and grain-fed beef. Nutrition Journal. 2010;**9**:10.DOI: 10.1186/1475-2891-9-10

[34] Shirreffs SM, Aragon-Vargas LF, Chamorro M, Maughan RJ, Serratosa L, Zachwieja JJ. The sweating response of elite professional soccer players to training in the heat. International Journal of Sports Medicine. 2005;**26**(2):90-95

[35] Laitano ORJBL. La ciencia de la hidratación y estrategias en fútbol. Sports Science Exchange. 2014;**27**(128):1-7

[36] Maughan RJ, Shirreffs SM, Leiper JB. Errors in the estimation of hydration status from changes in body mass. Journal of Sports Sciences. 2007;**25**(7):797-804

[37] Sawka MN, Burke LM, Eichner ER, Maughan RJ, Montain SJ, Stachenfeld NS. American College of Sports Medicine position stand. Exercise and fluid replacement. Medicine and Science in Sports and Exercise. 2007;**39**(2):377-390

[38] Viitasalo JT, Kyröläinen H, Bosco C, Alen M. Effects of rapid weight reduction on force production and vertical jumping height. International Journal of Sports Medicine.1987;**8**(4):281-285

[39] Watson G, Judelson DA, Armstrong LE, Yeargin SW, Casa DJ, Maresh CM. Influence of diuretic-induced dehydration on competitive sprint and power performance. Medicine and Science in Sports and Exercise. 2005;**37**(7):1168-1174

[40] Godek SF, Bartolozzi AR, Godek JJ. Sweat rate and fluid turnover in American football players compared with runners in a hot and humid environment. British Journal of Sports Medicine. 2005;**39**(4):205-211

[41] Maughan RJ, Merson SJ, Broad NP, Shirreffs SM. Fluid and electrolyte intake and loss in elite soccer players during training. International Journal of Sport Nutrition and Exercise Metabolism. 2004;**14**(3):333-346

[42] Luetkemeier MJ, Hanisko JM, Aho KM. Skin tattoos Alter sweat rate and Na+ concentration. Medicine and Science in Sports and Exercise. 2017;**49**(7):1432-1436

[43] Jeukendrup AE. How much do you sweat? [Internet]. 2017. Disponible en: http://www.mysportscience.com/single-post/2016/11/18/ Protein-intake-guidelines-for-athletes

[44] Noakes TD. Overconsumption of fluids by athletes. BMJ. 2003;**327**(7407): 113-114

[45] Moss HB. The impact of alcohol on society: A brief overview. Social Work in Public Health. 2013;**28**(3-4):175-177

[46] Shirreffs SM, Maughan RJ. Restoration of fluid balance after exercise-induced dehydration: Effects of alcohol consumption. Journal of Applied Physiology. 1997;**83**(4):1152-1158

[47] Barnes MJ. Alcohol: Impact on sports performance and recovery in male athletes. Sports Medicine. 2014;**44**(7):909-919

[48] Koziris LP, Kraemer WJ, Gordon SE, Incledon T, Knuttgen HG. Effect of acute postexercise ethanol intoxication on the neuroendocrine response to resistance exercise. Journal of Applied Physiology. 2000;**88**(1):165-172

[49] Murillo S. Diabetes tipo 1 y deporte: Para niños adolescentes y adultos jovenes. Barcelona: Edika Med; 2015

[50] Palacios N, Manonelles P, Blasco R, Bonafonte L, Gaztañaga T, Manuz B, et al. Ayudas ergogénicas nutricionales para personas que realizan ejercicio físico. Archivos de Medicina del Deporte. 2013;**XXIX**(Suplemento 1):5-80

[51] Outram S, Stewart B. Doping through supplement use: A review of the available empirical data. International Journal of Sport Nutrition and Exercise Metabolism. 2015;**25**(1):54-59

[52] Commission AS. Classification [Internet]. 2018. Available from: https:// www.ausport.gov.au/ais/nutrition/ supplements/classification

11

Hydrogen Water on Survival Rate after Fasting in Drosophila Model

Chung-Hsing Chao

Abstract

In this study, we use a Drosophila model to examine the effect of drinking hydrogen water on survival rate after fasting. The cells produce free radicals to help to absorb nutritious substances due to metabolism, which is a unique phenomenon for biological organisms. But if over the tension of free radicals can seriously affect the physiological functions, and even lead to death. Recently, scientists found that molecular hydrogen is a free radicals scavenger. However, no bio physiological mechanism and experiment have shown that by drinking hydrogen water, can eliminate the free radicals in animals and the evidence sufficient to influence the survival rate after fasting. Surprisingly, the results of the study support that hydrogen water may be helpful for the survival rate of the fasted fly. When the body loses oxygen free radicals due to food breakoff, hydrogen water may neutralize free radicals and reduce damage to cells. However, we also found that hydrogen water seems to be much help for relatively weak individuals, such as the mutant flies, and it is also favorable for individuals with stronger physique in wild *Drosophila melanogaster* females. In conclusion, the results show that flies can increase their survival rate by feeding hydrogen water under extreme oxidation stress.

Keywords: survival effect, hydrogen, Drosophila, fasting, free radicals, oxidative stress

Introduction

In recent years, there has been a great deal of attention toward the field of free radical chemistry. Our body generates free radicals of reactive oxygen species or reactive nitrogen species by various endogenous systems, exposure to different physiochemical conditions. To balance the free radicals and antioxidants is necessary for proper physiological function. If we can regulate free radicals to reduce the potential reactive oxygen species over tension on body's ability, it will not cause oxidative stress damage. Free radicals thus do not adversely alter lipids, proteins, DNA and trigger many diseases. As a result application of an external source of antioxidants likes oral hydrogen water can assist in coping this oxidative stress.

This metabolism phenomenon also occurs in many other animals or even insects that are less evolved. In 1946, the fruit flies were successfully carried out by National Aeronautics and Space Administration (NASA) for the biological experiments in space. About 75% of the genetic code of fruit flies has similarities to all human pathogenic genes. Insect life is much shorter than human. Drosophila flies also has found free radicals in their cells. The scientists take Drosophila to study aging effects much efficiently due to shortening the time in experiments. It is an important reason why studying *Drosophila melanogaster* in fruit flies is very popular among biological researchers. They also found many mutant species of fruit flies, which are related to the regulatory function of oxidative stress attacked by free radicals in cells. Therefore, we study the survival effects of drinking hydrogen-water on fruit flies after fasting.

According to past research reports, fasting or severely hungry animals will rapidly accumulate a large number of free radicals in cells because of lack of well physiological functions. Excessive free radicals, however, can damage the cell's genetic material and cell membranes, eventually killing the fruit fly. And the flies of the mutant species are more likely to accumulate free radicals in vivo because the chromosome of the Drosophila cell, an enzyme gene that removes peroxidase free radicals by hydrazine, is removed so that the number of free radicals is out of control. Although the fruit fly of this mutant species can still develop to adults, its lifespan is shorter than that of wild fruit flies. I used this kind of fruit fly to do experiments because they have accumulated many free radicals in the body, and alkaline hydrogen water (negatively charged) can neutralize positively charged free radicals, so feeding hydrogen-water on the mutant flies are more evident than wild species. In the course of the experiment, I found that the mutant flies fasting (stop feeding water), causing the flies to die. It proved that the fruit fly did have poor anti oxidative stress, so I did not fast-feed the fruit flies in advance during the experiment. Only for the wild flies, fasting beforehand.

In the study, the experimental result shows that the mutant fruit flies of *Drosophila melanogaster* have a much stronger response to hydrogen water than wild ones. It appears to support a possibility that hydrogen-water seems to be a definite help for individuals who are more likely to accumulate free radicals. Therefore, it is the best way to use the mutant flies directly for anti-free radicals experiments. There will be more significant results. It is also possible to test older flies that are more sensitive to alkaline electrolyzed water because the larger the flies, the more free radicals will accumulate in the body. In our experiments, we found that the older the flies, the more they can't afford the pressure of fasting. On the other hand, the open trial can also directly use strong alkaline hydrogen water to feed mutant flies. In addition, the moisture of the feeding environment in the test tube during the experiment is also vital; otherwise, the fruit flies will die a lot and affect the experimental result. In the same operation, the problem of escaping of the flies is also to avoid. Otherwise, if the trial flies are too few, they are not representative.

Materials and methods

The untreated tap water is almost neutral at about pH 7.0 with a positive oxidative potential of +150 mV. The tap water after filtered and electrolysis treated, the cathode hydrogen dissolving water belongs to be alkaline at a pH over 8.0 with a relatively high negative reductive potential of −150 to −300 mV. Recently, a lot of literatures [1–3] found that drinking hydrogen water increases the activity of a critical detoxifying enzyme of superoxide dismutase in the body. It protects against free radicals toxic damage on protein, enzyme, DNA, lipid, and membrane in cells (see **Figure 1**). Since the alkaline hydrogen water molecules with an extra amount of free electrons, which can neutralize the highly reactive free radicals before free radicals take away free electrons from intracellular molecules.

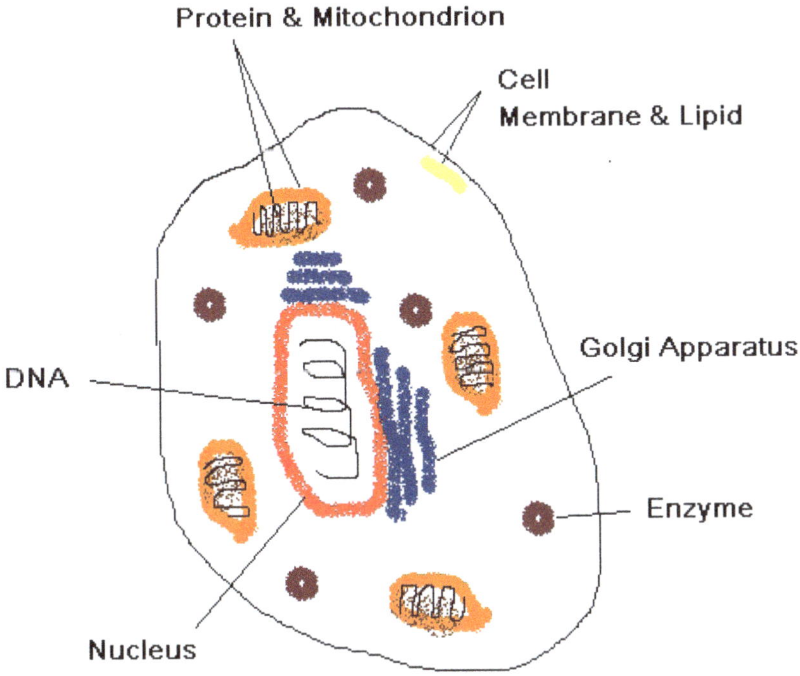

Figure 1. *Free radicals toxic damage on protein, enzyme, DNA, lipid, and membrane.*

Water, which constitutes over 70% of the body, is involved in virtually every function of life. It forms the bodily fluids, such as blood, lymph, cerebrospinal fluid, saliva, and digestive fluids to regulate the metabolism of joint lubrication, detoxification, and maintaining the blood pressure. While the water molecules around the cell membranes, they show a long-range ordering feature and like an epitaxial liquid crystal with distinct properties from the bulk state [1]. Shirahata et al. [2] showed that drinking hydrogen water increases the activity of a critical detoxifying enzyme, superoxide dismutase (SOD), which exists in humans, animals, plants, and micro-organisms, as an essential antioxidant to protect cell under oxidative stress damage in vitro. Superoxide is one of the primary reactive oxygen species in the cell. So SODs serves a key antioxidant role. This antioxidant function exerted by molecular hydrogen has been proved [3]. In the rat model, drinking hydrogen water showed signs in the decrease of the peroxided lipid level in their urine. When comparing to tap water to hydrogen-water, the rat drinks hydrogen-water can extended to live 20–50% longer [4]. Finally, we studied the survival rate of drinking hydrogen-water on Drosophila flies after fasting, which related to the regulatory function of oxidative stress attacked by free radicals in cells.

Drosophila lacking SOD1 has a dramatically shortened lifespan, whereas fly lacking SOD2 will die before birth. Lacking SOD3 does not show any visible defects and exhibit an average lifespan, though more sensitive to hyper oxidative injury. *Drosophila melanogaster* is a species of fruit flies. Drosophila fly is typically used in research because it can readily rear in the laboratory. Since Charles W. Woodworth used *Drosophila melanogaster* as modal organism, eight Nobel prizes have awarded to research using Drosophila. It continues to be widely applied to biological research in genetics, physiology, microbial pathogenesis, and lifespan [5]. Wild-type fruit flies are yellow-brown, with brick-red eyes and transverse black rings across the abdomen. Females are about 2.5 mm long, and males are slightly smaller with darker backs (see **Figure 2**).

The wild-type and mutant-type flies obtained from the *Drosophila melanogaster* stock center at the National Health Research Institutes in Taiwan. Peroxide reductase-1 is one of the mutant-type fruit flies. *Drosophila melanogaster* flies have every six tubes of females and males of 2 day-old-adult flies, 30 flies per tube. Four ones (20/tube) of females and four ones (30 tubes/tube) of males collect within 2 day- olds of adult flies. These flies gently placed to the bottom of the vial (9.5 cm tall × 2.4 cm diameter) and top with cotton swabs and balls with pure neutral water and alkaline hydrogen water (pH 8.5 and 9.5) in the standard medium supplement at room temperature of 50–70% relative humidity. Before experiments, each group carefully collected 2 day-old males and females of adult flies, respectively. The experimental procedures are as follows: 1. Wild-type flies have fasted for 12 hours and then feed water, while the munt flies do not. 2. Using wetted cotton swabs inserted into the test tube for two feeds a day. 3. Observe the death of the flies every 12 hours until all the flies have died. 4. All experiments treatments kept at the standard medium. 5. If the feeding tube wetted with water droplets and change it periodically.

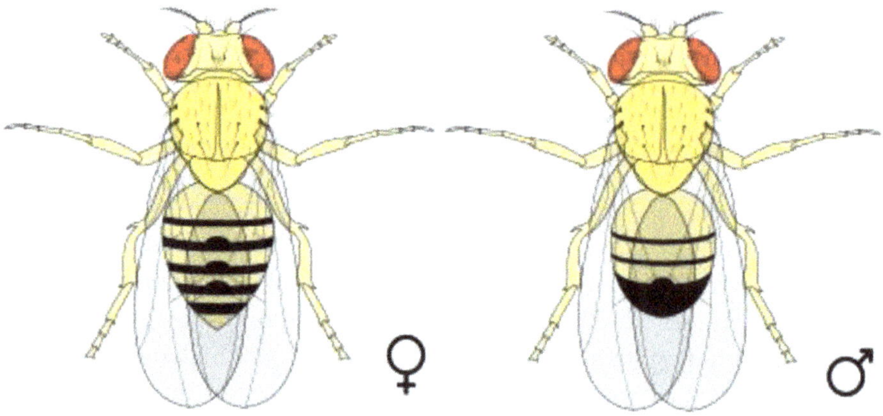

Figure 2. *Female (left) and male (right) of Drosophila melanogaster [6].*

Experimental results

For the control group, every two tubes are wild and mutant species of fruit flies feed with pure water of pH 7. One is female fly, and another is male fly. For the treatment group, every four tubes are wild and mutant species with the female and the male ones fed with alkaline hydrogen water of pH 8.5 and 9.5, respectively. Generally, regardless of whether it is a wild fruit fly or a mutant fruit fly, in the fasting state, feeding of hydrogen water has a significant increase in the survival rate (see **Figures 3–6**).

The mutant and wild species of Drosophila

If we compare with the results of the mutant and wild species, the mutant fruit fly of males to feed weak alkaline hydrogen water of pH 8.5 is the most significant change in survival among them (see **Figure 3** vs. **Figure 5**; **Figure 4** vs. **Figure 6**). In the case of feeding mutant flies with pure water of pH 7, for example, when fasting for more than 4 days, half number of deaths occur. If weak alkaline hydrogen water of pH 8.5 fed, it will delay to more than 9 days to happen it (see **Figure 3**). That is about a twice of increase in the lifespan. Therefore, a weak alkaline hydrogen water of pH 8.5 seems to have a positive effect on the survival rate of flies in the state of starvation.

The females and males of Drosophila

Past research results have shown that the average lifespan of females is longer than that of males. Our experimental results showed that the effect in response to the feeding of hydrogen water, the male-fly was significantly more than the female-fly for all the wild and mutant species. While the case of feeding wild flies with pure water, for example, fasting for more than four to 6 days, to dead a half (see **Figures 5** and **6**).

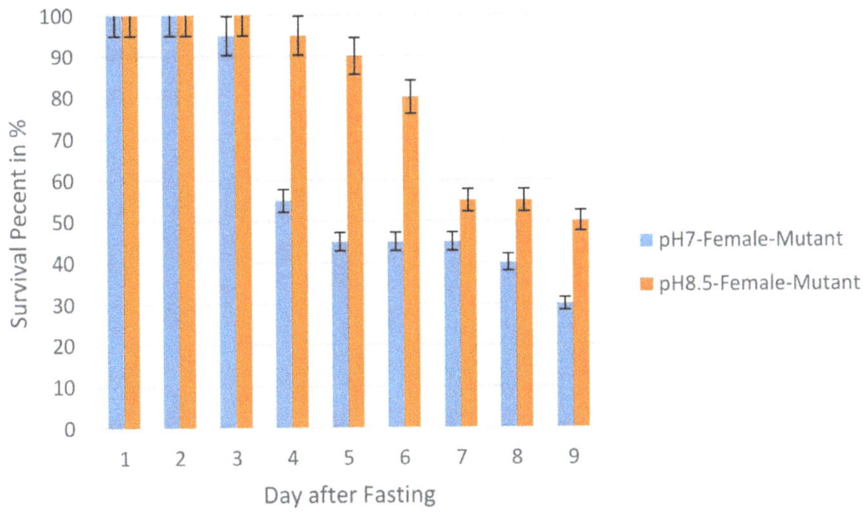

Figure 3. *Survival percent in % of female-mutant fruit flies vs. day after fasting. Note: pH 7: pure water; pH 8.5: weak-alkaline-H2-water.*

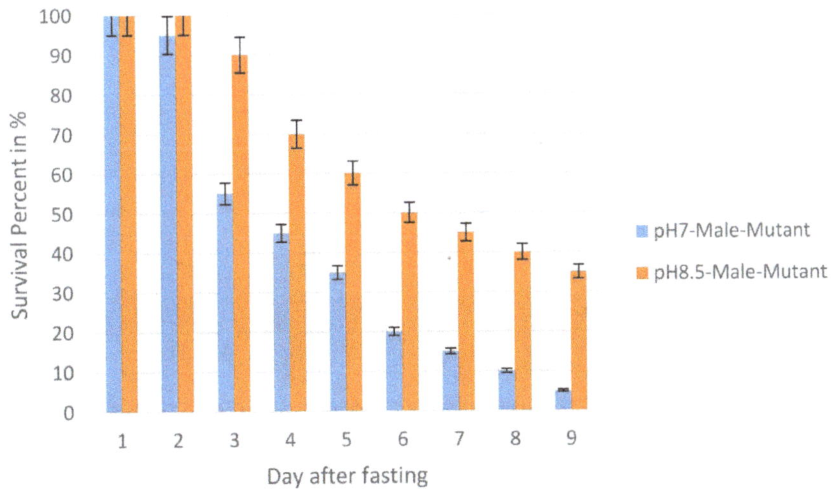

Figure 4. *Survival percent in % of male-mutant fruit flies vs. day after fasting. Note: pH 7: pure water; pH 8.5: weak-alkaline-H2-water.*

If hydrogen water supplied, fasting time of female fly and male fly extended for more than 7 days. However, hydrogen water seems to have a less help on the survival rate of wild female flies in the state of starvation (see **Figure 5**). This result implies that hydrogen water appears to be of much more help to individuals with weaker constitutions than to individuals who have stronger ones.

The alkaline hydrogen water for pH 8.5 and 9.5

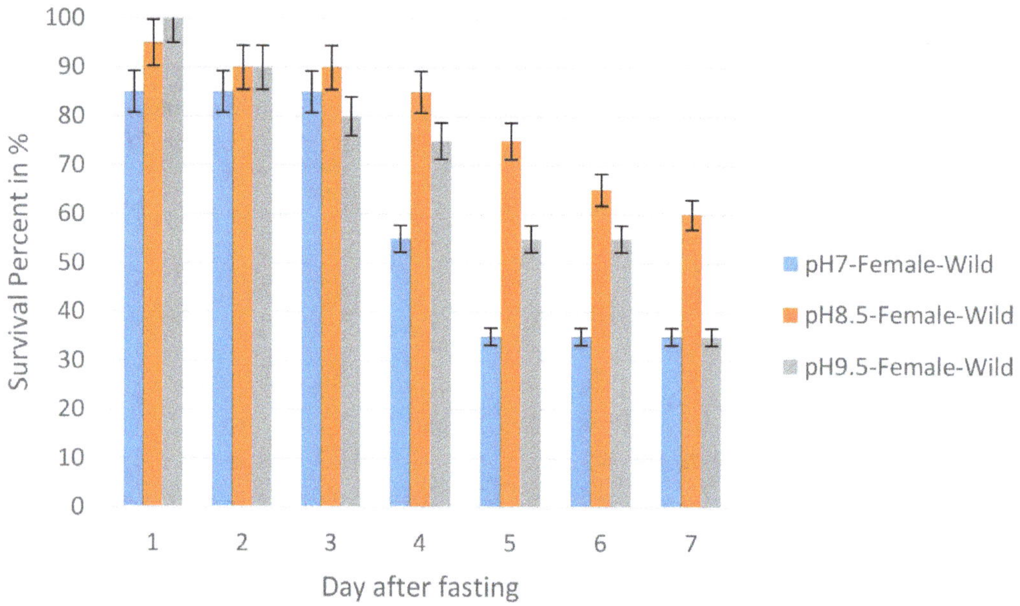

Figure 5. *Survival percent in % of female-wild flies vs. day after fasting. Note: pH 7: pure water; pH 8.5: weak-alkaline- H2-water; pH 9.5: medium-alkaline-H2-water.*

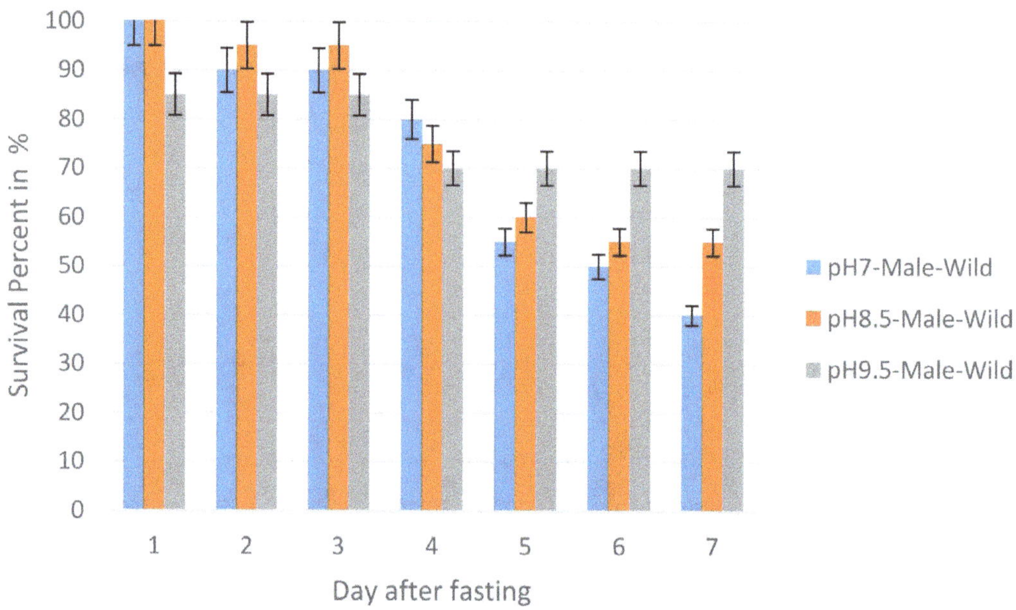

Figure 6. *Survival percent in % of male-wild flies vs. day after fasting. Note: pH 7: pure water; pH 8.5: weak-alkaline-H2-water; pH 9.5: medium-alkaline-H2-water.*

Tested for the relationship between the alkaline pH (pH 8.5 and 9.5) and the survival response. Our previous results have shown that drinking hydrogen water seems to be helpful for the survival rate of Drosophila in the case of starvation. Therefore, it is worthwhile to analyze hydrogen water in alkalinity further the impact on the survival rate of Drosophila. When the pH of the hydrogen water increased from 8.5 to 9.5, after fasting time more than 4 days the significant increase in the survival rate of the male fly observed in **Figure 6**. However, for the female fly, the result is not the same. Interestingly, although the wild species of female fruit fly, hydrogen water increased from pH 8.5 to 9.5, the survival response was slightly decreased. That is to say, further addition in alkalinity, however, has the opposite effect on the female flies, and the survival rate does not rise any longer.

Results and discussions

In the past, many works of literature have reported that human aging may be related to the function of free radicals to destroy cells. However, why do free radicals come? For example, the role of cells depends on the oxidation and decomposes the nutrients in the body. It is like gasoline, which burns oxygen to release heat energy and promote steam. However, in the process of redox, cells produce a byproduct, oxygen free radicals. The oxygen molecule (O_2) itself has 16 electrons, but it loses one electron in the process of the redox reaction, and the oxygen that becomes a single electron becomes very unstable, and it will destroy the function of the cell and even cause disease. Interestingly, if the neutral water is decomposed using a water electrolysis generator, the water molecules will change to negatively charged alkaline hydrogen water. If the electrolytic liquids are separated, acidic water will act like oxygen free radicals to destroy the cells. However, hydrogen water is the opposite, with an extra free electron, which can combine with free radicals to neutralize the ability to equilibrate free radicals before free radicals take away an electron from intracellular molecules. Therefore, hydrogen water may have anti- oxidant function and protect cells from free radical damage.

Conclusions

This experiment supports that drink hydrogen water may help the fasting fly survival rate. When oxygen free radicals in the intestine are out of balance, hydrogen water may neutralize free radicals and reduce damage to cells. Drosophila has an innate immune system similar to humans, and the structure and physiology of the fruit fly's gastro-intestine, cardiac, and neurological diseases resemble that of humans. Even if the genes and mechanisms that they are involved whether conserved or not, the biological process in a similar genes species often provides a valuable framework to study anti-oxidative stress effect and allow development of potential clinical applications.

When Drosophila intestinal oxygen free radicals increase due to fasting, the increased reactive oxygen species in the intestine pass through nitric oxide, erythrocytes, and another non-nitric oxide signal to activate transcription of NF-κB protein in the fat of Drosophila. The factor, Drosophila liver, promptly initiated in the response of cells to many stimuli, including oxidative stress, cytokines, free radicals, ultraviolet radiation, and immune response of the antibacterial peptide, causing a systemic immune response in the Drosophila. The biological model of

Drosophila used to simulate that the immune response of human organs is closely related to intestinal health [7].

However, this does not mean that drinking hydrogen water is beneficial to all healthy individual because, in the body, some enzymes that regulate free radicals, which can balance the problems caused by the accumulation of free radicals. Therefore, drinking a significant amount of hydrogen water in a healthy state may be interference to the body's natural regulation mechanism. In other words, as healthy people do not need and should not take medicine, only those who are sick need to follow the doctor's instructions. All in all, the function of hydrogen water on the human body needs further experiments to be further studied. This experiment can only support the flies in the extreme unfavorable environmental pressure; feeding hydrogen water may increase its survival rate.

Author details

Chung-Hsing Chao

Ta Hwa University of Science and Technology, Hsinchu County, Taiwan, ROC

*Address all correspondence to: dd500929@gmail.com

References

[1] Shirahata S, Hamasaki T, Teruya K. Advanced research on the health benefit of reduced water. Trends in Food Science & Technology. 2012;**23**(2): 124-131. DOI: 10.1016/j.tifs.2011.10.009

[2] Shirahata S, Kabayama S, Nakano M, Miura T, Kusumoto K, Gotoh M, et al. Electrolyzed-reduced water scavenges active oxygen species and protects DNA damage. Biochemical and Biophysical Research Communications. 1997;**234**:269-274. DOI: 10.1006/bbrc.1997.6622

[3] Hanaoka K, Sun D, Lawrence R, Kamitani Y, Fernades G. The mechanism of enhanced antioxidant effects against superoxide anion radicals of reduced water produced by electrolysis. Biophysical Chemistry. 2004;**107**(1): 71-82. DOI: 10.1016/j.bpc.2003.08.007

[4] Yanagihara T, Arai K, Miyamae K, Sato B, Shudo T, Yamada M, et al. Electrolyzed reduced water for drinking elicits an antioxidant effect: A feeding test with rats. Bioscience, Biotechnology, and Biochemistry. 2005;**69**(10):1985-1987. DOI: 10.1271/ bbb.69.1985

[5] Reiter LT, Potocki L, Chien S, Gribskov M, Bier E. A systematic analysis of human disease-associated gene sequences in Drosophila melanogaster. Genome Research. 2001;**11**(6):1114-1125. DOI: 10.1101/ gr.169101

[6] FlyBase. A Database of Drosophila Genes and Genomes, Genetics Society of America on August 15, 2009

[7] Wangler MF, Yamamoto S, Bellen HJ. Fruit flies in biomedical research. Genetics. 2015;**199**(3):653-639. DOI: 10.1534/genetics.114.171785

12

Increasing the Solubility and Recovery of Ara h3 Allergen from Raw and Roasted Peanut

Gary B. Smejkal, Srikanth Kakumanu and Amanda Cannady-Miller

Abstract

Ara h3 belongs to the glycinin family of seed storage proteins and is one of the major peanut allergens. It comprises over 20% of the total peanut protein mass, making it a logical target for the detection of trace quantities of undeclared peanut contamination in foods. Both Ara h1 and Ara h3 are detected in lower quantities in cooked foods, either because of the failure to completely resolubilize the denatured proteins or because of the disruption of conformational epitopes required for monoclonal antibody recognition. A new reagent containing a proprietary non- detergent sulfobetaine (NDSB) is described which solubilizes more total protein and yields more Ara h3 protein from both raw and roasted peanut than other commonly used ELISA-compatible reagents.

Keywords: Ara h1, Ara h3, ELISA, non-detergent sulfobetaine, peanut allergy, protein solubilization

Introduction

In the United States, an acute food allergy reaction sends someone to the emergency room every 3 minutes [1]. While over 170 foods are known to cause allergic reaction, only eight foods are responsible for over 90% of food allergies [2]. Between 1997 and 2008, the prevalence of peanut and tree nut allergies has more than tripled in the U.S. [3, 4]. Peanut allergies are a leading cause of fatal anaphylaxis [5, 6].

The U.S. Food and Drug Administration (FDA) and the European Union have imposed strict requirements for the labeling of food ingredients. However, warnings such as "May contain peanut" or "Manufactured in a facility that processes peanuts" are voluntary and considers the possibility of contamination with peanut residues [7]. Since traces of peanut may contaminate foods supposedly free of peanuts, methods capable of reliably detecting undeclared allergens are necessary to ensure food safety [8]. Highly sensitive enzyme-linked immunosorbent assays

(ELISAs) can detect low nanogram quantities of contaminating allergens in foods and biologics, whereas the rapid lateral flow assays available for consumers to test their foods are less sensitive. For example, the recently described Ara h3 ELISA [9] is about 2000 times more sensitive than the NIMA Peanut Sensor, which also targets Ara h3 [10]. To put into perspective, the ELISA could detect roughly 14 peanuts dissolved in an Olympic size swimming pool, having a volume of 2,499,330 L of water.

Proteins constitute 24–27% of the total peanut mass [11]. At least 13 different protein allergens have been identified in *Arachis hypogaea*. Of these, Ara h2 and Ara h6 are reportedly the most potent allergens [12, 13], whereas Ara h1 and Ara h3 are the two most abundant allergens, together comprising at least a third of the total peanut protein mass [14]. Ara h4 has 91.3% sequence homology with Ara h3 [8] and are considered to be the same allergen [15, 16].

Ara h3 exists as a trimer or hexamer consisting of identical 58.3 kDa subunits and having molecular masses of 180 and 360 kDa, respectively. Each subunit is derived from a single precursor which is posttranslationally cleaved to produce an acidic and a basic chain that are held together by a disulfide bond [17, 18]. Multiple subunits in the mature Ara h3 are associated via hydrophobic bonding.

The roasting of peanuts decreases the extractability of soluble protein by as much as 50% [19]. Upon heating, Ara h1 and Ara h3 may form aggregates, further decreasing their solubility [20]. Further, the denaturation of proteins drives conformational changes that can result in the loss of epitopes. Decreased antibody recognition in ELISA has been reported for both monoclonal and polyclonal antibodies [21, 22].

Lipid constitutes approximately 50% of the total peanut mass. There are conflicting reports on whether delipidation of peanuts increase protein recovery [22, 23]. Likewise, detergents such as Sarkosyl have been shown to increase protein solubility [24].

Sample preparation will be critical to the reliable quantitation of undeclared peanut allergens in foods by immunoassay, particularly in cooked foods where the denaturation of proteins renders them insoluble (e.g., imagine trying to resolubilize cooked egg whites). The failure to completely resolubilize target proteins results in their underestimation, a critical shortcoming where undeclared allergens may be present in only trace amounts.

This chapter reviews the solubility and the recovery of the Ara h3 allergen from raw and roasted peanuts extracted in several different buffers with consideration of ELISA compatibility. Since Ara h3 is one of the most abundant proteins, it is a logical target for the detection of trace quantities of peanut contamination in foods.

Methods

Sample preparation of raw and roasted peanuts

Raw Virginia peanuts (Hampton Farms, Severn, NC, USA) were dry roasted at 175°C for 20 minutes. Raw and roasted peanuts were shelled, and then course ground in a stainless steel coffee grinder. The resulting grounds were sifted through a 0.5 mm stainless steel mesh to provide uniform triturates.

The peanut triturates (53.9 ± 4.1 mg, n = 24) were weighed into the insert of a BioMasher centrifugal homogenizer (Omni International, Kennesaw, GA, USA). Biological replicates were extracted in 0.4 mL of each sample buffer. Sample buffers were (i) PBS pH 7.4, (ii) 0.05% Tween-20 in PBS pH 7.4, (iii), 8 M urea, 16 mM 3-[(3-cholamidopropyl)dimethylammonio]-1-propanesulfonate (CHAPS) in 40 mM Tris-HCl pH 8.8, and (iv) a proprietary non-detergent sulfobetaine (NDSB) from ProdigY Biosciences (Louisville, KY, USA).

Each sample was homogenized in the BioMasher for 20 seconds and the extract was collected by centrifugation at 15,000 RCF for 1 minute. The BioMasher insert was removed and centrifugation was continued at 15,000 RCF for an additional 5 minutes. Both an insoluble pellet and a floating lipid layer were observed in all samples. The supernatant was carefully aspirated from below the lipid layer and further clarified in an UltraFree MC centrifugal microfilter with 0.22 micron pore size (Millipore-Sigma, Burlington, MA, USA) at 12,000 RCF for 5 minutes.

The homogenizer bar was withdrawn from the BioMasher insert and an additional 0.4 mL of each reagent was added and the process was repeated a second time. This enabled estimates of extraction efficiency in first and second extractions of raw and roasted peanuts, and in 0.4 and 0.8 mL extraction volumes.

Analysis

Total protein concentration was estimated using the Bradford protein assay (BioRad, Hercules, CA, USA) calibrated with a qualified BSA standard (Pierce Biotechnology, Rockland, IL, USA). Ara h3 was quantified using the Ara h3 ELISA 2.0 Kit (Indoor Biotechnologies, Charlottesville, VA, USA) using the 1E8 and 4G9 monoclonal antibody pair and streptavidin-HRP reporter. Calibration was linear over the 2–125 ng/mL range (r^2 = 0.9998).

Calculation of grand average of hydropathicity (GRAVY) values

FASTA sequences of representative peanut proteins were procured from the UniProtKB Protein Knowledgebase [25, 26]. GRAVY values were based on amino acid hydropathy index [27] and calculated using the ProtParam software tools available from the ExPASy Bioinformatics Resource Portal [28].

Results and discussion

Total recoverable protein from raw peanut

In every case, more total protein was recovered in raw than in roasted peanut. The NDSB buffer recovered more total protein in a single 0.4 mL extraction than all of the other buffers tested. NDSB replicates averaged 14.8% total protein recovery from raw peanut triturates, nearly twice as much protein than what was extracted with urea-CHAPS. On average, NDSB extracted seven times more total protein than PBS-Tween (**Figure 1**).

Total recoverable protein from roasted peanut

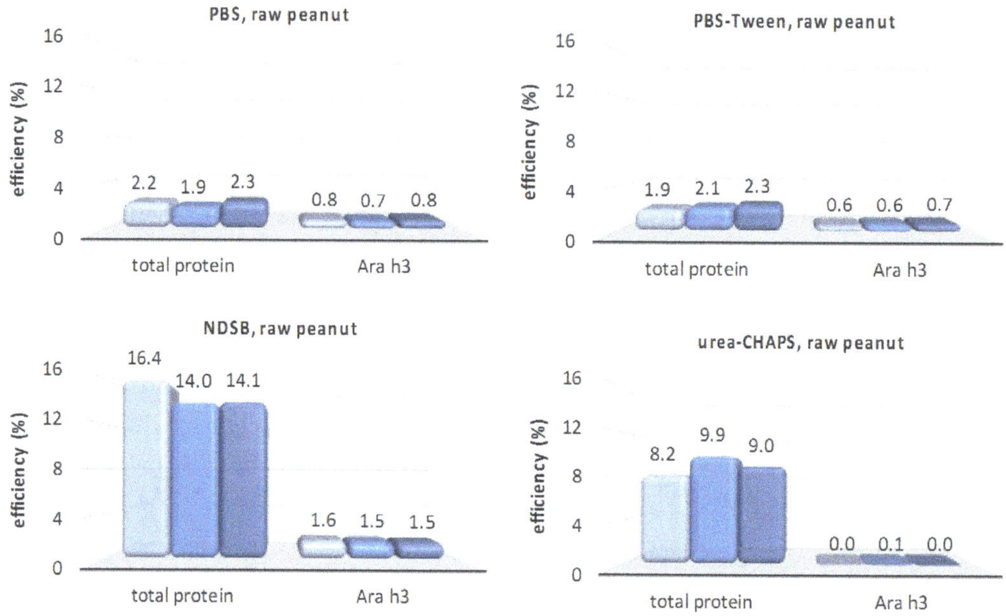

Figure 1. *Normalized recovery of total protein and Ara h3 from biological triplicates of raw peanut (53.6 ± 4.9 mg, n = 12) extracted in 0.4 mL of PBS, PBS-Tween, NDSB, or urea-CHAPS. For extraction efficiency, total protein and Ara h3 mass are expressed in terms of their percentage of the total peanut biomass.*

Lower total protein recoveries were observed from roasted peanut. NDSB yielded 4.0% total protein from roasted peanut, compared to 4.4% from urea- CHAPS. NDSB and urea-CHAPS yielded twice as much soluble protein from roasted peanut than PBS-Tween (**Figure 2**).

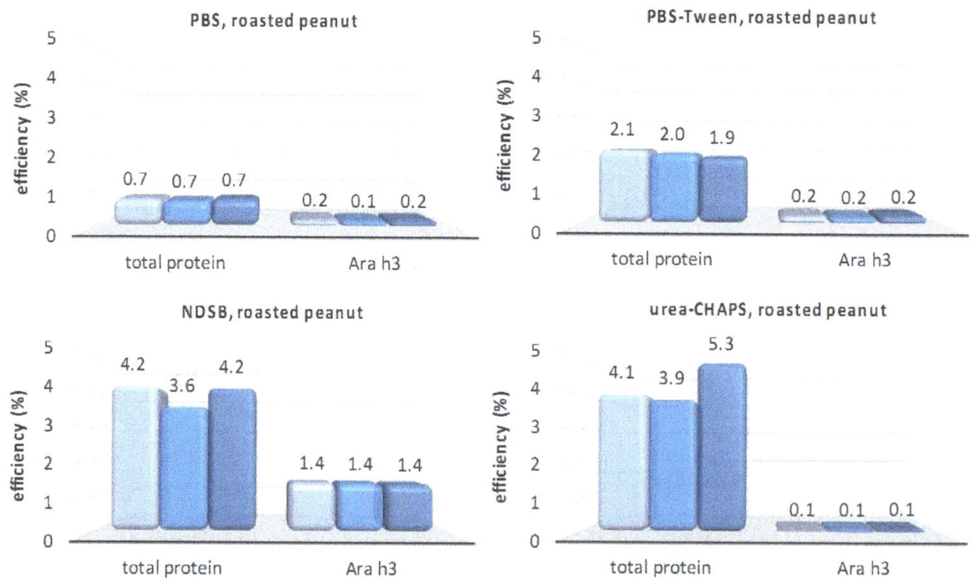

Figure 2. *Normalized recovery of total protein and Ara h3 from biological triplicates of roasted peanut (53.6 ± 4.9 mg, n = 12) extracted in 0.4 mL of PBS, PBS-Tween, NDSB, or urea-CHAPS. Total protein and Ara h3 mass are expressed in terms of their percentage of the total peanut biomass.*

Ara h3 yields from raw and roasted peanut

NDSB yielded the highest recoveries of specific Ara h3 protein in both raw and roasted peanut as measured by ELISA. On average, NDSB yielded more than twice the measurable Ara h3 from raw peanut than PBS-Tween (**Figure 1**). From roasted peanut, NDSB yielded nearly seven times more Ara h3 than PBS-Tween (**Figure 2**).

Ara h3 was not detected by ELISA in raw or roasted peanut samples extracted in urea-CHAPS. This is apparently due to the disruption of tertiary and secondary structure of the protein and the obliteration of conformational epitopes required for binding by the monoclonal antibodies used in the ELISA. While the urea-CHAPS was substantially diluted for ELISA, no restoration of antibody recognition was observed.

Increasing total protein yields by sequential extraction

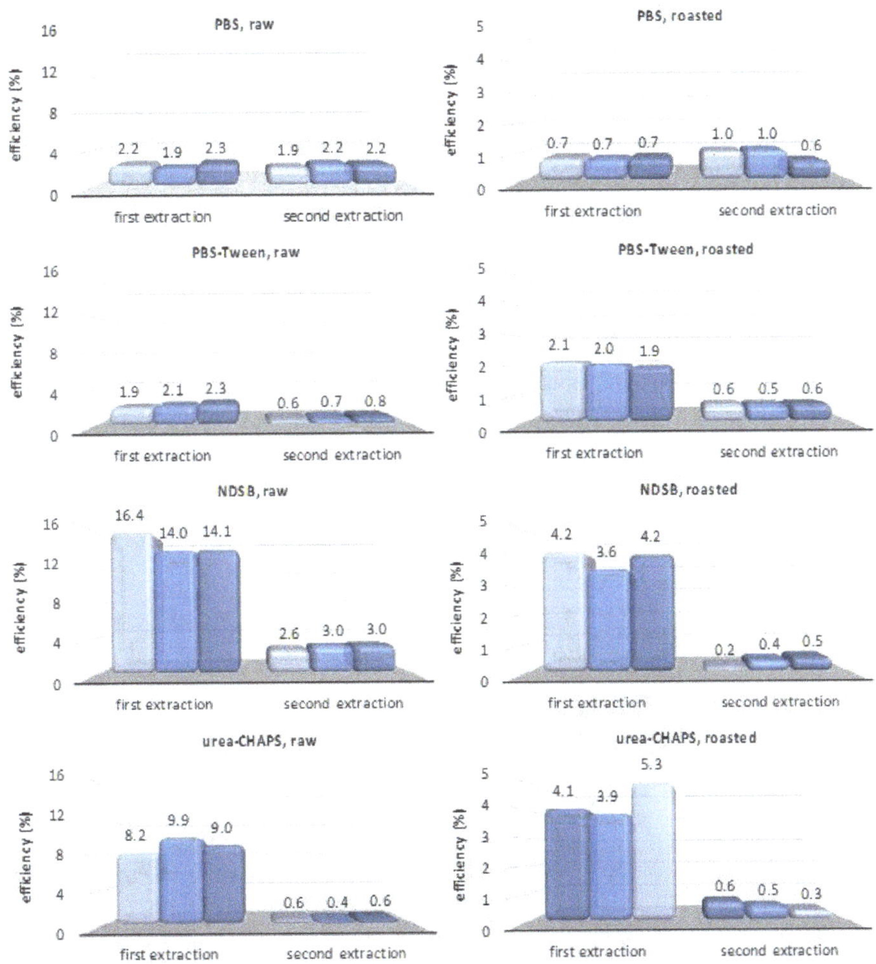

Figure 3. *Normalized recovery of total protein following sequential extractions in 0.4 mL of PBS, PBS-Tween, NDSB, or urea-CHAPS. Following an initial extraction in 0.4 mL, an additional 0.4 mL of buffer was added to the insoluble peanut triturate remaining in the BioMasher insert and the extraction process was repeated. Total protein is expressed in terms of its percentage of the total peanut biomass.*

To investigate whether a second extraction would significantly improve total protein yields, an additional 0.4 mL of each buffer was added to the insoluble peanut triturate remaining in each homogenizer insert following the first extraction.

PBS extracted 50.4 and 45.3% of the total PBS soluble protein in the first extraction for raw and roasted peanut, respectively. PBS-Tween extracted 75.6 and 78.2% of the total PBS-Teen soluble protein in the first extraction for raw and roasted peanut, respectively.

NDSB extracted 83.7 and 92.0% of the total NDSB soluble protein in the first extraction for raw and roasted peanut, respectively. For raw peanut, mean efficiency of NDSB was 14.8% for the first extraction, which was increased to 17.7% when a second extraction was performed. For roasted peanut, mean efficiency of NDSB was 4.0 ± 0.3% for the first extraction, which was increased to 4.4 ± 0.3% when a second extraction was performed (**Figure 3**). In practical terms, only about 10% more protein is recovered when a second extraction is performed, but at the cost of doubling the sample volume of the isolate.

Urea-CHAPS extracted 94.5 and 89.9% of the soluble protein in the first extraction for raw and roasted peanut, respectively. For raw peanut, mean efficiency of urea-CHAPS was 9.0 ± 0.9% for the first extraction which was increased to 9.6 ± 0.8% when a second extraction was performed. For roasted peanut, mean efficiency of urea-CHAPS was 4.4 ± 0.8% for the first extraction which was increased to 4.9 ± 0.6% when a second extraction was performed. While the total protein recovered from roasted peanut extracted in urea-CHAPS or NDSB were similar, the chaotrope rendered the samples incompatible with the capture ELISA used in these studies (**Figures 3** and **4**).

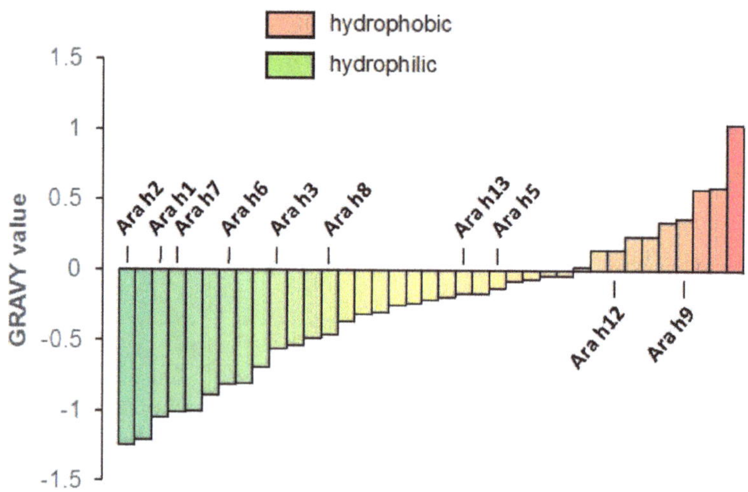

Figure 4. *Relative hydrophobicity of 37 published protein sequences including 10 known allergens from Arachis hypogaea. Grand average of hydropathicity (GRAVY) values were calculated from FASTA sequences where the sum of the hydropathy index values for each amino acid is divided by the total number of residues.*

Concluding remarks

Of the reagents tested, the NDSB reagent yielded the highest recovery of Ara h3, on average yielding seven times more allergen from roasted peanut than PBS- Tween. While the overall solubility of proteins is significantly diminished in roasted peanut, NDSB recovered nearly identical amounts of Ara h3 from both raw and roasted peanut.

ELISA and total protein values obtained from this cultivar indicated that Ara h3 comprised 34.9 ± 1.4% (CV = 0.039, n = 3), of the soluble protein derived from raw peanut and 34.6 ± 3.0% (CV = 0.085, n = 3) of the soluble protein from roasted peanut. Seed storage proteins may be overexpressed in response to growing conditions and can vary considerably between cultivars. This suggests that some cultivars may be more hyperallergenic than others. Moreover, the recovery of total soluble protein varies between cultivars, and extraction efficiencies as low as 9% based on the initial peanut mass have been reported for boiled runner peanuts [29]. The calculation of extraction efficiency, however, is influenced by variable water content. In these experiments, the NDSB reagent yielded 17.7 and 4.4% of the initial peanut mass as soluble protein from raw and dry roasted peanuts, respectively.

The described sample preparation method may be positively biased toward the solubility of this particular allergen. Further work is needed to investigate the solubility of other peanut proteins, particularly other clinically important peanut allergens.

Abbreviations

CHAPS 3-[(3-cholamidopropyl)dimethylammonio]-1-propanesulfonate

ELISA enzyme-linked immunosorbent assay

NDSB non-detergent sulfobetaine

PBS phosphate buffered saline.

Author details

Gary B. Smejkal[1]*, Srikanth Kakumanu[1] and Amanda Cannady-Miller[2] 1 Focus Proteomics, Hudson, New Hampshire, USA

2 ProdigY Biosciences, Louisville, Kentucky, USA

*Address all correspondence to: info@focusproteomics.com

References

[1] Clark S, Espinola J, Rudders SA, Banerji A, Camargo CA. Frequency of US emergency department visits for food-related acute allergic reactions. The Journal of Allergy and Clinical Immunology. 2011;**127**:682-683

[2] NIAID-Sponsored Expert Panel. Guidelines for the diagnosis and management of food allergy in the United States: Report of the NIAID- sponsored expert panel. The Journal of Allergy and Clinical Immunology. 2010;**126**:S1-S58

[3] Sicherer SH, Muñoz-Furlong A, Burks AW, Sampson HA. Prevalence of peanut and tree nut allergy in the US determined by a random digit dial telephone survey. The Journal of Allergy and Clinical Immunology. 1999;**103**:559-562

[4] Sicherer SH, Muñoz-Furlong A, Godbold JH, Sampson HA. US prevalence of self-reported peanut, tree nut, and sesame allergy: 11-year follow-up. The Journal of Allergy and Clinical Immunology. 2010;**125**:1322-1326

[5] Umasunthar T, Leonardi-Bee J, Hodes M, Turner PJ, Gore C, Habibi P, et al. Incidence of fatal food anaphylaxis in people with food allergy: A systematic review and meta-analysis. Clinical and Experimental Allergy. 2013;**43**:1333-1341

[6] Finkelman FD. Peanut allergy and anaphylaxis. Current Opinion in Immunology. 2010;**22**:783-788

[7] Taylor SL, Hefle SL. Food allergen labeling in the USA and Europe. Current Opinion in Allergy and Clinical Immunology. 2006;**6**:186-190

[8] Wen HW, Borejsza-Wysocki W, DeCory TR, Durst RA. Peanut allergy, peanut allergens, and methods for the detection of peanut contamination in food products. Comprehensive Reviews in Food Science and Food Safety. 2007;**6**:47-58

[9] Hoyt AEW, Chapman MD, King EM, Platts-Mills TAE, Steinke JW. Food allergen component proteins are not detected in early-childhood vaccines. The Journal of Allergy and Clinical Immunology. In Practice. 2018;**6**:677-679

[10] NIMA Labs. The Science behind NIMA: Understanding the device. 2018. Available from: https://nimasensor.com/ science-nima-understanding-device/

[11] Koppelman SJ, Vlooswijk RAA, Knippels LMJ, Hessing M, Knol EF, van Reijsen FC, et al. Quantification of major peanut allergens Ara h1 and Ara h2 in the peanut varieties runner, Spanish, Virginia, and Valencia, bred in different parts of the world. Allergy. 2001;**56**:132-137

[12] Zhuang Y, Dreskin SC. Redefining the major peanut allergens. Immunologic Research. 2013;**55**:125-134

[13] Koppelman SJ, Wensing M, Ertmann M, Knulst AC, Knol EF. Relevance of Ara h1, Ara h2 and Ara h3 in peanut-allergic patients as determined by immunoglobulin E Western blotting, basophilhistamine release and intracutaneous testing: Ara h2 is the most important peanut allergen. Clinical and Experimental Allergy. 2004;**34**:583-590

[14] Johnson PE, Sayers RL, Gethings LA, Balasundaram A, Marsh JT, Langridge JI, et al. Quantitative proteomic profiling of peanut allergens in food ingredients used for oral food challenges. Analytical Chemistry. 2016;**88**:5689-5695

[15] Koppelman SJ, Knol EF, Vlooswijk RA, Wensing M, Knulst AC, Hefle SL, et al. Peanut allergen Ara h3: Isolation from peanuts and biochemical characterization. Allergy. 2003;**58**:1144-1151

[16] Boldt A, Fortunato D, Conti A, Petersen A, Ballmer-Weber B, Lepp U, et al. Analysis of the composition of an immunoglobulin E reactive high molecular weight protein complex of peanut extract containing Ara h1 and Ara h3/4. Proteomics. 2005;**5**: 675-686

[17] Beardslee TA, Zeece MG, Sarath G, Markwell JP. Soybean glycinin G1 acidic chain shares IgE epitopes with peanut allergen Ara h3. International Archives of Allergy and Immunology. 2000;**123**:299-307

[18] Yusnawan E, Marquis CP, Lee NA. Purification and characterization of Ara h1 and Ara h3 from four peanut market types revealed higher order oligomeric structures. Journal of Agricultural and Food Chemistry. 2012;**60**:10352-10358

[19] Koppelman S, Apostolovic D, Warmenhoven H, Verbart D, Taylor S, Isleib T, et al. The content of allergens Ara h1, Ara h2, Ara h3, and Ara h6 in different peanut cultivars commonly consumed in Europe and the USA. Allergy. 2012;**67**:548

[20] Koppelman SJ, Smits M, Tomassen M, De Jong GAH, Baumert J, Taylor SL, et al. Release of major peanut allergens from their matrix under various pH and simulated saliva conditions: Ara h2 and Ara h6 are readily bio-accessible. Nutrients. 2018;**10**:1281

[21] Iqbal A, Shah F, Hamayun M, Ahmad A, Hussain A, Waqas M, et al. Allergens of *Arachis hypogaea* and the effect of processing on their detection by ELISA. Food and Nutrition Research. 2016;**60**:28945

[22] Comstock SS, Maleki SJ, Teuber SS. Boiling and frying peanuts decreases soluble peanut (*Arachis Hypogaea*) allergens Ara h1 and Ara h2 but does not generate hypoallergenic peanuts. PLoS One. 2016;**11**:0157849

[23] Walczyk NE, Smith PMC, Tovey ER, Roberts TH. Peanut protein extraction conditions strongly influence yield of allergens Ara h1 and 2 and sensitivity of immunoassays. Food Chemistry. 2017;**221**:335-344

[24] Lin HY, Huang CH, Park J, Pathania D, Castro CM, Fasano A, et al. Integrated magneto-chemical sensor for on-site food allergen detection. ACS Nano. 2017;**11**:10062-10069

[25] UniProt Consortium. UniProt: The universal protein knowledgebase. Nucleic Acids Research. 2018;**46**:2699

[26] Pundir S, Martin MJ, O'Donovan C. UniProt protein knowledgebase. Methods in Molecular Biology. 2017;**1558**:41-55

[27] Kyte J, Doolittle RF. A simple method for displaying the hydropathic character of a protein. Journal of Molecular Biology. 1982;**157**:105-132

[28] Gasteiger E, Hoogland C, Gattiker A, Duvaud S, Wilkins MR, Appel RD, et al. Protein identification and analysis tools on the ExPASy server. In: The Proteomics Protocols Handbook. New York, NY: Humana Press; 2005. pp. 571-607

[29] Yusnawan E. Study of variation in Ara h1 and Ara h3 expression in Australian and Indonesian peanut genotypes, based on the antibody-based phenotyping assays [thesis]. School of Chemical Engineering, University of New South Wales. 2012. Available from: https://www. unsworks.unsw.edu. au/fapi/datastream/ unsworks:10654/ SOURCE01

13

Role of Poultry Research in Increasing Consumption of PUFA in Humans

Hanan Al-Khalaifah and Afaf Al-Nasser

Abstract

In recent years, polyunsaturated fatty acids (PUFA) have received considerable attention in both human and animal nutrition. As a mean of increasing the low consumption of long chain n-3 PUFA by humans consuming diets, there has been some interest in the enrichment of poultry meat with these fatty acids for people seeking healthy lifestyles. Dietary supplementation with n-3 PUFA, such as these found in fish oil and linseed oil, were found to have nutritional benefits in humans. Modulation of fatty acid profiles as a result of n-3 PUFA incorporation is well documented in humans, rodents, and poultry. The current chapter focuses on enriching poultry meat with these beneficial fatty acids to increase its consumption by human beings.

Keywords: health, n-3 fatty acids, polyunsaturated fatty acids, poultry

Introduction

Recently, PUFA have received considerable attention in both human and animal nutrition, particularly those of the n-3 family; which are distinct due to the placement of the first double bond onto the third carbon atom from the methyl end of the fatty acid molecule. Long-chain fatty acids primarily those with more than 18 carbon atoms, derived mainly from fish oils are consumed quite less along with the other PUFAs. In order to increase their consumption through human diets, has led to studies for enriching the poultry meat infused with these fatty acids and thus enabling people to live healthier lifestyles. Dietary supplementation with n-3 PUFA, such as these found in fish oil and linseed oil, were found to have nutritional benefits in humans [1–5].

This chapter will shed light on the overview, sources, and metabolism of PUFA, their incorporation into cell membrane structure, their involvement in health and clinical problems, enrichment of poultry products with PUFA, and their involvement in immune system.

Overview of fatty acids

All fatty acids are carboxylic acids characterized by a chain-like structure with a carboxyl group (COOH) at one end, and a methyl group (CH3) at the other end. The rest of the chain consists of carbon atoms varying in length from 2 to 20 or more with hydrocarbon bonds (CH2). Fatty acids (FA) differ in the number of hydrogen atoms and the number and location of the double bonds between adjacent carbon atoms if hydrogen atoms are removed. If a fatty acid chain is fully loaded with hydrogen atoms, the FA is termed saturated. Consequently, saturated fatty acids form straight chains as there are no double bonds between carbon atoms. These usually contain between 12 and 24 carbon atoms. This kind of FA is abundantly present in adipose tissues of animals, including poultry and used as a source of energy if needed. An example of a saturated FA is stearic acid (C18:0). This is one way to name a fatty acid (C:D) where C is the number of carbon atoms in the fatty acid and D is the number of double bonds in the fatty acid. Sources of saturated FA include meat, dairy products, palm oil, coconut oil and vegetable shortening [6].

If a pair of hydrogen atoms is removed under the influence of specific enzymes, a double bond is formed between adjacent carbon atoms and the saturated FA becomes monounsaturated. An example of a monounsaturated FA is oleic acid (18:1), an n-9 FA that constitutes 74% of total FA in olives. n-x is a nomenclature of fatty acids where a double bond is located on the xth carbon–carbon bond, counting from the terminal methyl carbon (designated as n). Other sources of monosaturated FA are avocados, rapeseed, peanuts and soybeans [7]. If two or more double bonds are formed due to removal of more than a pair of hydrogen atoms, the FA is termed polyunsaturated. The more double bonds a fatty acid has, the more unsaturated it is [8–10]. The main sources of PUFA are seeds and seed oils, oily fish and fish oils [10].

Moreover, the orientation of the fatty acid chain at the site of a double bond determines and characterizes a fatty acid. For example, a FA called cis-configured when both segments of the molecule lie at the same side. On the other hand, in the trans configuration, the two parts of the molecule face opposite with respect to the bond directions (see Figure 1). Most PUFA in plants and sea foods are of cis configuration [11].

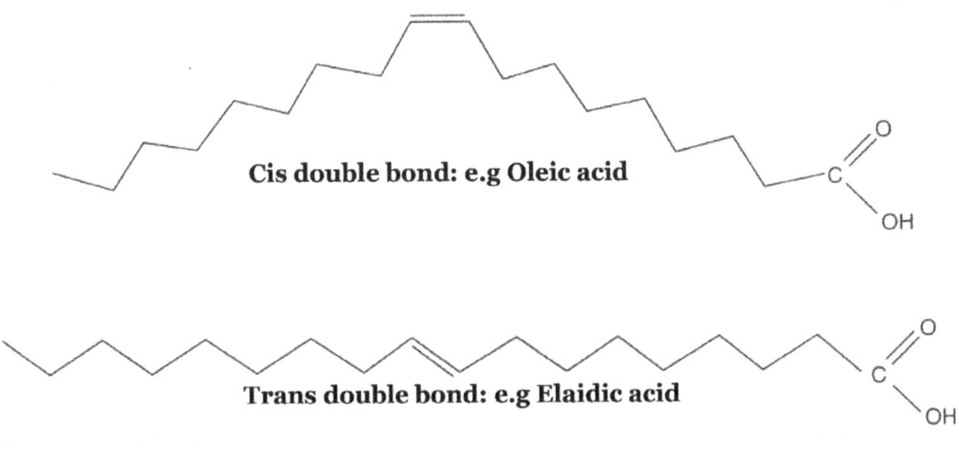

Figure 1. *cis and trans configuration of FA molecules.*

The two major types of PUFA which play a crucial role in the biological functioning of both, humans and animals are the n-3 and n-6 PUFA. The n-3 PUFA consists of linolenic acid (LNA, C18:3), eicosapentaenoic acid (EPA, C20:5) and docosahexaenoic acid (DHA, C22:6) whereas the n-6 PUFAs comprise mainly linoleic acid (LA, C18:2) and arachidonic acid (AA, C20:4). LA and α-LNA are classified as essential fatty acids (EFA) due to their inability to be synthesized by the body. However, these EFAs should be consumed through the diet because of shortage of specific desaturation enzymes. AA can be synthesized in from LA when the diet is consumed. In a similar manner, EPA along with DHA can be synthesized from α-LNA although synthesis between them is inadequate in most conditions. Due to the absence of specific desaturase enzymes, the n-3 and n-6 fatty acids are not inter-convertible. On the other hand, saturated FA such as palmitic acid (C16:0) and stearic acid (C18:0) and most monounsaturated FA such as oleic acid (C18:1 n-9) can be synthesized in the human body from precursors such as glucose or amino acids [12, 13]. Table 1 shows a list of the common saturated and unsaturated fatty acids.

Table 1. *List of common saturated and unsaturated fatty acids.*

Common name	FA name
Butyric	C4:0
Caproic	C6:0
Caprylic	C8:0
Capric	C10:0
Undecanoic	C11:0
Lauric	C12:0
Tridecanoic	C13:0
Myristic	C14:0
Myristoleic	C14:1
Pentadecanoic acid	C15:0
c10 Pentadecanoic acid	C15:1
Palmitic	C16:0
Palmitoleic	C16:1
cis-10-heptadecanoic	C17:1
Stearic	C18:0
Elaidic	C18:1n9t
Oleic	C18:1n9c
Linolelaidic	C18:2n6t
Linoleic	C18:2n6c
Arachidic	C20:0
γ-Linolenic	C18:3n6
α-Linolenic	C18:3n3
Heneicosanoic	C21:0
c11, 14 Eicosadienoic	C20:2
Behenic	C22:0
c8,11,14 Eicosatrienoic	C20:3n6
Erucic acid	C22:1 n9
c11,14,17 Eicosatrienoic	C20:3n3
Arachidonic	C20:4n6
Tricosanoic	C23:0
c13,16 Docosadienoic	C22:2
Eicosapentaenoic acid (EPA)	C20:5n3
Lignoceric	C24:0
Nervonic	C24:1
Docosapentaenoic acid (DPA)	C22:5n3
Docosahexaenoic acid (DHA)	C22:6n3

Sources and metabolism of fatty acids

General speaking, there are small amounts of AA in fish. However Brown et al. [14] have reported that there is 4.8–14.3% AA in some Australian fish species. However, fish oil contains high amounts of EPA and DHA. These fatty acids are synthesized by phytoplankton that are consumed by fish. Some fish species may contain more than 30% n-3 PUFA about 50% of the FA in fish is PUFA, of which about 30% are n-3 FA [15, 16].

Conversely, the presence of α–LNA in seafood is almost nil; although plant sources like chia, linseed, rapeseed, perilla and blackcurrant possess high amounts of this FA, this is because these plant sources have Δ12-desaturase that converts oleic acid into LA, this is further converted into α-LNA under the influence of Δ 15- desaturase [10]. Linseed is one of the richest know sources of α-LNA, as it contains almost 60% of this fatty acid in its oil [17].

Some algal oil and algal biomass obtained from marine regions are known to be good sources of DHA and EPA and thus can be used as a means to enrich meats and eggs using these long chain fatty acids. This has proved to be successful and is well documented in literature, even though DHA is mostly obtained from these algal biomasses [18–26].

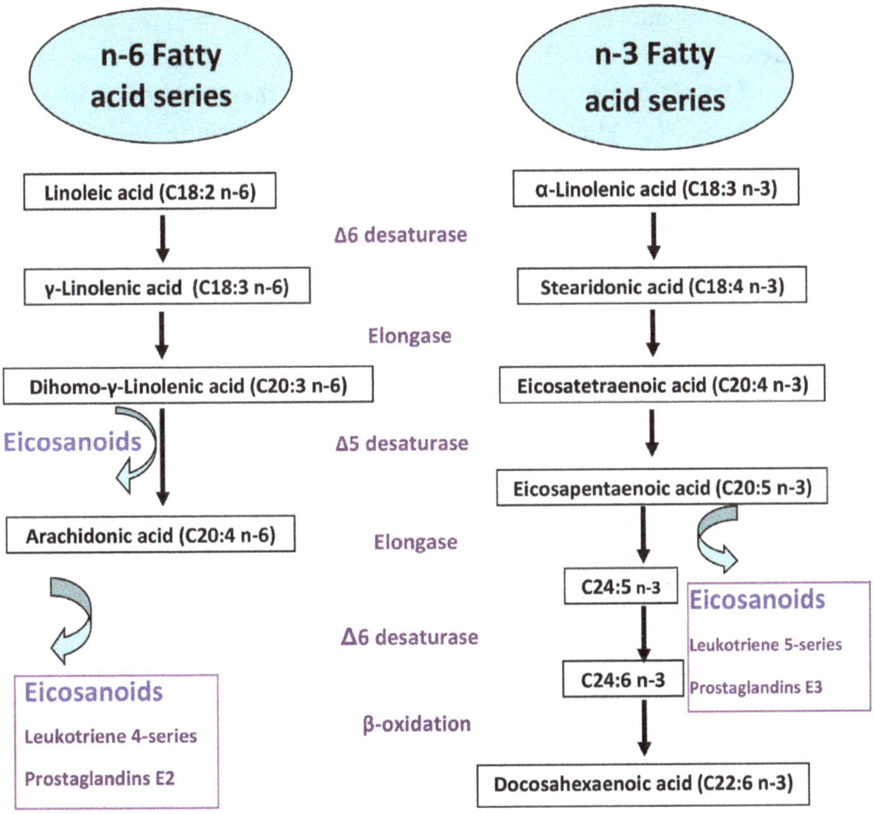

2. Metabolic pathways of the long chain n-3 and n-6 PUFA.

In addition, echium oil from the plant *Echium plantagineum* has been recognized as an ideal source of stearidonic acid (C18:4n-3) that is naturally converted to the important long-chain n-3 fatty acid, EPA, when metabolized in the body [27, 28]. In addition, there are considerable amounts of α-linolenic acid and γ-linolenic acid in the echium oil as well. Rymer et al. [29] showed that γ-linolenic acid is accumulated as stearidonic acid increases in the chicken's diet.

N-3 PUFA, particularly EPA and DHA, are reported to compete with AA for incorporation in the phospholipid bilayer of cell membranes of all body cells, especially erythrocytes, platelets, neutrophils, monocytes and liver cells [30, 31]. Both AA and EPA are parent precursors of different kinds of eicosanoids that play a crucial role in the inflammatory responses in both humans and animals, including poultry.

Initially, the dietary essential fatty acid α-LNA is converted to EPA and DHA while LA is converted to AA by elongation and desaturation reactions [32–34]. These conversion reactions are mediated in humans by three desaturases, Δ9, Δ6, and Δ5. The desaturases work by introducing a double bond at a specific position of the carbon backbone. Nakamura and Nara [35] have reported that desaturases in mammals are regulated at the transcriptional level and their transcription is genetically controlled. However, regulation of Δ9 desaturase differs from Δ6 and Δ5 desaturases because the Δ 9-desaturase converts the nonessential stearic acid (18:0) to oleic acid (18:1 n-9). Oleic acid can go through the same steps of desaturation and elongation as LA and α-LNA, resulting in the synthesis of the fatty acids 20:3 n-9 and 22:4 n-9. Consequently, the Δ 9-desaturation provides an alternative to Δ6 and Δ5 desaturation when the cell is subject to essential fatty acid deficiency. However in the case of availability of sufficient amounts of essential fatty acids, AA and EPA act as precursors for eicosanoid synthesis, although EPA metabolism predominates [32, 33, 36, 37]. When sources rich in stearidonic acid (SDA) such as echium oil are consumed, the body deposits EPA directly in tissues such as plasma, blood leukocytes, liver, breast and legs of human, rodents and chicken because SDA does not require Δ6 desaturase activity to form EPA [28, 38–43].

Under the influence of Δ6 desaturase, free α-LNA is converted to SDA (18:4 n-3) then to eicosatetraenoic acid (20:4 n-3) by an elongase. Next, Δ5 desaturase acts on eicosatetraenoic acid and converts it into EPA (20:5 n-3). Elongase converts EPA into the FA (24:5 n-3) that is converted into the FA (24:6 n-3) by the action of Δ6 desaturase. Then, oxidation of (24:6 n-3) by β-oxidase produces DHA. During this metabolic pathway, eicosanoids such as leukotriene 5-series, prostaglandins E3 and thromboxane A3 are derived from EPA [37, 41, 44–50]. 2 shows the metabolic pathway of the long chain n-3 and n-6 PUFA [35].

Incorporation into cell membrane structure

Cell membranes consist of a variety of molecules that enable cells to survive via various biological interactions. Proteins and lipids are the main elements of cell membranes. Different cell types have different cell membrane lipids and proteins that reflect different biological functions and specializations of cells.

Lipids in the cell membranes are arranged in a bilayer structure with the hydrophobic moieties in the center of the membrane and the hydrophilic heads at the two surfaces, facing the inner cytoplasm and the outside surrounding. There are three main types of lipids in the cell membranes, namely: phospholipids, glycolipids, and steroids. Both saturated and unsaturated FA are attached to the glycerol moiety in the cell membrane, with the saturated FA attached to the first carbon atom in the glycerol backbone (sn-1), while PUFA occupy the sn-2 position [17]. Membrane fluidity is highly affected by the length and the degree of unsaturation of FA chains. Lipid moieties within the cell membrane determine different biological cellular functions such as intracellular pathways and receptors formation. In humans, EPA, DHA, AA and oleic acid are the main PUFA incorporated into the cell membranes. Interestingly, changes in these lipid moieties leads to changes in biological functions of different cell types due to the production of different cellular intermediates such as leukotrienes, prostacyclins and prostaglandins. These intermediates are involved in the immunomodulatory effect of PUFA [42, 49, 51–60].

Involvement in health and clinical problems

Vitality of living cells depends profoundly on dietary lipids that are incorporated into phospholipid layers of cellular membranes as a result there is a constant competition between the omega-3 fatty acids; eicosapentaenoic acid (EPA) and docosahexaenoic acid (DHA), with arachidonic acid (AA) for this incorporation. As AA controls the upregulation of eicosanoids such as leukotrienes, this competitive inhibition downregulates inflammation responses related to man, which are associated to numerous diseases and disorders such as cardiovascular disease, increased triglycerides, blood pressure, thrombosis, atherosclerosis, stress, mental problems, asthma and rheumatoid arthritis [21, 50, 61–79]. These benefits of an optimal ratio of n-3/n-6 PUFAs on health are just a few examples of a wide range of clinical problems that are improved by consumption of the very long chain n-3 fatty acids.

n-3 enrichment of poultry diet

Traditionally, fish and fish oil are the main sources of essential, long chain n-3 PUFA that induce modifications in the lipid composition of poultry products because marine sources in general contain high levels of EPA and DHA PUFA. Of less nutritional importance are plant sources such as linseed that is rich in α- linolenic acid (α-LNA). α-LNA is an 18 carbon n-3 fatty acid that is the precursor to the long chain n-3 PUFA, but because the efficiency of conversion is so low in humans, the accumulation of α-LNA is of little real nutritional benefit.

In chickens, there are number of studies that investigated effects of PUFA on fatty acid profile of different tissues, if sources rich in these fatty acids are added to the poultry feed. Bou et al. [80] reported that supplementing the diet of broilers with 2.5% fish oil produced double the amount of EPA and DHA in their carcass than diets supplied with 1.25% fish oil. In another study, Ratnayake et al. [81] fed broiler chickens increasing levels of redfish meal (40–120 g/kg) for a period of 42 days. The effect of this dietary manipulation on fatty acid composition of breast and thigh muscles was investigated. Authors of this study observed a linear relationship between the level of the dietary fish meal and the proportions of DHA, DPA and EPA in the meat muscles. Givens and Rymer [82] also conducted an experiment to investigate the effect of poultry species and genotype on the efficiency of incorporation of n-3 PUFA in poultry meat. The two genotypes of turkeys (Wrolstad and BUT T8) and broilers (Ross 308 and Cobb 500) were fed one or four diets that contained 50 g/kg added oil; either vegetable oil (control), partially replaced with linseed

(20 or 40 g/kg), FO (20 or 40 g/kg), or mixture of linseed and FO (20 g linseed and 20 g FO/kg diet). It was observed that on replacement of the control diet with either low or high levels of FO caused a significant increase in the concentration of EPA and DHA in all the meats whereas feeding linseed-enriched diet significantly increased the concentration of α-linolenic acid. No significant difference was noted with the incorporation of n-3 PUFA between the two broiler genotypes. Turkey genotypes were only different in the case of α-linolenic acid incorporation. It was also seen that there was a greater incorporation of DHA in white than in dark meat. In order to confirm the effect of dietary fatty acid modulation in broiler chickens, another study was conducted by Lopez-Ferrer et al. [83]. Here, a diet enriched with 8.2% FO was fed to broilers for duration of 5 weeks, after this it was replaced by diets containing 8.2% linseed or rapeseed in three different periods: the last week before slaughtering, the last 2 weeks and throughout the experiment. The end results for the fatty acid analysis of thigh and breast showed that the total amounts of n-3 PUFA were significantly decreased after removal of FO diet. Upon replacement of FO with the linseed diet caused a substantial increase in α-linolenic acid, furthermore there was an increase in the total amounts of n-6 PUFA and a decrease in the DHA proportions due to its limited conversion to longer n-3 PUFA. When FO was replaced by rapeseed there was an increase in the total amounts of monounsaturated fatty acids, especially oleic acid.

Recently, Zelenka et al. [84] studied the effect of increasing levels of linseed oil in the diets of chickens and its influence on the fatty acid content in breast and thigh meat of chickens. Linseed oil at levels of 1, 3, 5 or 7% were fed to broiler chickens from 25 to 40 days of age. Oils were derived from the linseed cultivar Atalante with a high content of α-linolenic acid or the cultivar Lola with a high content of linoleic acid. Results showed that feeding a diet with a high content of α-linolenic acid significantly increased all n-3 PUFA, decreased n-6 PUFA and decreased the ratio of n-6/n-3 PUFA. On the contrary, when the birds were fed a diet with a high content of linoleic acid, this caused a significant increase in the levels of all n-6 PUFA in thigh and breast of chickens. Similarly, a study by Kartikasari et al. [85] showed that feeding broilers on diets with a high content of α-linolenic acid, while keeping a constant linoleic acid level, significantly increased the incorporation of all n-3 PUFA into breast and thigh meat by 5 and 4-fold compared to chickens fed low α-linolenic acid content. In another experiment [86], the authors fed broiler chickens on diets with constant level of α-linolenic acid (2.1%) and different levels of linoleic acid, which included 2.9–4.4%, and consisted of pure or blended vegetable oils such as macadamia, flaxseed and sunflower oils. The overall lipid content was kept at a constant of 5%. Post analysis it was observed that chickens when fed diets the lowest linoleic acid content (2.9%) contributed towards higher incorporation of total n-3 PUFA in the breast by 16% compared with feeding the highest linoleic acid content (4.4%). When the chickens were fed with a diet with a high content of linoleic acid, this resulted in a significant reduction in EPA levels in both thigh and breast tissues. The levels for DPA and DHA were not affected by dietary linoleic acid. Authors suggested that this could be due to fact that linoleic acid competes with α-linolenic acid for Δ^6 desaturase. In other words, high dietary level of linoleic acid might reduce the conversion of α- linolenic to n-3 PUFAs. In a further study [87], the authors fed broiler chickens on diets containing 0, 2, or 4% linseed oil plus tallow to make 8% added fat throughout 38 growth period. The total amounts of saturated and monounsaturated fatty acids were significantly decreased after feeding increased levels of linseed. Conversely, the total amounts of PUFA were significantly increased. A recent study [88] showed that upon supplementing n-3 PUFA, in the form of linseed oil (3/100 g mixed feed), in the diet of laying hens resulted in a significant increase in α-linolenic of the plasma. The same study also revealed that, FO administration (same dose as linseed) caused a significant increase in the proportion of plasma EPA and DHA.

Involvement in avian immune function

The immunomodulatory effect of PUFA in broiler chickens occurs by affecting intercellular communications and signals that change the reactivity of leukocytes upon antigenic stimulation. This effect is highly associated with down-regulation or up-regulation of different cytokines that are believed to affect the avian immune function such as IL-1β, IFNγ, MGF, IL-1, IL-4, IL-2 [89–92].

There is some concern that diets enriched with n-3 PUFA have detrimental effects on chicken immunity and impair resistance to infection. However, it is not clear whether this concern is justified, since some studies show no effect [93], some show a detrimental effect [94] while some show an improvement [89, 90, 93, 95–97] in chicken immune response following feeding of n-3 PUFA.

Conclusion

Consumption of omega-3 fatty acids should be increased in human diets to get the beneficial effects of these fatty acids. One way to achieve this goal is by enriching poultry meat and eggs with omega-3 fatty acids, which is proved to be very successful. This role of poultry production in enhancing health aspects of human needs more research and interest from nutritionists and poultry producers.

Acknowledgements

The authors would like to extend their gratitude and appreciation to the management of Kuwait Institute for Scientific Research for their continuous technical and financial support of scientific research.

Conflict of interest

There is no conflict of interest related to the current work.

Author details

Hanan Al-Khalaifah* and Afaf Al-Nasser

Environment and Life Sciences Research Centre, Kuwait Institute for Scientific Research, Safat, Kuwait

*Address all correspondence to: hkhalifa@kisr.edu.kw

References

[1] Al-Khalifa H. Production of added- value poultry meat: Enrichment with n- 3 polyunsaturated fatty acids. World's Poultry Science Journal. 2015;71(2): 319-326

[2] Al-Khalifa H, Al-Nasser A, Al- Bahouh M, Ragheb G, Al-Qalaf S, Al- Omani N, et al. The effect of polyunsaturated fatty acids on avian immune cell subpopulations in peripheral blood, spleen, and thymus. World's Poultry Science Journal. 2016;1: 1-4

[3] Abbaci K, Joachirn S, Garric J, Boisseaux P, Exbrayat JM, Porcher JM, et al. Anatomical and histological characterization of the gametogenesis of Radix balthica (linnaeus, 1758) in comparison with Lymnaea stagnalis (linnaeus, 1758). Journal of Histology & Histopathology. 2017;4:5

[4] Apperson KD, Cherian G. Effect of whole flax seed and carbohydrase enzymes on gastrointestinal morphology, muscle fatty acids, and production performance in broiler chickens. Poultry Science. 2017;96(5): 1228-1234

[5] Colussi G, Catena C, Novello M, Bertin N, Sechi LA. Impact of omega-3 polyunsaturated fatty acids on vascular function and blood pressure: Relevance for cardiovascular outcomes. Nutrition, Metabolism, and Cardiovascular Diseases. 2017;27(3):191-200

[6] Rees AM, Austin MP, Parker G. Role of omega-3 fatty acids as a treatment for depression in the perinatal peiod. Australian and New Zealand Journal of Psychiatry. 2005;39(4):274-280

[7] Reeves JB, Weihrauch JL. Composition of Foods. Fats and Oils. Agriculture Handbook. Washington, DC: USDA; 1979

[8] Castro-Gonzalez MI. Omega 3 fatty acids: Benefits and sources. Interciencia. 2002;27(3):128-136

[9] Budowski P. Oils rich in omega-3 fatty acids—health implications. Harefuah. 1995;128(2):121-125

[10] Nettleton JA. omega -3 fatty acids: Comparison of plant and seafood sources in human nutrition. Journal of the American Dietetic Association. 1991; 91(3):331-337

[11] Ackman RG, Marine lipids and omega-3 fatty acids. In: Akoh CC, editor. (Functional Foods and Nutraceuticals Series), in Handbook of functional lipids. Boca Raton: Taylor & Francis; p. 311-324

[12] Landmark K. Alpha-linolenic acid, cardiovascular disease and sudden death. Tidsskrift for den Norske Lægeforening. 2006;126(21):2792-2794

[13] Herbaut C. Omega-3 and health. Revue Médicale de Bruxelles. 2006; 27(4):355-360

[14] Brown AJ, Robrts DCK, Truswell AS. Fatty acid composition of australian marine finfish: A review. Food Australia. 1989;1:655-666

[15] Kris-Etherton MKP, Harris WS, Appel LJ. Fish consumption, fish oil, omega-3 fattyacids, and cardiovascular disease. Journal of the American Heart Association. 2002;106:2747-2773

[16] Kartal M, Kurucu S, Aslan S, Ozbay O, Ceyhan T, Sayar E, et al. Comparison of n-3 fatty acids by GC-MS in frequently consumed fish and fish oil preparations on the turkish market. FABAD Journal of Pharmaceutical Sciences. 2003;28:201-205

[17] Alexander JW. Immunonutrition: The role of omega -3 fatty acids. Nutrition. 1998;14(7/8):627-633

[18] Holub BJ. Clinical nutrition: 4. Omega-3 fatty acids in cardiovascular care. Canadian Medical Association Journal. 2002;166(5):608-615

[19] Simopoulos AP. Health effects of [Omega]3 polyunsaturated fatty acids in seafoods. In: World Review of Nutrition and Dietetics. Vol. 66. Basel; London: Karger; 1991

[20] Simopoulos AP. Human requirement for n-3 polyunsaturated fatty acids. Poultry Science. 2000;79(7): 961-970

[21] Simopoulos AP. Importance of the ratio of omega-6/omega-3 essential fatty acids: Evolutionary aspects. (World Review of Nutrition and Dietetics). In: Simopoulos AP, Cleland LG, editors. Omega-6/Omega-3 Essential Fatty Acid Ratio: The Scientific Evidence. Vol. 92. Basel, Switzerland: Karger AG; 2003. pp. 1-22

[22] Singer P, Wirth M. Omega-3 fatty acids of marine and vegetable origin: State of the art. Ernahrungs-Umschau. 2003;50(8):296-304

[23] Rymer C, Givens DI. N-3 fatty acid enrichment of edible tissue of poultry: A review. Lipids. 2005;40(2):121-129

[24] Cheng CH, Shen TF, Chen WL, Ding ST. Effects of dietary algal docosahexaenoic acid oil supplementation on fatty acid deposition and gene expression in laying leghorn hens. The Journal of Agricultural Science. 2004;142:683-690

[25] Cachaldora P, Grcia-Rebollar P, Alvarez C, Mendez J, de Blas JC, Mendez J. Effect of type and level of basal fat and level of fish oil supplementation on yolk fat composition and n-3 fatty acids deposition efficiency in laying hens. Animal Feed Science and Technology. 2008;141:104-114

[26] WooCheol J, Jeong Yeoul L, Sangho K, Sangjin L, ByeongDae C, SeokJoong K. Production of DHA-rich meats and eggs from chickens fed fermented soybean meal by marine microalgae (Schizochytrium mangrivei MM103). Korean Journal of Poultry Science. 2008; 35:255-265

[27] Miller MR, Nichols PD, Carter CG. Replacement of dietary fish oil for atlantic salmon parr (Salmo salar L.) with a stearidonic acid containing oil has no effect on omega-3 long-chain polyunsaturated fatty acid concentrations. Comparative Biochemistry and Physiology. Part B, Biochemistry & Molecular Biology. 2007;109:1226-1236

[28] Kitessa SM, Young P. Echium oil is better than rapeseed oil in enriching poultry meat with n-3 polyunsaturated fatty acids, including eicosapentaenoic acid and docosapentaenoic acid. British Journal of Nutrition. 2009;101:709-715

[29] Rymer C, Gibbs RA, Givens DI. Comparison of algal and fish sources on the oxidative stability of poultry meat and its enrichment with omega-3 polyunsaturated fatty acids. Poultry Science. 2010;89(1):150-159

[30] Simonpoulos AP. Is insulin resistance influenced by dietary linoleic acid and trans fatty acids? Free Radical Biology and Medicine. 1994;17(4): 367-372

[31] Surai PF, Sparks NHC. Tissue- specific fatty acid and alpha -tocopherol profiles in male chickens depending on dietary tuna oil and vitamin E provision. Poultry Science. 2000;79(8): 1132-1142

[32] Voss A, Reinhart M, Sankarappa S, Sprecher H. The metabolism of 7,10,13,16,19-docosapentaenoic acid to 4,7,10,13,16,19-docosahexaenoic acid in rat liver is independent of a 4- desaturase. The Journal of Biological Chemistry. 1991;266:19995-20000

[33] Mohammed B, Sankarappa S, Geiger M, Sprecher H. Reevaluation of the pathway for the metabolism of 7,10,13, 16-docosatetraenoic acid to 4,7,10,13,16 docosapentaenoic acid in rat liver. Archives of Biochemistry and Biophysics. 1995;317:179-184

[34] Yaqoob P, Calder PC. N-3 polyunsaturated fatty acids and the immune system. Recent Research Developments in Lipids - Research. 1997;1:31-61

[35] Nakamura MT, Nara TY. Structure, function, and dietary regulation of Delta 6, Delta 5, and Delta 9 desaturases. Annual Review of Nutrition. 2004;24: 345-376

[36] Calder PC. N-3 polyunsaturated fatty acids and mononuclear phagocyte function. In: Kremer J, editor. Medical Fatty Acids in Inflammation. Switzerland: Birkhauser Verlag Basel; 1998

[37] Calder PC, Bond JA, Harvey DJ, Gordon S, Newsholme EA. Uptake and incorporation of saturated and unsaturated fatty acids into macrophage lipids and their effect upon macrophage adhesion and phagocytosis. The Biochemical Journal. 1990;269(3): 807-814

[38] Surette ME, Edens M, Chilton FH, Tramposch KM. Dietary echium oil increases plasma and neutrophil long- chain (n-3) fatty acids and lowers serum triacylglycerols in hypertriglyceridemic humans. The Journal of Nutrition. 2004; 134(6):1406-1411

[39] Yang Q, O'Shea TM. Dietary echium oil increases tissue (n-3) long-chain polyunsaturated fatty acids without elevating hepatic lipid concentrations in premature neonatal rats. The Journal of Nutrition. 2009;139(7):1353-1359

[40] Whelan J. Dietary stearidonic acid is a long chain (n-3) polyunsaturated fatty acid with potential health benefits. The Journal of Nutrition. 2009;139:5-10

[41] Whelan J, Rust C. Innovative dietary sources of n-3 fatty acids. Annual Review of Nutrition. 2006;26: 75-103

[42] Miles EA, Banerjee T, Dooper MM, M'Rabet L, Graus YM, Calder PC. The influence of different combinations of gamma-linoleinic acid, stearidonic acid and EPA on immune function in healthy young male subjects. The British Journal of Nutrition. 2004;91:893-903

[43] James MJ, Ursin VM, Cleland LG. Metabolism of stearidonic acid in human subjects: Comparison with the metabolism of other n-3 fatty acids. The American Journal of Clinical Nutrition. 2003;77:1140-1145

[44] Lopez-Ferrer S, Baucells MD, Barroeta AC, Grashorn MA. Metabolism and nutrition. n-3 Enrichment of chicken meat using fish oil: Alternative substitution with rapeseed and linseed oils. Poultry Science. 1999;78(3):356-365

[45] Bibus DM, Stitt PA. Metabolism of alpha -linolenic acid from flaxseed in dogs. In: The Return of Omega 3 Fatty Acids into the Food Supply. 1. Land- Based Animal Food Products and Their Health Effects. Basel, Switzerland: S Karger AG; 1998. pp. 186-198

[46] Drevon CA, Baksaas I, Krokan H. Omega-3 fatty acids: Metabolism and Biological Effects. Basel, Boston: Birkhéauser Verlag; 1993;1:389

[47] Fischer S, Von Schacky C, Siess W, Strasser T, Weber PC. Uptake, release and metabolism of docosahexaenoic acid in human platelets and neutrophils. Biochemical and Biophysical Research Communications. 1984;120:907-918

[48] Calder PC. Polyunsaturated fatty acids and inflammation. Prostaglandins, Leukotrienes and Essential Fatty Acids. 2006;75:197-202

[49] Calder PC. The relationship between the fatty acid compostion of immune cells and their function. Prostaglandins, Leukotrienes and Essential Fatty Acids. 2008;79:101-108

[50] Calder PC, Yaqoob P, Thies F, Wallace FA, Miles EA. Fatty acids and lymphocyte functions. British Journal of Nutrition. 2002;87(Supplement 1: S31-S48

[51] Calder PC. n-3 Polyunsaturated fatty acids, inflammation, and inflammatory diseases. The American Journal of Clinical Nutrition. 2006; 83(1):1505-1519

[52] Kew S, Banerjee T, Minihane AM, Finnegan YE, Williams CM, Calder PC. Relation between the fatty acid composition of peripheral blood mononuclear cells and measures of immune cell function in healthy, free- living subjects aged 25-72 y. The American Journal of Clinical Nutrition. 2003;77(5):1278-1286

[53] Yaqoob P, Pala HS, Cortina-Borja M, Newsholme EA, Calder PC. Encapsulated fish oil enriched in alphatocopherol alters plasma phospholipid and mononuclear cell fatty acid compositions but not mononuclear cell functions. European Journal of Clinical Investigation. 2000;30(3): 260-274

[54] Calder PC. Dietary fish oil appears to prevent the activation of phospholipase c -gamma in lymphocytes. Biochimica et Biophysica Acta. 1998;1392:300-308

[55] Calder PC. N-3 polyunsaturated fatty acids, inflammation and immunity: Pouring oil on troubled waters or another fishy tale? (Special issue: Celebrating exciting nutrition research in the next century). Nutrition Research. 2001;21(1/2):309-341

[56] Calder PC. Fatty acids and lymphocytes functions. British Journal of Nutrition. 2002;87(1):31-48

[57] Calder PC. Long-chain polyunsaturated fatty acids and inflammation. Scandinavian Journal of Food and Nutrition. 2006;50(1 sup. 2): 54-61

[58] Yaqoob P, Calder P. Effects of dietary lipid manipulation upon inflammatory mediator production by murine macrophages. Cellular Immunology. 1995;163(1):120-128

[59] Yaqoob P, Newsholme EA, Calder PC. The effect of fatty acids on leucocyte subsets and proliferation in rat whole blood. Nutrition Research. 1995;15(2):279-287

[60] Yaqoob P, Newsholmee EA, Calder PC. The effect of dietary lipid manipulation on rat lymphocyte subsets and proliferation. Immunology. 1994; 82:603-610

[61] Bavelaar FJ, Hovenier R, Lemmens AG, Beynen AC. High intake of linoleic or alpha -linolenic acid in relation to plasma lipids, atherosclerosis and tissue fatty acid composition in the Japanese quail. International Journal of Poultry Science. 2004;3(11):704-714

[62] Cyrus T. Disruption of the 12/15- lipoxygenase gene diminishes atherosclerosis in apo E-deficient mice. The Journal of Clinical Investigation. 1999;103:1597-1604

[63] Calder PC. Dietary modification of inflammation with lipids. Proceedings of the Nutrition Society. 2002;61(3): 345-358

[64] Volker DH. Fat manipulation in the treatment of rheumatoid arthritis: A review. Journal of Nutraceuticals, Functional & Medical Foods. 2000;3(1): 5-31

[65] Arm P, Horton C, Mencia-Huerta J. Effect of dietary supplementation with fish oil lipids on mild asthma. Thorax. 1988;43:84-92

[66] Arm I, Horton C, Spur B, Mencia- Huerta J, Lee T, Am T. The effects of dietary supplementation with fish oil lipids on the airways response to inhaledallergen in bronchial asthma. American Review of Respiratory Diseases. 1989;139:1395-1400

[67] Simopoulos AP. Omega-3 fatty acids in inflammation and autoimmune diseases. Journal of the American College of Nutrition. 2002;21(6): 495-505

[68] Sellmayer A, Schrepf R, Theisen K, Weber PC. Role of omega-3 fatty acids in cardiovascular disease prevention. Deutsche Medizinische Wochenschrift. 2004;129(38):1993-1996

[69] Schwalfenberg G. Omega-3 fatty acids: Their beneficial role in cardiovascular health. Canadian Family Physician. 2006;52(JUN):734-740

[70] Nettleton JA. Omega-3 Fatty Acids and Health. New York; London: Chapman & Hall; 1995. p. 359

[71] Leaf A, Kang JX. Omega-3 fatty acids and cardiovascular disease (World Review of Nutriton and Dietetics, Vol. 89). In: Simopoulos AP, Pavlou KN, editors. Nutrition and Fitness 1: Diet, Genes, Physical Activity and Health. Basel Switzerland: S Karger AG; 2001. pp. 161-172

[72] Connor WE. Omega -3 Fatty acids and heart disease. In: Kritchevsky D, Carroll KK, editors. Nutrition and Disease Update: Heart Disease. Champaign: American Oil Chemists' Society (AOCS); 1994. pp. 1-137

[73] Budowski P. Omega 3-Fatty acids in health and disease. World Review of Nutrition and Dietetics. 1988;57:214-274

[74] Woods A, Brull D, Humphries S, Montgomery H. Genetics of inflammation and risk of coronary artery disease: The central role of interleukin-6. European Heart Journal. 2000;21:1574-1583

[75] Connor WE, Neuringer M, Lin DS. Dietary effects on brain fatty acid composition: The reversibility of n-3 fatty acid deficiency and turnover of docosahexaenoic acid in the brain, erythrocytes and plasma of rhesus monkeys. Journal of Lipid Research. 1990;31:237-247

[76] Nkondjock A, Shatenstein B, Maisonneuve P, Ghadirian P. Specific fatty acids and human colorectal cancer: An overview. Cancer Detection and Prevention. 2003;27(1):55-66

[77] Prasad KN, Kumar B, Yan XD, Hanson AJ, Cole WC. Alpha - Tocopheryl succinate, the most effective form of vitamin E for adjuvant cancer treatment: A review. Journal of the American College of Nutrition. 2003; 22(2):108-117

[78] Cotter PF, Sefton AE, Lilburn MS. Manipulating the immune system of layers and breeders: Novel applications of mannan oligosaccharides. In: Lyons TP, Jacques KA editors. Nutritional Biotechnology in the Feed and Food Industries. UK, Stamford: Alltech; 2002. p. 21-27

[79] Koller M, Senkal M, Kemen M, Konig W, Zumtobel V, Muhr G. Impact of omega-3 fatty acid enriched TPN on leukotriene synthesis by leukocytes after major surgery. Clinical Nutrition. 2003;22(1):59-64

[80] Bou R, Guardiola F, Tres A, Barroeta AC, Codony R. Effect of dietary fish oil, alpha-tocopherl acetate, and zinc supplementation on the composition and consumer acceptability of chicken meat. Poultry Science. 2004; 83:282-292

[81] Ratnayake WMN, Ackman RG, Hulan HW. Effect of redfish meal enriched diets on the taste and n-3 pufa of 42-day-old broiler chickens. Journal of the Science of Food and Agriculture. 1986;49(1):59-74

[82] Givens DI, Rymer C. Effect of species and genotype on the efficiency of enrichment of poultry meat with n-3 polyunsaturated fatty acid. Lipids. 2006;41(5):445-451

[83] Lopez-Ferrer S, Baucells MD, Barroeta AC, Grashorn MA. N-3 enrichment of chicken meat using fish oil: Alternative substituation with rapeseed and linseed oils. Poultry Science. 1999;78:356-365

[84] Zelenka J, Schneiderova D, Mrkvicova E, Dolezal P. The effect of dietary linseed oils with different fatty acid pattern on the content of fatty acids in chicken meat. Veterinary Medicine. 2008;53(2):77-85

[85] Kartikasari LR, Hughes RJ, Geier MS, Makrides M, Gibson RA. World Congress on Oils and Fats 28th ISF Congress; 2009. pp. 62-63

[86] Kartikasari LR, Hughes RJ, Geier MS, Makrides M, Gibson RA. Diets high in linoleic acid reduce omega-3 long chain polyunsaturated fatty acids in chicken tissues. In: Aust. Poult. Sci. Symp. Australia; 2010. pp. 64-67

[87] Lopez-Ferrer S, Baucells MD, Barroeta AC, Galobart J, Grashorn MA. n-3 Enrichment of chicken meat. 2. Use of precursors of long-chain polyunsaturated fatty acids: Linseed oil. Poultry Science. 2001;80(6):753-761

[88] Svedova M, Vasko L, Trebunova A, Kastel R, Tuckova M, Certik M. Influence of linseed and fish oil on metabolic and immunological indicators of laying hens. Acta Veterinaria. 2008; 77:39-44

[89] Yang X, Yuming G. Modulation of intestinal mucosal immunity by dietary polyunsaturated fatty acids in chickens. Food and Agricultural Immunology. 2006;17(2):129-137

[90] Korver DR, Klasing KC. Dietary fish oil alters specific and inflammatory immune responses in chicks. Journal of Nutrition. 1997;127(10):2039-2046

[91] Leshchinsky TV, Klasing KC. Vitamin E and leukocytic cytokine expression in broilers. Poultry Science. 2000;79(1):37

[92] Koutsos EA, Klasing KC. Effect of intra-abdominal injection of lipopolysaccharide or muramyl dipeptide on the acute phase response in Japanese quail (Coturnix coturnix japonica). Poultry Science. 2000; 79(1):37

[93] Puthpongsiriporn U, Scheideler SE. Effects of dietary ratio of linoleic to linolenic acid on performance, antibody production, and in vitro lymphocyte proliferation in two strains of Leghorn pullet chicks. Poultry Science. 2005; 84(6):846-857

[94] Adam O. Dietary fatty acids and immune reactions in synovial tissue. European Journal of Medical Research, 2003;8(8):381-387

[95] Phipps RP, Stein SH, Roper RL. A new view of prostaglandin regulation of the immune response. Immunology Today. 1991;12:349-352

[96] Parmentier HK, Nieuwland MGB, Barwegen MW, Kwakkel RP, Schrama JW. Dietary unsaturated fatty acids affect antibody responses and growth of chickens divergently selected for humoral responses to sheep red blood cells. Poultry Science. 1997;76(8): 1164-1171

[97] Sijben JWC, Groot Hd, Nieuwland MGB, Schrama JW, Parmentier HK. Dietary linoleic acid divergently affects immune responsiveness of growing layer hens. Poultry Science. 2000;79(8): 1106-1115

Permissions

All chapters in this book were first published in NHDOCNFT, by InTech Open; hereby published with permission under the Creative Commons Attribution License or equivalent. Every chapter published in this book has been scrutinized by our experts. Their significance has been extensively debated. The topics covered herein carry significant findings which will fuel the growth of the discipline. They may even be implemented as practical applications or may be referred to as a beginning point for another development.

The contributors of this book come from diverse backgrounds, making this book a truly international effort. This book will bring forth new frontiers with its revolutionizing research information and detailed analysis of the nascent developments around the world.

We would like to thank all the contributing authors for lending their expertise to make the book truly unique. They have played a crucial role in the development of this book. Without their invaluable contributions this book wouldn't have been possible. They have made vital efforts to compile up to date information on the varied aspects of this subject to make this book a valuable addition to the collection of many professionals and students.

This book was conceptualized with the vision of imparting up-to-date information and advanced data in this field. To ensure the same, a matchless editorial board was set up. Every individual on the board went through rigorous rounds of assessment to prove their worth. After which they invested a large part of their time researching and compiling the most relevant data for our readers.

The editorial board has been involved in producing this book since its inception. They have spent rigorous hours researching and exploring the diverse topics which have resulted in the successful publishing of this book. They have passed on their knowledge of decades through this book. To expedite this challenging task, the publisher supported the team at every step. A small team of assistant editors was also appointed to further simplify the editing procedure and attain best results for the readers.

Apart from the editorial board, the designing team has also invested a significant amount of their time in understanding the subject and creating the most relevant covers. They scrutinized every image to scout for the most suitable representation of the subject and create an appropriate cover for the book.

The publishing team has been an ardent support to the editorial, designing and production team. Their endless efforts to recruit the best for this project, has resulted in the accomplishment of this book. They are a veteran in the field of academics and their pool of knowledge is as vast as their experience in printing. Their expertise and guidance has proved useful at every step. Their uncompromising quality standards have made this book an exceptional effort. Their encouragement from time to time has been an inspiration for everyone.

The publisher and the editorial board hope that this book will prove to be a valuable piece of knowledge for researchers, students, practitioners and scholars across the globe.

List of Contributors

Milka Nashar, Yoana D. Kiselova-Kaneva and Diana G. Ivanova
Medical University of Varna, Varna, Bulgaria

Isabel Sospedra, Aurora Norte, José Miguel Martínez-Sanz, Enrique de Gomar, José Antonio Hurtado Sánchez and María José Cabañero-Martínez
Nursing Department, Faculty of Health Sciences, University of Alicante, Alicante, Spain

Gyula Mózsik
First Department of Medicine, University of Pécs, Hungary

Mária Figler
Second Department of Medicine, The Institute of Dietitian and Nutritional Science, University of Pécs, Hungary

Aleksandra Badora, Karolina Bawolska, Jolanta Kozłowska-Strawska and Jolanta Domańska
Department of Agricultural and Environmental Chemistry, The University of Life Sciences in Lublin, Lublin, Poland

Monyeki K. Daniel and Ramoshaba N. Elfas
Department of Physiology and Environmental, University of Limpopo, Sovenga, South Africa

Siweya H. James
Faculty of Science and Agriculture, University of Limpopo, Sovenga, South Africa

Kemper C.G. Han
Health and Activity, Amsterdam Public Health Academic Research Institute, Vrije Universiteit, Amsterdam, The Netherlands

Lingwen Zeng, Lei Peng, Dazhi Wu and Baoguo Yang
Institute of Environment and Safety, Wuhan Academy of Agricultural Sciences, Wuhan, China

Javier Marhuenda, Débora Villaño, Begoña Cerdá and María Pilar Zafrilla
Bachelor in Pharmacy, Health Sciences Faculty, Catholic University of Murcia, Murcia, Spain

Valente Velázquez-Ordoñez, Benjamín Valladares-Carranza, Esvieta Tenorio-Borroto, Martín Talavera-Rojas, Jorge Antonio Varela-Guerrero and Jorge Acosta-Dibarrat
Facultad de Medicina Veterinaria y Zootecnia, Centro de Investigación y Estudios Avanzados en Salud Animal, Universidad Autónoma del Estado de México (CIESA-FMVZ-UAEM), Toluca, Mexico

Florencia Puigvert and Lucia Grille
Departamento de Ciencia y Tecnología de la Leche, Facultad de Veterinaria, Universidad de la Republica, CENUR-Litoral Norte, Paysandú, Uruguay

Álvaro González Revello
Departamento de Ciencia y Tecnología de la Leche, Facultad de Veterinaria, Universidad de la Republica, Montevideo, Uruguay

Lucia Pareja
Facultad de Química, Universidad de la Republica, Estación Experimental Dr. Mario A. Cassinoni, Paysandú, Uruguay

João Silva Dias
Instituto Superior de Agronomia, University of Lisbon, Lisbon, Portugal

Raúl Arcusa Saura, María Pilar Zafrilla Rentero and Javier Marhuenda Hernández
Faculty of Health Sciences, Universidad Católica San Antonio de Murcia (UCAM), Spain

Chung-Hsing Chao
Ta Hwa University of Science and Technology, Hsinchu County, Taiwan, ROC

Gary B. Smejkal and Srikanth Kakumanu
Focus Proteomics, Hudson, New Hampshire, USA

Amanda Cannady-Miller
ProdigY Biosciences, Louisville, Kentucky, USA

Hanan Al-Khalaifah and Afaf Al-Nasser
Environment and Life Sciences Research Centre, Kuwait Institute for Scientific Research, Safat, Kuwait

Index

www.ingramcontent.com/pod-product-compliance
Lightning Source LLC
LaVergne TN
LVHW080602210926
848485LV00003B/93
* 9 7 8 1 6 3 9 8 9 3 8 9 8 *